Oxford Specialist Handbooks in Surgery
Oral and Maxillofacial Surgery

Second Edition

Edited by

Cyrus Kerawala

Consultant Maxillofacial/Head and Neck Surgeon,
The Royal Marsden Hospital,
London, UK

Carrie Newlands

Consultant Maxillofacial Surgeon,
Royal Surrey County Hospital,
Guildford, UK

OXFORD
UNIVERSITY PRESS

OXFORD
UNIVERSITY PRESS

Great Clarendon Street, Oxford, OX2 6DP,
United Kingdom

Oxford University Press is a department of the University of Oxford.
It furthers the University's objective of excellence in research, scholarship,
and education by publishing worldwide. Oxford is a registered trade mark of
Oxford University Press in the UK and in certain other countries

© Oxford University Press 2014

The moral rights of the authors have been asserted

First edition published in 2010
Second edition published in 2014

Impression: 1

Published in the United States of America by Oxford University Press
198 Madison Avenue, New York, NY 10016, United States of America

British Library Cataloguing in Publication Data

Data available

Library of Congress Control Number: 2013952031

ISBN 978–0–19–968840–1

Printed in China by
C&C Offset Printing Co. Ltd

Foreword

However much some of us may bemoan the tendency to rely heavily on examinations as a means of assessing knowledge and competence, they are firmly embedded as part of British surgical education, even though they risk giving the impression that testing is more important than training. Sadly, whether trainees like it or not, there is a lot of 'stuff' they simply have to learn to underpin the development of their clinical, surgical, and professional skills. Fortunately help is at hand in the form of this admirable text, even if the sheer scale of the facts and figures that have to be assimilated as a trainee or candidate for the exit FRCS is initially quite daunting—just the extensive list of symbols and abbreviations given at the start of the book is enough to make this writer tremble!

Written by a group of active surgeons who are all heavily involved in teaching and training, the information contained in these pages is pure gold dust for trainees in the specialty. Pedants are sometimes critical of books which consist of summaries and guidelines, preferring larger textbooks that allow a fuller explanation of a subject in order to bring some perspective to the discussion. However, I believe that each has a distinct and different role. Both are needed; and whether in the hurly burly of daily clinical practice, or in the frantic weeks before an impending examination, I can recommend no better aide memoire than this to have at your fingertips. The editors and their team are to be congratulated on packing so much solid information into a pocket (or handbag) sized book—even including to my delight as a medical history buff six pages of eponyms relevant to OMFS!

Andrew Brown
Formerly Consultant Maxillofacial Surgeon,
Queen Victoria Hospital, East Grinstead, UK
Past-President,
British Association of Oral and Maxillofacial Surgeons

Preface to the second edition

Since the first edition of this book the editors have maintained their strong interest in teaching and examining candidates for the exit FRCS in OMFS. They are definitely older, and possibly a little wiser. Like many specialties, oral and maxillofacial surgery develops over time so this new edition builds on the success and popularity of the first with updates by previous and new authors. We hope you find it useful.

Cyrus Kerawala and Carrie Newlands, 2014

Preface to the first edition

This handbook is edited by two young consultants in oral and maxillofacial surgery, who both maintain a strong interest in teaching and are involved in examining for the exit FRCS. The content closely follows the syllabus of higher surgical training in oral and maxillofacial surgery in the UK. We hope it will prove useful and stimulating for trainees in the specialty, both throughout their training and at that potentially worrying time when the exit exam approaches. It may even contain snippets that our more senior colleagues will find of interest.

Oral and maxillofacial surgery is an evolving and unique surgical specialty, with increasing numbers of young dentists and doctors continually attracted by its charms. We trust this book will further whet their appetites. It may also find a place on the bookshelves of those who are working and training in other allied surgical disciplines, or accident and emergency.

We have tried to present the information contained within, in a familiar and accessible format, with an emphasis on current evidence where available. In those many surgical situations where the literature does not provide an evidence base, we have outlined current UK practice and thinking. We would like to think that some of our readers will be inspired to help improve the scientific rationale for what we do where gaps are apparent.

Feedback and comments are welcomed and will be gratefully acknowledged, should this first attempt prove popular enough to give birth to further editions.

Carrie Newlands and Cyrus Kerawala, 2009

Acknowledgements

We would like to thank the following for their advice and assistance:

Our fellow authors as outlined in the contributors' section.

Many respected OMFS colleagues, trainers, and trainees, past and present, especially for their useful comments about the first edition.

Colleagues in other specialties, with whom we are always glad and often fortunate to collaborate.

The team at Oxford University Press for helpful guidance.

Our loved ones for their support, understanding, and occasional floral gifts.

Max and Miles for being generally fabulous.

Kate for doing all the gardening and cooking, and Ben for the games of golf he continues to miss.

And, of course, our readers—we hope you enjoy this book as much as we have.

Contents

Contents

Contributors

Brian Bisase (Chapters 12 and 13)
Consultant Oral and Maxillofacial Surgeon,
Queen Victoria Hospital,
East Grinstead, UK

Jeremy Collyer (Chapter 4)
Consultant Oral and Maxillofacial Surgeon,
Queen Victoria Hospital,
East Grinstead, UK

Stephen Dover (Chapter 10)
Consultant Oral and Maxillofacial Surgeon,
Queen Elizabeth and Birmingham Children's Hospitals,
Honorary Senior Lecturer,
University of Birmingham,
Birmingham, UK

Simon van Eeden (Chapter 5)
Consultant Cleft and Maxillofacial Surgeon,
Alder Hey and Aintree University Hospitals,
Liverpool, UK

Katharine Fleming (Chapter 11)
Consultant Oral and Maxillofacial Surgeon,
Countess of Chester Hospital,
Chester and Aintree University Hospitals,
Liverpool, UK

Ben Gurney (Chapter 3)
Specialist Registrar in Oral and Maxillofacial Surgery,
Queen Victoria Hospital,
East Grinstead, UK

Ian Holland (Chapter 1)
Consultant Oral and Maxillofacial Surgeon,
Southern General Hospital,
Glasgow, UK

Paul Johnson (Chapter 8)
Consultant Oral and Maxillofacial Surgeon,
Royal Surrey County Hospital,
Guildford, UK

Cyrus Kerawala (Chapters 2 and 3)
Consultant Maxillofacial/Head and Neck Surgeon,
The Royal Marsden Hospital,
London, UK

David Koppel (Chapter 6)
Consultant Craniofacial and Maxillofacial Surgeon and Lead Clinician,
Southern General Hospital,
Glasgow, UK

Jayanth Kunjur (Chapter 9)
Specialist Registrar in Oral and Maxillofacial Surgery,
King's Dental Institute,
King's College Hospital,
London, UK

Nigel Shaun Matthews (Chapter 9)
Consultant Oral and Maxillofacial Surgeon,
King's Dental Institute,
King's College Hospital,
London, UK

Ian Martin (Chapter 2)
Consultant Oral and Maxillofacial Surgeon and Medical Director,
Sunderland Royal Hospital,
Sunderland, UK

Carrie Newlands
(Chapters 3, 9, and 10)
Consultant Oral and Maxillofacial
Surgeon,
Royal Surrey County Hospital,
Guildford, UK

Ragu Sangra (Chapter 6)
Consultant Neurosurgeon,
Southern General Hospital,
Glasgow, UK

Kenneth Sneddon
(Chapter 5)
Consultant Oral and Maxillofacial
Surgeon,
Queen Victoria Hospital,
East Grinstead, UK

Nigel Taylor (Chapter 5)
Consultant Orthodontist,
Royal Surrey County Hospital,
Guildford, UK

Thian Keh Ong (Chapter 2)
Consultant Oral and Maxillofacial
Surgeon,
Leeds Teaching Hospitals,
Leeds, UK

Helen Witherow
(Chapter 8)
Consultant Oral and Maxillofacial
Surgeon,
St George's Hospital,
London, UK

**Thanks to contributors to first
edition:**

James McCaul (Chapter 2)
Consultant Maxillofacial/Head and
Neck Surgeon,
Bradford Teaching Hospitals,
Bradford, UK

Symbols and abbreviations

➲	cross reference
♂	male
♀	female
💣	bomb (controversial topic)
→	leading to
↓	decreased
↑	increased
🐭	website
3D	three-dimensional
ACC	adenoid cystic carcinoma
ACE	angiotensin-converting enzyme
ACE-27	Adult Co-morbidity Evaluation
ACJ	amelo-cemental junction
ADA	American Dental Association
ADP	adenosine diphosphate
AFB	acid-fast bacilli
AJCC	American Joint Committee on Cancer
ALA	aminolevulinic acid
ALARP	as low as reasonably possible
ALFH	anterior lower facial height
ALP	alkaline phosphatase
ANB	point A to nasion to point B
ANUG	acute necrotizing ulcerative gingivitis
AOB	anterior open bite
AP	antero-posterior
ARDS	acute respiratory distress syndrome
ASA	American Association of Anaesthesiologists
ATLS	advanced trauma life support
AUFH	anterior upper facial height
AVPU	Alert, Voice, Pain, Unresponsive
BAD	British Association of Dermatologists
BCC	basal cell carcinoma
BCL3	a protein coding gene
BCLP	bilateral cleft lip and palate
bd	twice a day
BDA	British Dental Association
BLCP	bilateral cleft lip and palate

BMI	body mass index
BMJ	*British Medical Journal*
BP	blood pressure
BSSO	bilateral sagittal split osteotomy
C&S	culture and sensitivity
CAD	computer-aided design
CAM	computer-aided manufacturing
CBCT	cone beam computed tomography
CBT	cognitive behavioural therapy
CCF	congestive cardiac failure
CEOC	calcifying epithelial odontogenic cyst
CEOT	calcifying epithelial odontogenic tumour
CL	cleft lip
CLAPA	Cleft Lip and Palate Association
CLP	cleft lip and palate
CMCC	chronic muco cutaneous candidosis
CMM	cutaneous malignant melanoma
CMV	cytomegalovirus
CNS	central nervous system
CO_2	carbon dioxide
COPD	chronic obstructive pulmonary disease
COX	cyclo-oxygenase
CP	cleft palate
CSF	cerebrospinal fluid
CT	computed tomography
CTA	computed tomography angiography
CTD	connective tissue disorder
CVA	cardiovascular accident
CVS	cardiovascular system
CXR	chest X-ray
dB HL	decibels hearing level
DCIA	deep circumflex iliac artery
DM	diabetes mellitus
DUSS	duplex ultrasound scanning
DVT	deep venous thrombosis
EAM	external auditory meatus
EAT	extra-alveolar time
EBV	Epstein–Barr virus
ECG	electrocardiogram
ELND	elective lymph node dissection
EM	erythema multiforme

EMLA	eutectic mixture of local anaesthetics
END	elective neck dissection
ENT	ear, nose, and throat
EORTC	European Organisation for Research Treatment of Cancer
ESR	erythrocyte sedimentation rate
ET	endotracheal
ETT	endotracheal tube
EUA	examination under anaesthesia
EUT	Eustachian tube
FACT-HNS	Functional Assessment of Cancer Therapy, H + N Scale
FBC	full blood count
FDG	fluoro-deoxy-glucose
FESS	functional endoscopic sinus surgery
FFP	fresh frozen plasma
FGFR	fibroblast growth factor receptor
FH	family history
FNA	fine needle aspiration
FNAB	fine needle aspiration biopsy
FNAC	fine needle aspiration cytology
FOXE1	forkhead box E1
FSS	frozen section substitute
FTA-ABS	fluorescent treponemal antibody absorption
FTSG	full-thickness skin graft
GA	general anaesthetic
GCS	Glasgow Coma Scale
GDC	General Dental Council
GDP	general dental practitioner
GIT	gastrointestinal tract
GL12	a transcription factor encoding gene
GMC	General Medical Council
GMP	general medical practitioner
GN	glossopharyngeal neuralgia
GP	general practitioner
GPP	gingivoperiosteoplasty
GTN	glyceryl trinitrate
H&E	haematoxylin and eosin
HADS	Hospital Anxiety and Depression Scale
HAI	health-care associated infections
HAI	hospital-acquired infection
HBO	hyperbaric oxygen
HIV	human immunodeficiency virus

HPT	hyperparathyroidism
HPV	human papilloma virus
HRQOL	health-related quality of life
HRT	hormone replacement therapy
HSV	herpes simplex virus
IBS	irritable bowel syndrome
ICP	intra-cranial pressure
ICR	idiopathic condylar resorption
ID	inferior dental
IDB	inferior dental bundle
IE	infective endocarditis
IgA	immunoglobulin A
IHC	immunohistochemistry
IHD	ischaemic heart disease
IJV	internal jugular vein
IM	intramuscular
IMF	intermaxillary fixation
IMRT	intensity-modulated radiotherapy
INR	international normalized ratio
IRF6	interferon regulatory gene 6
IRM	intermediate restorative material
IRMER	Ionising Radiation (Medical Exposure) Regulations
ITU	intensive care
IV	intravenous
IVS	intravenous sedation
LA	local anaesthesia
LDH	lactate dehydrogenase
LMA	laryngeal mask airway
LMN	lower motor neurone
LMWH	low-molecular-weight heparin
LN	lymph node
LOH	loss of heterozygosity
LP	lichen planus
MACS	minimal-access cranial suspension
MAL	methyl aminolevulinate
MDP	methylene diphosphonate
MDT	multidisciplinary team
MH	medical history
MI	myocardial infarction
MM	malignant melanoma
MRA	magnetic resonance angiography

MRG	median rhomboid glossitis
MRI	magnetic resonance imaging
MRND	modified radical neck dissection
MRSA	methicillin-resistant *Staphylococcus aureus*
MS	multiple sclerosis
MSX1	MSH homeobox 1
MTA	mineral trioxide aggregate
MTHFR	methylenetetrahydrofolate reductase
MVD	microvascular decompression
NAM	naso-alveolar moulding
NBM	nil by mouth
ND	neck dissection
NG	nasogastric
NGT	nasogastric tube
NHL	non-Hodgkin lymphoma
NICE	National Institute for Health and Care Excellence
NMSC	non-melanoma skin cancer
NO	nitrous oxide
NPSA	National Patient Safety Agency
OA	osteoarthritis
OAF	oro-antral fistula
OCP	oral contraceptive pill
od	once a day
OH	oral hygiene
OHI	oral hygiene instruction
OM	occipitomental
OME	otitis media with effusion
OMENS	Orbital distortion, Mandibular hypoplasia, Ear anomaly, Nerve involvement, Soft tissue deficiency
OMFS	oral and maxillofacial surgery
ON	osteonecrosis
ONJ	osteonecrosis of the jaws
OPG/OPT	orthopantomogram
ORIF	open reduction internal fixation
ORN	osteoradionecrosis
PA	postero-anterior
PCR	polymerase chain reaction
PDS	polydioxanone suture
PDT	photodynamic therapy
PE	pulmonary embolus
PEG	percutaneous endoscopic gastrostomy

PET	positive emission tomography
PGL	persistent generalized lymphadenopathy
PMMF	pectoralis major myocutaneous flap
PMOL	potentially malignant oral lesions
PMR	polymyalgia rheumatica
po	by mouth
PPI	proton-pump inhibitor
PRP	platelet-rich plasma
PSA	pleomorphic salivary adenoma
PSO	pre-surgical orthopaedics
PTH	parathyroid hormone
PUVA	psoralen and ultra-violet A
PVL	proliferative verrucous leukoplakia
QLQ	quality of life questionnaire
QOL	quality of life
RA	rheumatoid arthritis
RARA	retinoic acid receptor alpha
RAPD	relative afferent papillary defect
RCT	randomized controlled trial
RED	rigid external distractor
REM	rapid eye movement
RIG	radiologically inserted gastrostomy
RND	radical neck dissection
ROU	recurrent oral ulceration
RPE	rapid palatal expansion
RRF	retrograde root filling
RS	respiratory system
RSTL	relaxed skin tension line
RT	radiotherapy
SACT	systemic anti-cancer therapies
SALT	speech and language therapy/therapist
SAN	spinal accessory nerve
SARPE	surgically assisted rapid palatal expansion
SATB2	special AT-rich sequence-binding protein
SC	subcutaneous
SCC	squamous cell carcinoma
SCM	sternocleidomastoid muscle
SEND	selective elective neck dissection
SIDS	sudden infant death syndrome
SK1	small conductance calcium gated potassium channel
SLE	systemic lupus erythematosus

SMAS	superficial musculo-aponeurotic system
SMV	submento-vertex
SNA	point S to nasion to point A
SNB	sentinel node biopsy/point S to nasion to point B
SND	selective neck dissection
SPECT	single photon emission tomography
SPRY2	sprouty homolog 2
SS	Sjögren's syndrome
SSG	split-skin graft
STD	sodium tetradecyl sulphate
TB	tuberculosis
TCA	trichloroacetic acid
TED	thromboembolic deterrent
TENS	transcutaneous electrical nerve stimulator
TGFA	transforming growth factor alpha
TGFB	transforming growth factor beta
TLA	three-letter abbreviation
TMJ	temporomandibular joint
TMJDS	temporomandibular joint dysfunction syndrome
TN	trigeminal neuralgia
TNF	tumour necrosis factor
TNM	tumour, lymph nodes, distant metastases system
TPD	transpalatal distractor
TPHA	*Treponema pallidum* haemagglutination assay
TTP	tender to percussion
Tx	treatment
UCLP	unilateral cleft lip and palate
UMN	upper motor neurone
URT	upper respiratory tract
URTI	upper respiratory tract infection
USS	ultrasound scanning
UV	ultraviolet
VCF	velocardiofacial syndrome
VDRL	veneral disease reference laboratory
VPI	velopharyngeal incompetence
VSS	vertical subsigmoid osteotomy
VZV	varicella zoster virus
WHO	World Health Organization
WLE	wide local excision
ZN	Ziehl–Neelsen

1

Trauma

Introduction

Maxillofacial trauma can affect any part of the face and frequently occurs in conjunction with ophthalmic and neurosurgical injuries. There has been a change in the aetiology of this form of trauma in the UK following the introduction of seatbelt legislation in the 1980s and more recently safety features in automotive design such as airbags. Prior to these changes there were large numbers of high-energy road traffic accidents with drivers and passengers sustaining injuries from unrestrained impacts on dashboards or windscreens. Such injuries are now rare. Unfortunately, at the same time as road traffic injuries have reduced, there has been an increase in injuries as a result of interpersonal violence. This pattern of injury is mirrored in most of Western Europe and North America. In many parts of the developing world, road traffic injuries still predominate.

The other major historical change in the management of facial trauma has been the development of internal fixation, which was popularized in the 1980s with the introduction of titanium miniplates. At the time of publication there is a plethora of internal fixation devices available for craniomaxillofacial trauma. The limit on a surgeon's ability to correct fractures is no longer the devices available, but the ability to adequately expose the fracture sites and the healthcare system to absorb the costs of the devices used.

Initial assessment

Principles of assessment

History: the importance of the mechanism of injury, medical, and drug histories
The history of any injury is important and indirectly provides a guide not
only to its treatment, but also the potential surgical outcome. Important
factors relate to the patient and nature of the injury itself.

Patient factors
- **Medical history**: details of the patient's medical history should be sought
  in case they influence treatment pathways.
- **Social history**: a significant proportion of patients with facial injuries
  have some social problems which may influence post-operative
  management. Recreational drugs and alcohol use may also influence
  treatment outcomes. Patients with addictions to alcohol or
  recreational drugs are frequently malnourished and can be relatively
  immunocompromised. Domestic violence is often an aetiological
  factor in women who sustain facial trauma and this may influence
  post-operative management.

Injury factors
- **Sharp or blunt trauma**: exclusively sharp trauma produces an incised
  wound, the nature of the injury indicating if there is likely to be
  contamination of the wound, e.g. glass.
- **Energy transfer of trauma**: although energy transfer is a concept
  originally used to understand ballistic damage, it is relevant to all types
  of injury. High-energy transfer is exemplified by an object that is either
  low mass and moving very fast, or has a large inherent mass moving
  slowly, colliding with an object and stopping. This occurs in road traffic
  accidents and is also the case with blunt trauma imparted by an object
  such as a baseball bat or the force from a kick. By contrast, the energy
  transfer in a punch is lower, as a fist has less mass and moves more
  slowly.
- **Contamination of wounds**: cuts with knives are frequently clean and
  non-contaminated. Lacerations are often contaminated with particles
  from the surface that have produced the injury. The latter often require
  thorough debridement under general anaesthesia (GA).

'Advanced trauma life support' and facial trauma

Life-threatening conditions

- **Airway with cervical spine control**: if the airway is compromised in facial injuries it is frequently due to:
  - debris obscuring the airway, such as blood, and fragments of teeth and bone;
  - oedema in the pharyngeal tissues as result of injury;
  - rarely a grossly displaced mandibular injury may result in lack of tongue support and secondary obstruction of the airway.
- **Breathing**: foreign bodies such as teeth or fractures dentures can compromise respiration.
- **Circulation**: the head and neck has a rich blood supply. This can cause problems with acute haemorrhage. Patients with circulatory compromise and facial injuries should, however, have other possible sources of blood loss actively looked for. Torrential haemorrhage from the head and neck is likely to arise from:
  - the maxillary artery and pterygoid venous plexus in grossly displaced maxillary fractures;
  - branches of the carotid artery and tributaries of the internal jugular vein in penetrating neck trauma.
- **Disability**.
- **Exposure**.
- **Head injury**: cerebral injury is frequently associated with facial injury. Head injury in the presence of severe facial injuries may be milder than expected as, to some extent, the face acts as a 'crumple zone' protecting the cranial contents from injury. Patients should be assessed using the Glasgow Coma Scale (GCS). Many patients with facial injury will have consumed alcohol or drugs that can mask the symptoms of head injury. This needs to be borne in mind when assessing the patient. There needs to be a low threshold for computed tomography (CT) scanning to exclude intra-cranial injury or mass effects.

Sight-threatening conditions

The eyes lie in the centre of the face surrounded inferiorly by the maxilla, laterally by the zygoma, and medially by the frontal, nasal, and lacrimal bones. Orbital trauma is frequently associated with ocular injury. All patients with a suspected orbital injury should have their visual acuity documented at their time of initial assessment. Loss of visual acuity should raise the question of whether there is intra-ocular injury, primary optic nerve injury, or ↑ pressure within the orbit leading to secondary injury of the optic nerve. Retrobulbar haemorrhage is an example of a condition that causes acute compression of the optic nerve. (See ➲ Initial management of ocular injuries, p. 16.)

Priority setting in polytrauma

Multidisciplinary considerations

Life- or sight-threatening facial injuries should be treated immediately. Facial lacerations and unstable mandibular fractures should be treated within 24h. Most other bony facial injury can be treated on a delayed basis. The delay involved is dependent upon the amount of facial oedema present. Mid-face and orbital injuries should either be treated before the onset of facial oedema or after facial oedema has settled. The decision of definitive timing to treat injuries is also affected by other injuries, and the need to treat major chest, abdominal, pelvic, and limb trauma.

Imaging

Polytrauma patients are often immobilized or supine due to potential spinal injuries.

Plain film radiographs for facial injuries include:
- Occipito-mental (OM) views.
- Orthopantomogram (OPG).
- Postero-anterior (PA) mandible.

Unfortunately, all three of these views require the patient to be upright. In the multiple-injury patient this is not possible. If the patient cannot stand and has clinical indicators that suggest significant bony facial injury, a fine-cut (0.5mm) CT scan of the area should be considered. Every effort should be made to incorporate facial imaging into trauma protocols. If a patient is having a CT of their head and cervical spine and they have facial injuries, they should have simultaneous imaging of the face.

'How to do' emergency procedures

Airway management

Except in the management of battlefield trauma, where control of cata-strophic haemorrhage takes priority, the airway always takes first priority and should be managed in association with protection of the cervical spine. Airway management can be summarized as follows:

- Clear debris from the airway.
- Posture. In the absence of associated spinal injuries it is appropriate to sit the patient up. Patients with grossly displaced mandibular injuries, such as those from gunshot wounds, should be allowed to sit leaning forward so that the tongue and any debris from the oral cavity is allowed to fall away from the airway.
- Neck extension and jaw thrust also helps to clear the airway, although neck extension is not permitted in the case of suspected injuries to the cervical spine.
- A Guedel airway can be used to help maintain the airway temporarily in a patient with reduced consciousness (Fig. 1.1). The majority of these patients will need a definitive airway, i.e. one in which there is a tracheal cuff to prevent debris escaping into the lungs. The best example of this is the endotracheal tube (ETT, Fig. 1.2).

Vomiting in the immobilized patient

Patients immobilized on a spinal board who vomit are in grave danger of aspiration as they cannot sit up to clear their airway. If such a patient is about to vomit they should be immediately turned on their side on the spinal board.

Surgical airways

An emergency surgical airway can be achieved in one of two ways.

Needle cricothyroidotomy

This provides a temporary surgical airway. In essence, it supplies the patient with oxygen, but without a definitive surgical airway there is an inevitable build-up of CO_2 which limits the usefulness of this technique.

Technique

- Make sure there is an oxygen supply and tubing available.
- Place patient in a supine position.
- Assemble a 12G or 14G needle with a 5mL syringe.
- Surgically prepare the neck using antiseptic swabs.
- Identify the cricothyroid membrane, between the cricoid cartilage and the thyroid cartilage. Stabilize the trachea with the thumb and forefinger of one hand to prevent lateral movement of the trachea during performance of the procedure.
- Puncture the skin in the midline with the needle attached to the syringe, directly over the cricothyroid membrane. A small incision with a No. 11 blade may facilitate passage of the needle through the skin.

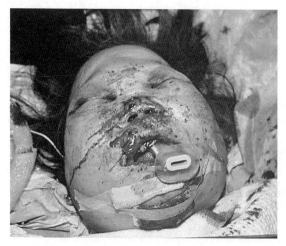

Fig. 1.1 Initial airway management of multiple facial injuries with Guedel airway.

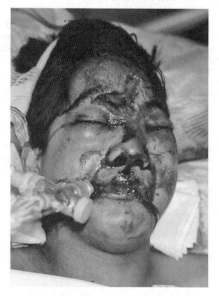

Fig. 1.2 Initial airway management of multiple facial injuries with the ETT.

- Direct the needle at a 45° angle inferiorly, while applying negative pressure to the syringe, and carefully insert the needle through the lower half of the cricothyroid membrane. Aspiration of air signifies entry into the tracheal lumen.
- Remove the syringe and attach the oxygen tubing over the needle hub. Intermittent ventilation can be achieved by occluding the open hole cut into the oxygen tubing with your thumb for 1s and releasing it for 4s.

Cricothyroidotomy

Surgical cricothyroidotomy provides a definitive surgical airway. It is a procedure that can be performed extremely rapidly and, in an emergency, any rigid tube with a hollow lumen can be used. Specially designed cricothyroidotomy tubes are available.

Technique

- Place the patient in a supine position with the neck in a neutral position. Palpate the thyroid notch, cricothyroid membrane, and the sternal notch for orientation. Surgically prepare and anaesthetize the area (if there is time and the patient is conscious).
- Stabilize the thyroid with the left hand. Make a transverse skin incision over the cricothyroid membrane. Carefully incise through the membrane. Insert the scalpel handle into the incision and rotate it 90° to open the airway. Insert an appropriately-sized, cuffed ETT or tracheostomy tube into the cricothyroid membrane incision, directing the tube inferiorly into the trachea. Inflate the cuff and ventilate the patient (Fig. 1.3 and Fig. 1.4).

Conscious patients with a compromised airway will often shows signs of agitation and will not want to lie supine as this causes the tongue to fall back into the airway. There may also be stridor present and signs of ↑ respiratory effort. Hypoxia may reveal itself by:

- Agitated patient.
- Varying level of consciousness.
- Inappropriate behaviour.
- Signs of airway compromise.
- Combination of these points.

Spinal immobilization

Patients with suspected spinal injuries or patients who are unconscious should be immobilized in the in-line spinal position. The cervical spine can be immobilized at the same time as establishing an airway.

Moving the patient

Multiple-injury patients should be immobilized on a spinal board for the purposes of transfer.

Intravenous access

Intravenous (IV) access should be established with two large-bore cannula (brown 14G or grey 16G) at two peripheral sites, such as the ante-cubital fossae.

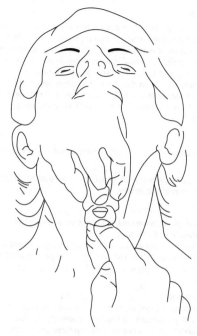

Fig. 1.3 Cricothyroidotomy: surface landmarks.

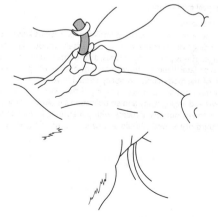

Fig. 1.4 Cricothyroidotomy: airway secured with ETT.

Facial bleeding

Sitting the patient up not only improves the airway and breathing, but also reduces venous pressure with a consequent beneficial effect on bleeding from injury. Most facial bleeding from soft tissue injuries can be controlled with direct pressure. Torrential haemorrhage from mid-facial fractures is not so easily controlled. Anterior and posterior nasal packing is used to staunch haemorrhage from the nose. It is often also helpful to prop the mouth open, impacting the maxilla against the skull base and compressing bleeding vessels. Hypovolaemia may be clinically apparent by:

- Tachycardia.
- Tachypnoea.
- Anxiety.
- Peripheral vasoconstriction (cool clammy periphery, prolonged capillary refill).

The first priority in the presence of appreciable facial haemorrhage always remains protection of the airway.

Bleeding from the neck

- Bleeding from penetrating neck trauma is potentially serious.
- Neck is divided into three zones:
  - zone I *(base)*—thoracic inlet to cricoid cartilage (highest mortality);
  - zone II *(mid-portion)*—cricoid cartilage to angle of mandible;
  - zone III *(superior)*—angle of mandible to skull base (difficult to access surgically).

External haemorrhage

If the haemorrhage is external, then local temporary measures such as iso-lating the bleeding point with a haemostat are appropriate. Bleeding from the tissues overlying the mandible from the facial artery can be controlled by pressure. Bleeding from the major vessels in the neck, such as the internal jugular vein, cannot be so easily controlled by pressure and will need prompt surgical exploration.

Concealed haemorrhage

Penetrating neck trauma from sharp implements, such as knives, can cause internal bleeding from damage to the great vessels without signs of external haemorrhage. This is potentially serious, as the consequences of rapid neck swelling can be fatal. Patients showing signs of neck swelling or patients who show signs of haemodynamic instability should have protection of the airway and control of haemorrhage. Imaging of the neck may be appropriate if time allows and angiography and embolization should be borne in mind as possible treatment options. Patients with penetrating injuries at the upper and lower third of the neck should also have imaging of the chest.

Imaging
- Plain films of neck.
- Chest X-ray (CXR).
- Computed tomography angiography (CTA).
- Conventional angiography.
- Magnetic resonance imaging (MRI)/magnetic resonance angiography (MRA).
- Ultrasound scanning (USS).

Initial management of head injuries

Patients with head injuries can initially be assessed using the 'Alert, Voice, Pain, Unresponsive' (AVPU) system before formal GCS assessment.

AVPU

A   Alert.
V   Voice, able to respond to verbal command.
P   Does not respond to verbal command, will respond to pain.
U   Unresponsive.

The first priority is to prevent secondary brain injury from inadequate cerebral circulation.
- Airway:
  - provide 100% oxygen;
  - consider intubation in the presence of hypoxia, hypercapnia, respiratory distress, or in a patient unable to protect their own airway.
- Breathing: assess and treat chest injuries.
- Circulation:
  - evaluate and treat hypovolaemia;
  - identify and control haemorrhage;
  - use isotonic fluids (crystalloid now shown to be fluid of choice usually 0.9% saline);
  - increasing use of permissive hypotension.

Glasgow Coma Scale

↓ level of consciousness as assessed by GCS.

Best eye response (E)
There are four grades starting with the most severe:
- **Grade 1**: no eye opening.
- **Grade 2**: eye opening in response to pain (patient responds to pressure on fingernail bed; if this does not elicit a response, supraorbital and sternal pressure or rub may be used).
- **Grade 3**: eye opening to speech (not to be confused with an awaking of a sleeping person; such patients receive a score of 4, not 3).
- **Grade 4**: eyes opening spontaneously.

Best verbal response (V)
There are five grades, starting with the most severe:
- **Grade 1**: no verbal response.
- **Grade 2**: incomprehensible sounds (moaning, but no words).
- **Grade 3**: inappropriate words (random or exclamatory articulated speech, but no conversational exchange).
- **Grade 4**: confused (patient responds to questions coherently, but there is some disorientation and confusion).
- **Grade 5**: orientated (patient responds coherently and appropriately to questions such as name and age, etc.).

Best motor response (M)
There are six grades, starting with the most severe:
- **Grade 1**: no motor response.
- **Grade 2**: extension to pain (adduction of arm, internal rotation of shoulder, pronation of forearm, extension of wrist—decerebrate response).
- **Grade 3**: abnormal flexion to pain (adduction of arm, internal rotation of shoulder, pronation of forearm, flexion of wrist—decorticate response).
- **Grade 4**: flexion/withdrawal to pain (flexion of elbow, supination of forearm, flexion of wrist when supraorbital pressure applied, pulls part of body away when nail bed pinched).
- **Grade 5**: localizes to pain (purposeful movements towards painful stimuli, e.g. hand crosses mid-line and gets above clavicle when supraorbital pressure applied).
- **Grade 6**: obeys commands (patient carries out simple requests).

A fully conscious patient scores 15. A patient scoring <8 should be considered to be in a coma and, as such, unable to protect their own airway. The minimum score is 3.

Computed tomography imaging in head injury

Criteria for immediate request for CT scan of the head (adults; National Institute for Health and Care Excellence (NICE)):
- GCS <13 on initial assessment in the emergency department.
- GCS <15 at 2h after the injury on assessment in the emergency department.
- Suspected open or depressed skull fracture.
- Any sign of basal skull fracture (haemotympanum, 'panda' eyes, cerebrospinal fluid (CSF) leakage from the ear or nose, Battle's sign).
- Post-traumatic seizure.
- Focal neurological deficit.
- More than one episode of vomiting.
- Amnesia for events >30min before impact.

Criteria for immediate request for CT scan of the head provided patient has experienced some loss of consciousness or amnesia since the injury (adults):
- Age 65 years or older.
- Coagulopathy (history of bleeding, clotting disorder, current treatment with warfarin).
- Dangerous mechanism of injury (a pedestrian or cyclist struck by a motor vehicle, an occupant ejected from a motor vehicle, or a fall from a height of >1m or five stairs).

Criteria for immediate request for CT scan of the head (children):
- Loss of consciousness lasting >5min (witnessed).
- Amnesia (antegrade or retrograde) lasting >5min.
- Abnormal drowsiness.
- Three or more discrete episodes of vomiting.
- Clinical suspicion of non-accidental injury.

- Post-traumatic seizure but no history of epilepsy.
- GCS <14, or for a baby <1 year GCS (paediatric) <15, on assessment in the emergency department.
- Suspicion of open or depressed skull injury or tense fontanelle.
- Any sign of basal skull fracture (haemotympanum, 'panda' eyes, CSF leakage from the ear or nose, Battle's sign).
- Focal neurological deficit.
- If <1 year, presence of bruise, swelling, or laceration of >5 cm on the head.
- Dangerous mechanism of injury (high-speed road traffic accident either as pedestrian, cyclist, or vehicle occupant; fall from a height of >3m; high-speed injury from a projectile or an object).

Initial management of ocular injuries

A high proportion of patients with orbital injuries will have coexisting ocular injuries. It is essential to make an initial basic assessment of ocular function. In a conscious patient, this should consist of an assessment of visual acuity using a pocket Snellen chart. If the patient cannot read the bottom line on the Snellen chart, then assessment is as follows:

- Can the patient count fingers?
- Can the patient see hand movement?
- Has the patient any light perception?

Relative afferent pupillary defect (RAPD) is an indication of damage to the visual system that is useful in an unconscious patient. It is assessed by the swinging light test in which a pen torch is alternatively shone into one eye and then the other. Swinging the torch from the normal eye to the affected eye results in bilateral pupillary dilatation (Marcus Gunn sign). The presence of a RAPD usually indicates damage to the retina or optic nerve.

Directly examine the eye for the following clinical features:

- **Hyphema:** blood in anterior chamber.
- **Irregular pupil:** sign of underlying ocular injury.
- **Constricted pupil:** consider coexisting opiate abuse.
- **Dilated pupil:** suspect optic nerve or retinal injury or cocaine abuse.

Retrobulbar haemorrhage

Retrobulbar haemorrhage is best thought of as an example of acute orbital compression syndrome as a result of an intraconal bleed. The commonest causes are orbital trauma or as a complication of orbital surgery. Haemorrhage causes ↑ pressure within the orbit, reducing flow in the retinal artery (an anatomical end-artery), which in turn leads to irreversible vascular changes within the optic nerve, resulting in visual loss. Consider retrobulbar haemorrhage if:

- **Tense proptosed eye:** eye pushed forward under pressure compared with contralateral eye.
- **Ophthalmoplegic eye:** no eye movement.
- **Chemosis** and **orbital pain.**
- **RAPD.**
- **Raised intra-ocular pressure.**
- **Retinal signs:**
  - papilloedema;
  - lack of central retinal artery pulsation;
  - pale optic disc (occurs late);
  - cherry red macula.

Treatment of retrobulbar haemorrhage needs to be prompt in order to avoid permanent visual loss.

Treatment options
Medical decompression
- Mannitol (osmotic diuretic) 20% 2g/kg IV over 5min.
- Dexamethasone 8mg IV.
- Acetazolamide (carbonic anhydrase inhibitor, reduces production of aqueous humour), 500mg IV and then 1000mg orally over 24h.

Surgical decompression
Lateral canthotomy and cantholysis.

Canthotomy technique
- Clean the area with sterile saline.
- Inject local anaesthetic (LA) into the lateral canthus.
- Apply a haemostat/clamp with one side anterior and one side posterior to the lateral canthus and advance until the rim of the bony orbit is felt.
- Clamp for 30–60s.
- Perform the lateral canthotomy by carefully cutting through the crushed, demarcated line to the orbital rim/lateral fornix to avoid traumatizing the orbit.

Cantholysis technique
- Grasp lower eyelid with forceps and pull outwards/downwards away from eye.
- Identify the canthal ligament by either inspection or palpation. Incise the inferior crus of the lateral canthal ligament with scissors to avoid traumatizing the orbit.
- Recheck the orbit for reduction in intra-orbital and intra-ocular pressure. If pressure is still high, dissect the superior limb of the canthal ligament in a similar fashion. Care should be taken to avoid any trauma to the lacrimal gland.

'First aid', antibiotics, and tetanus

Antibiotic usage

Indications for prophylactic usage of antibiotics in trauma include:
- Contaminated soft tissue injury.
- Mandibular fractures which are compound to the mouth.
- Surgical emphysema.
- Peri-operative surgical prophylaxis in ORIF.

The importance of prompt surgical debridement cannot be over-emphasized in the management of contaminated wounds and compound fractures. Without surgical debridement infection will eventually occur even with antibiotic prophylaxis. Antibiotic prophylaxis should therefore start promptly and continue until surgical debridement has occurred.

In the case of grossly infected wounds and systemic signs, such as rigor, pyrexia, and tachycardia, antibiotics should continue for at least 5 days.

The choice of antibiotic will depend upon local policy.

Bite injuries should be covered with co-amoxiclav.

Antibiotic prophylaxis is no longer routinely recommended for patients with CSF leaks.

Tetanus prophylaxis

Consideration of tetanus prophylaxis depends upon the status of the wound and immunization status of the patient (Table 1.1).

Adsorbed tetanus vaccine
- Adsorbed tetanus vaccine is given as 0.5mL by deep subcutaneous (SC) or intramuscular (IM) injection into the deltoid or gluteal muscle.
- A full course of adsorbed tetanus vaccine consists of three doses of 0.5mL at intervals of not less than 4 weeks, followed by two further doses.
- Tetanus vaccine must not be given to anyone who has received a reinforcing dose in the preceding year.
- Patients with impaired immunity who suffer a tetanus-prone wound may not respond to vaccine and may therefore require anti-tetanus immunoglobulin in addition.

Human tetanus immunoglobulin for prophylaxis
- Human tetanus immunoglobulin is given as 250IU in 1mL by IM injection into the deltoid or gluteal region.
- If >24h have elapsed since injury, or there is risk of heavy contamination, or following burns, the recommended dose is 500IU.

Tetanus vaccine and immunoglobulin must be given by separate syringes into separate sites.

Penicillin/metronidazole is the drug of choice for treatment of tetanus.

Table 1.1 Wound type and immunization status

Immunization status	Clean wound	Tetanus-prone wound	
	Vaccine	Vaccine	Human tetanus immunoglobulin
Fully immunized, i.e. has received a total of five doses of vaccine at appropriate intervals	None required	None required	Only if high risk
Primary immunization complete, boosters incomplete but up to date	None required (unless next dose soon and convenient to give now)	None required (unless next dose soon and convenient to give now)	Only if high risk
Primary immunization incomplete or boosters not up to date	A reinforcing dose of vaccine and further doses required to complete the recommended schedule (to ensure future immunity)	A reinforcing dose of vaccine and further doses required to complete the recommended schedule (to ensure future immunity)	Yes one dose of human tetanus immunoglobulin in a different site
Not immunized or immunization status not known or uncertain	An immediate dose of vaccine followed, if records confirm the need, by completion of a full five-dose course to ensure future immunity	An immediate dose of vaccine followed, if records confirm the need, by completion of a full five-dose course to ensure future immunity	Yes one dose of human tetanus immunoglobulin in a different site

Definitive diagnosis

Full assessment of the maxillofacial region requires careful examination of the soft and hard tissues.

Inspection: facial

Soft tissue

Facial soft tissue injuries should be carefully recorded.

A laceration is caused by blunt trauma—an incised wound caused by a sharp object.

The use of clinical photography is to be commended especially for complex lacerations. Such photographs may be needed for medicolegal purposes and are always a useful adjunct to planning revision surgery. Each laceration should have the following recorded:

- **Contamination**: the greatest influence on management is the presence or absence of wound contamination. Heavily contaminated wounds, regardless of size and depth, need debridement, which often needs to be completed under GA.
- **Condition of wound margins:**
  - *sharp clean cut edge*—this results from sharp injury such as injury on a metal edge. These are simple to repair after appropriate debridement;
  - *serrated edge*—this can implicate glass fractured in the aetiology of the wound; if so, exploration of the wound to locate and remove them is required;
  - *rounded edge*—if the edge of wound is rounded then it is likely that the wound has arisen as a result of friction over a bony protuberance. This is the case for the common paediatric injuries, such as cuts on the forehead, eyebrows, and chin;
  - *necrotic edge*—higher energy transfer to the wound causes irreversible damage to the soft tissue edge, such that it is dusky or black. Judicious trimming of wound edges needs to be considered in such cases.
- **Size**: measure length of the laceration with a ruler.
- **Depth:**
  - *up to dermal depth*—abrasion;
  - *up to fat depth*—laceration likely to require suture;
  - *muscle involvement*—consider the possibility of facial nerve or parotid involvement (surface anatomy of parotid duct is middle third of line drawn from the tragus to the corner of the mouth). The buccal branch of facial nerve is always closely associated with the parotid duct. Repair of the facial nerve is indicated in wounds lateral to the lateral canthus.
  - *bony involvement.*
- **Orientation to relaxed skin tension lines**: lacerations which are orientated in the direction of relaxed skin tension lines are likely to heal better than lacerations orientated away from relaxed skin tension lines.

The following signs of bruising raise suspicion of an underlying fracture:

• **Bruising over the skin of the mastoid bone**: 'Battle's sign' (can indicate a base of skull fracture).
• **Bilateral periorbital bruising**: 'Raccoon eyes' (can indicate a fracture of base of the skull, naso-ethmoid region, frontal sinus, or Le Fort II/III fracture).
• **Bilateral inner canthus bruising**: can indicate of nasal bone fracture.
• **Bruising overlying the lower border of the mandible**: can indicate a mandibular fracture.

The presence of facial swelling should be noted, although it correlates poorly with the severity of the underlying bony injury. Swelling often masks underlying bony deformity as described:

Bony/cartilaginous deformity
• Evidence of deformity in the frontal and naso-ethmoid area:
  • *frontal bone deformity*—this is most commonly seen in patients with fractures of the anterior wall of the frontal sinus. The appearance is of a midline depression in the area immediately above the supraorbital ridge;
  • *naso-ethmoidal deformity*—this is often associated with frontal deformity. The classic appearance includes telecanthus, depression of nasal bridge, and elevation of the nasal tip.
• **Nasal bone deformity**: the nose is frequently disrupted in facial injuries. Anatomically, only the upper third of nose is bony. Nasal fractures often present with deviation of the nose.
• **Evidence of malar flattening**: the zygomatic bone forms most of the lateral and inferior orbital rim. Inferolateral to this is the prominence of the zygoma. Displaced fractures of the zygoma produce flattening of this area that it is easy to underestimate in the acute setting as facial swelling obscures the appearance.
• Evidence of zygomatic arch deformity:
  • *in-fracture of the arch of the zygoma*—may be an isolated fracture of the arch or may be associated with an externally rotated zygomatic fracture;
  • *out-fracture of the arch of the zygoma*—seen as bowing of the zygomatic arch. Often associated with posterior displacement and an internally rotated zygomatic fracture. This is an important clinical sign as bowing of the zygomatic arch is hard to correct surgically and, if left untreated, leads to persistent bony swelling overlying the zygomatic arch.

Inspection: oral

An examination of the mouth is mandatory since clinical signs indicating fractures of the maxilla and mandible are often reflected in intraoral changes that are not obscured by general facial swelling.

• **Bruising**: sublingual haematoma (Coleman's sign) is highly suggestive of a mandibular fracture.
• **Gingival lacerations**: laceration of the gingivae in the lower jaw is suggestive of a mandibular fracture, and in the upper jaw is suggestive of a segmental maxillary fracture.

- **Palatal bruising**: indicates either a split palate or Le Fort fracture.
- **Gross deformity of mandible.**
- **Disorders of occlusion** (Fig. 1.5):
  - *anterior open bite*—either bilateral mandibular condylar fracture or a posteriorly displaced Le Fort fracture;
  - *lateral open bite*—the patient's teeth meet normally on one side, but on the opposite side there is no contact. The most common cause for this is a mandibular condylar fracture on the *contralateral side* to the open bite.

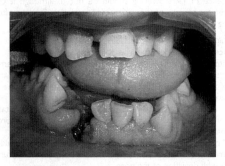

Fig. 1.5 Step in occlusion with mandibular fracture.

Inspection: orbital

Swelling may obscure a full view of the patient's eye. If this is the case, it is still important to obtain a basic assessment of visual function (see ➜ Initial management of ocular injuries, p. 16). Systematic examination of the orbit is as follows:

- **Pupillary level**: is the pupil at the same level as the opposite eye? If one eye is lower then a vertical orbital dystopia exists that may be the result of a zygomatic or orbital floor fractures.
- **Antero-posterior eye position**: are the eyes in the same position? Enophthalmos can be associated with internal orbital wall injury. Exophthalmos is one sign of retrobulbar haemorrhage (see ➜ Initial management of ocular injuries, p. 16).
- **Intercanthal distance (normally same width as palpebral fissure)**: an increase in the intercanthal width (normal range in Caucasians 28–35mm) results from lateral displacement of the medial canthal tendon. The result is telecanthus. The usual cause is a naso-ethmoidal fracture.

Inspection: nasal

The nose should be examined externally and internally. Internal examination of the nose is facilitated by the use of a Thuddicum's speculum.

- **External nasal examination**: look for deviation of the nose and asymmetry of nasal bones.

- Internal nasal examination:
  - *septal haematoma*—this is seen as a bulge on both sides of the nasal septum that often totally obscures the nasal airway. It is a surgical emergency and requires immediate drainage to prevent long-term damage to the septal cartilage;
  - *septal deviation/dislocation*—this is common and should be elicited during the initial examination. Acute management may be required.
- CSF rhinorrhoea: this is seen as clear fluid leaking from the nose (detected by beta-2 transferrin assay). It occurs in high-level mid-face injuries, as well as naso-ethmoidal and frontal bone injury. The fluid is often seen tram lining—blood leaking from the nose forms clotted streaks of blood down the face with CSF washing away the central portion of clotted blood.

Inspection: ear

Inspect the pinna for signs of laceration and haematoma.

- Haematoma of the pinna can compromise the blood supply to the underlying cartilage producing a 'cauliflower' ear. These haematomas need drainage.
- CSF otorrhoea.
- Bleeding from the external auditory meatus: this can result from a number of injuries:
  - *base of skull fracture*—Battle's sign usually coexists;
  - *laceration of the cartilaginous auditory meatus*—can be a sign of mandibular condylar injury;
  - *bleeding from tympanic membrane*—usually associated with rupture of the tympanic membrane.

Active range of movement

Mandibular

Normal mandibular opening is around 35–45mm. Reduced mandibular opening is not a reliable indicator of mandibular fracture, since it can be secondary to soft tissue injuries and effusions of the temporomandibular joint. A more accurate clinical sign is the amount of protrusion of the mandible (activity of the lateral pterygoid muscles attached to head of the mandibular condyles).

Ocular

Examine the eyes in primary gaze (looking straight ahead), as well as the other eight positions of gaze (left and right central; left, central, and right upward gaze; left, central, and right downward gaze). Patients may report double vision.

- Monocular: lens dislocation or retinal detachment.
- Binocular:
  - entrapment of extraocular muscles and orbital contents;
  - haematoma;
  - dysfunction of extraocular muscles;
  - periglobular oedema;
  - neuropathy of cranial nerves supplying extraocular muscles (III, IV, and VI).

Diplopia on upward gaze is a clinical sign of orbital floor entrapment with the false imaging originating in the injured eye. Diplopia in downward gaze can be associated with dysfunction of the inferior rectus usually due to muscle bruising. Consider ophthalmology or orthoptic referral.

Sensory changes and facial fractures

Assessment should be made of the three divisions of the trigeminal nerve:

- **Supraorbital/supratrochlear nerves:** rarely injured. If sensory abnormality exists, it is most likely to be localized injury to the nerve itself (i.e. neuropraxia) without underlying fracture.
- **Infraorbital nerve:** commonly injured in orbital floor and zygomatic fractures.
- **Mental nerve/inferior dental (ID) nerve:** commonly injured in fractures of the mandible. Usually indicates an angle, body, or parasymphyseal fracture.

Specific signs of abnormal mobility

These signs should be elicited carefully in a conscious patient, since they can be painful.

Maxillary

Hold the maxilla in a gloved hand and attempt to move it, whilst restraining the forehead. See if movement can be elicited at:

- Nasal bones and lateral orbital rims—Le Fort III level fracture.
- Nasal bones and infraorbital rims—Le Fort II fracture.

Mandible

Press bilaterally at both mandibular angles and see if movement in the region anterior the angles can be elicited. If no movement can be appreciated and the patient can protrude their mandible normally, a fracture is unlikely. The test should not be pursued in the presence of an obvious fracture as it will elicit pain.

Investigations

Radiography

Plain film radiographs are sometimes undertaken as a screening tool. In simple fractures they are often the only necessary investigation, e.g. fractures of the tooth-bearing portion of the mandible or single-piece fractures of the zygoma.

Occipitomental views

Otherwise known as 'Water's view', the OM view is taken with the film at the chin and the radiographic source at the occiput. High-quality films need the patient to extend their neck, which is not always possible in the acute setting. The angulation of the OM view is recorded in degrees and refers to the extension of the neck that is present when the film is taken—a 30° OM is commonly ordered, which is a film taken with a 30° neck extension. OM views are indicated if a fracture of the zygoma or zygomatic arch is suspected.

Orthopantomogram

This is a tomogram of the mandible and is effectively two lateral views of the mandible joined together. A second view of the mandible (usually PA) is required.

Postero-anterior mandible

This is a PA view of the mandible with the film placed at the patient's chin.

Computed tomography

CT has been available since 1972. The use of cross-sectional imaging has revolutionized the diagnosis of complex facial trauma. Modifications such as helical and multi-slice scanning mean that CT can be acquired quickly. There is also no need for the patient to stand to gain adequate CT images. CT images can be reformatted in any plane and three-dimensional reconstructions can be derived from the original scan data. The other main advantage of CT scanning is that good quality images can be gained from patients in cervical spine immobilization who are supine.

Indications for CT scanning for facial trauma include:
- Any unconscious patient who is having CT for head injury with an associated facial injury.
- Injuries of the frontal sinus and naso-ethmoidal area.
- Injuries of the middle third of the face.
- Imaging of orbital floor and orbital wall injuries.
- Bilateral injuries of the mandibular condylar region.
- High-energy transfer injuries to facial region, e.g. gun shots.
- Pan-facial fractures.

Cone beam computed scanning

The main disadvantage of CT scanning is the radiation dose involved. Since CT scanning for facial injuries is finer cut than brain CT, there is a higher radiation dose per patient volume (risk of iatrogenic cataracts) hence the development of low-dose cone beam computed tomography (CBCT) scanning. The reduction in radiation dose (see ➜ Ionizing Radiation (Medical Exposure) Regulations, p. 491) results in a loss of the number of Hounsfield units that the scanner can detect. Soft tissue definition of the images are therefore inferior to conventional CT scanning. However, for diagnostic and reconstructive use in hard tissue facial trauma CBCT scanning is adequate for mandibular and basic orbital imaging.

MRI

May be of use in orbital trauma. Detects CSF leaks well.

Ultrasound

Of limited value in diagnosing fractures of the facial skeleton. There are some proponents of its use in hard and soft tissue orbital trauma.

Imaging of specific areas

Upper third

- **Plain films:** of limited value.
- **CT:** significant risk of intracranial injury.
- **MRI:** CSF leaks.

Middle third

- **Plain films:** simple fractures (OMs).
- **CT:** orbits, consider stereolithography/navigation.
- **MRI:** orbits.

Lower third

- **Plain films:** usually sufficient.
- **CT:** condylar fractures and polytrauma.

Soft tissue

- **Plain films:** foreign bodies.
- **CT:** metallic foreign bodies.
- **MRI:** non-metallic foreign bodies.
- **Sialography:** parotid duct injuries.
- **Dacrocystography:** nasolacrimal injuries.
- **Angiography:** penetrating neck trauma (see ➜ 'How to do' emergency procedures, p. 6).

Orthoptic

Orthoptic examination is the specialized assessment of eye movement. This examination requires individual items of equipment and the patient has to be able to open both eyes. As a result this form of assessment is only practical when any facial swelling has resolved. An orthoptic assessment includes a Hess chart and documentation of fields of binocular vision.

Definitive surgery

Soft tissue management

The facial soft tissues should be repaired as soon as possible after the injury. Contaminated wounds need debridement within 24h of injury. Consider use of Steri-Strips™ or glue.

Choice of anaesthetic

Many clean small lacerations can be treated under LA. Indications for GA include:

- Lacerations in some children.
- Large or multiple lacerations.
- Lacerations that require exploration of deeper structures.
- Contaminated wounds that need significant debridement.

Primary treatment

All contamination of the wound must be addressed before the wound is closed. Facial injuries resulting from direct abrasions on road surfaces impregnate debris deep into the dermis. The tattooing effect that results from inadequate primary debridement of such wounds is difficult to correct with scar revision.

Choice of suture material and technique

- Close wounds in layers using resorbable sutures in the deeper layers.
- Shelving wounds that need differential suturing (larger bite on thicker wounds edge).
- Use non-resorbable sutures (5/0 to 6/0) unless it is impractical to remove sutures, in which case 6/0 to 7/0 resorbable sutures should be employed.

Specialized sites

Lips

- Lips need careful repair, paying particular attention to realignment of the vermillion border (Fig. 1.6).
- Full-thickness lip lacerations demand three-layer closure and consideration to antibiotic prophylaxis.

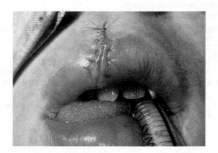

Fig. 1.6 Careful approximation of vermillion border in lip laceration.

Parotid duct

The surface marking of the parotid duct is the middle third of a line drawn between the tragus of the ear and the midpoint between the upper lip and alar base. It is always closely associated with the buccal branch of the facial nerve that is often injured along with injuries of the parotid duct.

- Any deep facial wound crossing this area should be explored under GA and examined under magnification.
- Parotid duct injuries can sometimes be diagnosed preoperatively by inspecting the wound for a salivary leak. Alternatively retrograde injection of methylene blue into the parotid duct can be employed.
- The distal cut end of the parotid duct can be identified by cannulating the duct from the mouth.
- The proximal end is more difficult to identify—milk the gland and watching its cut surface under magnification for saliva pooling.
- The duct is repaired by loosely tacking the ends around a stent passed via the mouth through the distal and proximal ends of the duct.
- The stent, e.g. plastic IV cannula is left *in situ* for 7 days.

Facial nerve

The facial nerve exits the stylomastoid foramen at the base of the skull and enters the parotid gland. After a short distance it divides into an upper and lower division that then further divides into five main branches (temporal, zygomatic, buccal, marginal mandibular and cervical). The facial nerve is afforded a degree of protection in blunt facial trauma, since its lies embedded within the parotid gland.

Anatomical notes relevant to injury:

- The facial nerve has an intratemporal course, as well as an extratemporal course. Intrabony injuries of the facial nerve can occur in skull base fracture, extratemporal lesions tend to occur in penetrating neck and facial injuries.
- The facial nerve has rich cross-innervation between the zygomatic and buccal branches that mediates the effects of injury to these branches.
- The temporal and marginal mandibular branches have less cross-innervation and if injured will frequently require repair.
- The temporal branch crosses the zygomatic arch at least 1cm in front of the root of the arch.
- The buccal branch is closely associated with parotid duct.
- The marginal mandibular branch crosses the neck and lies up to 1.5cm below the lower border of the mandible. Its lowest point is posterior to the facial artery.

Primary nerve repair should be undertaken if there is obvious muscle weakness and there is a nerve injury proximal to a line down vertically from the lateral canthus of the eye (Fig. 1.7).

Delayed nerve repair is still worth attempting, since it can take several months after the original injury for the motor end plates to atrophy.

Nerve repair should be performed under magnification using a microscope and 10/0 sutures. Both epineural and perineural repair can yield good results if the nerve is correctly opposed. If there is a segment of nerve missing it is advisable to include a nerve graft in the repair to prevent over-stretching.

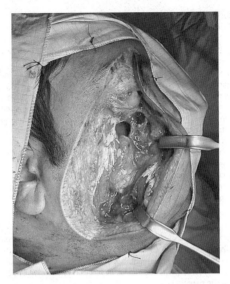

Fig. 1.7 Facial incised wound caused by knife.

Eyelids
Eyelid lacerations can be a marker for the presence of underlying injuries to the globe, orbit, and brain. Beware the possibility of an already ruptured globe. Eyelid lacerations can also herald the presence of foreign body. Local structures that may be injured include:
• Lacrimal apparatus (laceration in the medial canthal area).
• Levator apparatus (within the upper eyelid)—check for ptosis of the upper eyelid.
• Corneal injury (frequently found in association with lid lacerations crossing the free margin of the lower eyelid).

Injuries to these three areas should be managed in conjunction with an ophthalmic surgeon. Small lacerations of the eyelid skin not associated with globe injury and not involving the three areas as outlined can often be managed conservatively with debridement alone or, if large, addressed with 6/0 suture material.

Management of tissue loss

Wounds should be carefully assessed for tissue loss at the time of debridement. Options for management of tissue loss will depend upon:
- Quantity of tissue loss.
- Degree of contamination.
- Site of tissue loss.
- Damage to/loss of deep structures—bone/cartilage.

The options for management of tissue loss broadly follow the reconstructive ladder:
- Used in primary injury:
  • dressings/healing be secondary intention;
  • primary closure;
  • delayed closure;
  • split-thickness graft;
  • full-thickness graft.
- Used in secondary reconstruction:
  • tissue expansion;
  • local flap (random-pattern/axial, pedicled);
  • distant flap (random-pattern/axial, pedicled);
  • free flap.

For most acute injuries it is better to use as simple a method of reconstruction as possible for treatment, since tissue loss is most commonly associated with heavy contamination, such as animal and human bites, or high-energy trauma. Unresolved infection and tissue necrosis under a complex soft tissue reconstruction will likely lead to failure of the reconstruction.

Dressings/healing by secondary intention

Small areas of tissue loss at sites where there is no underlying exposed bone or cartilage can be allowed to granulate. The process of wound healing occurs in three stages—inflammatory, fibroplasia, and remodelling. The remodelling phase commences at around 3 weeks and involves maturation of myofibroblasts with contraction of the wound.

Primary/delayed closure

Facial skin is elastic and can be used to advance over areas of tissue loss. The best example of this is the heavily contaminated wound with necrotic edges. The wound is debrided, necrotic edges excised, the wound advanced, and then closed primarily. Delayed primary closure is rarely required in the face.

Split-thickness graft/full-thickness graft

Skin grafts are useful in the management of tissue loss as they can provide cover for large exposed areas of muscle, perichondrium, and pericranium. Skin grafts are particular useful in areas where there is little tissue movement that would otherwise influence graft take. Skin grafts are therefore appropriate in areas such the nose and scalp as opposed to the mobile lips. Skin grafting has the added advantage of wound contracture that reduces the size of the graft area in cases subsequently requiring secondary reconstruction.

Flaps

Flap surgery is frequently avoided in the acute setting. However, certain circumstances necessitate the use of flaps:

- Areas of exposed bone or cartilage that cannot be closed primarily.
- Gross incompetence of the lips as a result of tissue loss (as a delayed primary procedure following initial debridement).
- Composite tissue loss in gunshot injury (as a delayed primary procedure following initial debridement).

After care

Patients require wound care following soft tissue injury. Facial lacerations should have all non-resorbable sutures removed at 5 days. Wounds which have been left to granulate should ideally be dressed with a non-adherent, absorbent dressing. This is not possible with tissue loss on the lips, to which simple petroleum jelly can be applied. Dressings over skin grafts should initially be removed at 5 days to inspect the take of the graft.

Secondary procedures

Since maturation of skin scars can takes up to 2 years it is usually inadvisable to consider early secondary revision. The exception to this is the early excision of a skin graft or area left to heal by secondary intention.

Hypertrophic scars

These are usually apparent within 2 months of primary procedure. Since pressure accelerates maturation of the scar, pressure garments or massage might reduce their occurrence. Hypertrophic scars are more likely to occur in deeper wounds, contaminated wounds, and those allowed to heal by secondary intention. Silicone sheets or gels can minimize the impact of such scars.

Principles of hard tissue management

Fractures

Types
- **Simple**: single fracture.
- **Compound**: communicates with body surface.
- **Comminuted**: several pieces.
- **Complicated**: involving vascular or neurological structure.
- **Greenstick**: involves only one cortex.
- **Pathological**.

Phases of bone healing
- Haematoma and acute inflammation.
- **Osteolytic phase**: eburnation of bone ends and formation of granulation tissue.
- **Osteogenic phase**: early callus formation and lamellar bone production.
- Remodelling.

Problems with bone healing
- General, e.g. diabetes, scurvy, immunocompromise, smoking.
- Local, e.g. infection, soft tissue interposition.
- Delayed union.
- Mal-union—fracture healing with misalignment.
- Non-union—failure to heal.

Principles of management
- Reduction.
- Immobilization/fixation.
- Rehabilitation.

Osteosynthesis principles

Fracture healing in facial bones is rapid and reliable. Non-union is unusual, but mal-union is a frequent result of inadequate primary treatment. Unlike long bones, fracture healing does not require absolute rigid immobilization. A limited amount of micro-movement in a clean uninfected fracture with healthy periosteum does not impede healing.

Osteosynthesis was revolutionized with the introduction of titanium miniplates that can be used to fix almost all fractures in the facial skeleton. The advantages of miniplates include:
- Variety of small sizes available with both monocortical and bicortical fixation.
- Titanium is extremely well biotolerated and rarely requires a secondary removal procedure.
- Titanium is malleable to ensure passive fit of plates at the fracture site.

Choice of anaesthesia

The majority of facial fractures will require treatment under a GA. The occasional exception to this rule is the mandible and dento-alveolar process of the maxilla and mandible. The latter tooth-bearing region is easily anaesthetized with regional nerve blocks and can be repaired under LA as long as there are no other associated injuries.

Mandibular fractures

The mandible is the densest bone in the human body. It is 'U'-shaped with a temporomandibular joint at either end. Mandible fractures can be anatomically divided into regions:

- **Symphysis:** the midline of the mandible.
- **Parasymphysis:** either side of the midline proximal to the mental foramen.
- **Body:** area anterior to the mandibular angle and posterior to the mental foramen.
- **Angle:** junction of body and ramus.
- **Ramus:** below sigmoid notch and above the angle.
- **Coronoid process:** a fracture above the base of the sigmoid notch affecting the coronoid process.
- **Condylar area:**
  - *condylar base*—runs from the posterior border of the mandible into the sigmoid notch;
  - *condylar neck*—superior to condylar base;
  - *intracapsular*—within the joint capsule.

Mandibular fractures are often multiple. The commonest fracture patterns are the parasymphysis and angle fracture, or the parasymphysis and condylar fracture.

Mandibular fractures should be assessed for:

- **Inferior alveolar nerve injury:** must be documented before fracture treatment.
- **Presence of decayed or fractured teeth:** teeth that cannot be restored either as a result of the injury or pre-existing dental disease should be extracted at the time of surgery.
- **Displacement:** undisplaced fractures should be considered for conservative management.
- **Stability:** displacement of the fracture is the key indicator of fracture stability: a grossly displaced fracture tears the periosteum that otherwise adds stability to the fracture.
- **Dental occlusion:** an abnormal occlusion indicates displacement and mobility of the fracture that requires correction.
- **Height of alveolar bone:** the greater the effective height of the mandible the greater the potential stability of the fracture.
- **Comminution:** this suggests a high-energy injury that is difficult to treat and prone to infection and non-union.

Tooth-bearing regions: symphysis, parasymphysis, body, and angle

Indications for treatment

- Displaced fracture with abnormal occlusion.
- Unresolving pain from undisplaced fracture.

Mandibular fractures can be treated conservatively if they are undisplaced. Patients have to be compliant and able to tolerate a strictly liquid/soft diet for 4 weeks. They need careful monitoring to check for failure of treatment that is usually heralded by a change in occlusion or increasing pain.

Historically, many patients with mandibular fractures were treated with rigid intermaxillary fixation. This is now rarely carried out except in instances of exceptionally complex fractures when the full remit of reconstructive techniques is not available.

Surgical access

These fractures can be accessed via transmucosal incisions made in the buccal sulcus or around the necks of the teeth. A mucoperiosteal flap is raised taking care to protect the mental nerve at the junction of the parasymphysis and body of the mandible. Incisions need to be designed avoiding a suture line directly over osteosynthetic material which should ideally be covered by the muscle, such as buccinator and mentalis.

It is advisable to expose all the potential fractures of the mandible before reduction and fixation. Incorrect fixation of one fracture site will make it impossible to reduce the fracture at other sites.

Reduction

It is essential that there is adequate reduction of the bony fragments, particularly at the level of the teeth so that a normal occlusion is returned. Small discrepancies in bony reduction can be tolerated but even small discrepancies in the dental occlusion should not be accepted.

Reduction of the fracture can be achieved by:

- Hand-held reduction.
- Temporary intermaxillary fixation:
  - eyelet wire;
  - Leonard buttons and wires;
  - intermaxillary fixation (IMF) screws;
  - arch bars.
- **Direct bony reduction:** this can sometimes be obtained in the anterior mandible by applying a temporary wire between two monocortical screws. There is a tendency to close the fracture on the buccal aspect of the mandible and, consequently, to open it on its lingual aspect.

Fixation

The bony ends are fixed according to the principles set out by Michelet–Champy:

- Monocortical fixation with 2.0mm diameter screws through the outer cortex only to avoid damage to the roots of the teeth. A minimum of two screws either side of the fracture line should be placed per plate.
- All plates to be pre-bent so that they fit passively on to the surface of the mandible.
- Two plates used anterior to the mental foramen to resist the torsional effects of the anterior mandibular musculature. Plates to be placed at least 5mm apart.
- One plate along the line of maximal tension in the body and angle. This line approximates to the external oblique ridge of the mandible.
- Osteosynthesis at the mandibular angle can be placed on the lateral aspect of the external oblique ridge, utilizing a transbuccal trochar to maintain the screw direction perpendicular to the plate and the underlying bone (Fig. 1.8 and Fig. 1.9).

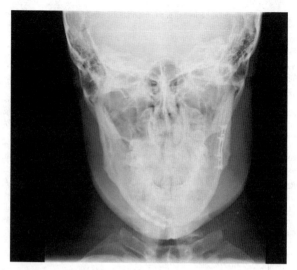

Fig. 1.8 PA view of treated fractured mandible.

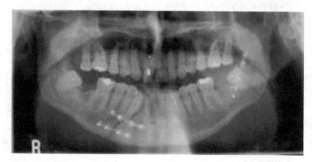

Fig. 1.9 OPG view of treated fractured mandible.

When Michelet–Champy principles do not apply

Michelet and Champy originally published their articles on miniplate fixation recommending that patients be placed in intermaxillary fixation post-operatively for 6 weeks for additional stability. Current trauma management focuses on early return to function so patients are not placed in IMF post-operatively.

Michelet–Champy is essentially a 'load-sharing' osteosynthesis, relying on optimal fracture healing conditions and good bony contact. This can be lacking under the following circumstances:

- Comminution.
- Body fractures.
- Multiple edentulous segments.
- Multiple carious teeth.
- Irradiation, bisphosphonate therapy, or other cause for pathological fracture.
- Infected fracture.
- Poor patient compliance.
- Diabetes, alcoholism, smoking, immunosuppression.

These factors tend to occur in combination. If they are present then consideration should be given to 'load-bearing' osteosynthesis. This is fundamentally different to 'load-sharing osteosynthesis' in the following respects:

- Rigid fixation with thick profile plate capable of taking most of muscular load of the mandible. This is placed along the lower border of the mandible to give maximal mucosal coverage, and minimize the risk to the inferior dental nerve and teeth roots.
- Bi-cortical fixation usually >2.0mm screws, at least three screws either side of the fracture line, with all screws perpendicular to bone surface. Modern designs of plates utilize locking screws that lock into the plate eliminating any micromovement between the plate and screw, which is otherwise a cause of metalwork loosening and subsequent failure of fixation.
- Greater access to mandible usually required. This may mean a trans-cutaneous approach through an extended submandibular incision.

Post-operative care
Post-operatively patients need to be advised of care of their fracture:

- **Soft diet:** irrespective of the type of fixation. Patients need to avoid full masticatory force for between 4 and 6 weeks after fixation.
- **Oral hygiene:** patients need to be diligent and keep the mouth clean.

Complications
- Iatrogenic inferior alveolar nerve injury.
- Infection.
- Late metalwork loosening leading to late infection.
- Occlusal changes (inadequate reduction/malunion).
- Non-union.

Edentulous mandible
The fractured edentulous mandible is challenging to treat for a variety of reasons:

- Reduced mandibular height as a result of loss of alveolar bone—particularly a problem with <10mm of mandibular height.
- Fractures often tend to occur in the mandibular body where muscle pull displacing the fracture is at its greatest.

- Potential vascular compromise if significant periosteal stripping is undertaken.
- Old age and other patient co-morbidity reduce capacity for fracture healing.

Treatment options
- Undisplaced fractures: treat conservatively.
- Displaced fractures:
  - conservative if significant co-morbidity;
  - ORIF with mucosal flap;
  - ORIF with transmucosal screws and supramucosal locking plate;
  - ORIF with extra-oral approach (bi-cortical reconstruction plate or sandwich technique with split rib) (Fig. 1.10 and Fig. 1.11);
  - extra-oral pin fixation.

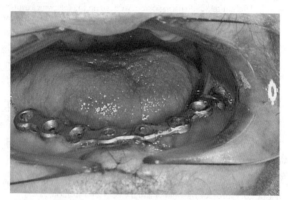

Fig. 1.10 Transmucosal plate.

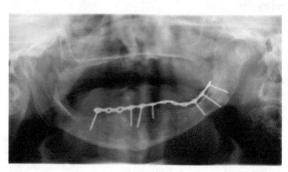

Fig. 1.11 Post-operative image of transmucosal plate.

Mandibular condyle

In addition to the anatomical area of the condyle, affected fractures can be further described in terms of:

- Displacement: overlap of proximal and distal fragment.
- Angulation—anteroposteriorly.
- Angulation—mediolaterally.
- Dislocation of condylar head.
- Comminution.

Displaced unilateral fractures of the mandibular condyle region that cause an abnormality of occlusion usually demand treatment. The options are:

- Conservative.
- Closed reduction.
- Open reduction.

Conservative

- Appropriate for:
  - intracapsular fractures (particularly need early mobilization to prevent ankylosis);
  - most fractures in children (often intracapsular);
  - undisplaced fractures;
  - minimally displaced fractures with no malocclusion;
  - edentulous patients;
  - patients with significant co-morbidity.
- Achieved by:
  - soft diet;
  - close follow-up.

Closed reduction

- Appropriate for:
  - displaced fractures in children;
  - cases with malocclusion where ORIF contraindicated.
- Achieved by:
  - arch bars and elastic traction (unilateral fracture) or wire fixation (bilateral fracture);
  - suspension wires + IMF in mixed dentition.
- Advantages:
  - no surgical scar or nerve complications;
  - simple technique.
- Disadvantages:
  - reliant on good patient compliance;
  - arch bars and associated wiring may cause periodontal damage to teeth;
  - limitation of mouth opening leads to long-term reduction in mandibular movement (can take months to recover);
  - requires a second procedure to remove the arch bars.
- Complications:
  - occlusal abnormality;
  - ↓ range of mandibular movement;
  - damage to teeth, caries, periodontal disease.

Open reduction
- Indications:
  - lateral extracapsular displacement;
  - bony overlap of over 5mm—ramus shortening;
  - open joint wound with foreign body or gross contamination;
  - dislocation of condylar head into middle cranial fossa or external auditory meatus (EAM);
  - associated maxillary fracture so that closed reduction with intermaxillary traction is not possible;
  - patient preference/poor patient compliance (many patients are unwilling to undergo elastic traction).

In patients with bilateral fractures each side should be assessed independently and treatment undertaken in light of the indication on each side.

Surgical access
- Retromandibular with transparotid approach (most frequently used approach).
- Submandibular.
- Pre-auricular with temporal extension.
- Transmeatal through EAM (popular in Europe).
- Intraoral.
- Intra-/extra-oral approach with endoscopic visualization.

Transparotid approach
- Cutaneous incision 2–3cm long just below the ear lobule in a skin crease directly overlying the posterior border of the mandible.
- Sharp dissection through parotid capsule.
- Blunt dissection through the parotid gland between branches of the facial nerve until mandible is visible.
- Periosteum of mandible incised and widely stripped to give access to the condylar base and condylar neck region.
- Fixation using:
  - two 4-hole miniplates (controlled position with initial fixation to proximal fragment);
  - specially-designed condylar plates;
  - bi-cortical/lag screws.

Complications
- Facial nerve injury: most studies reveal a low rate of temporary injury with permanent injury being rare.
- Salivary fistula.
- Facial scar.
- Frey's syndrome.
- Mal-union (inadequate reduction).
- Fixation failure (inadequate fixation).

Guardsman's fracture

Caused by direct impact to the chin producing:
- Bilateral condylar injury.
- Symphyseal fracture.
- Chin laceration.
- ± Injuries to dentition.

Results in:
- Retrognathia.
- Anterior open bite.
- ↑ mandibular width (particularly with medial displaced condyles).

These can be corrected with appropriate treatment.

Mid-face fractures

Le Fort fracture levels

There are three levels of maxillary fracture classically described as Le Fort fracture levels. Fractures at these levels rarely occur in isolation. They may also occur at different levels on both sides. Comminuted fractures are commonplace due to the thin nature of the maxillary bone. Le Fort classification is used to describe the highest level of the fracture.

Le Fort I

This fracture runs from the pterygoid plates anteriorly through the lateral wall of the maxillary antrum to the piriform aperture of the nose (Fig. 1.12).

Le Fort II

This fracture runs from the pterygoid plates anteriorly and superiorly, through the inferior orbital rim, and into the inferomedial orbital floor. The fracture then runs across the bridge of the nose. As a result, the whole of the tooth-bearing portion of the maxilla and the nose is in involved (Fig. 1.13).

Le Fort III

This is craniofacial dysjunction with the whole of the mid-face separated from the skull base. The fracture lines run from the superior aspect of the pterygoid plates, through the lateral wall of the orbit, and out into the base of the zygomatic arch and fronto-zygomatic suture, as well as the nasal bridge in the midline (Fig. 1.14).

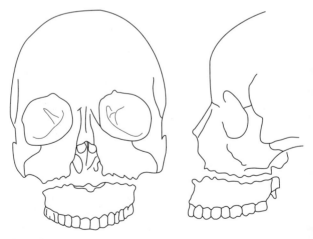

Fig. 1.12 Le Fort I fracture.

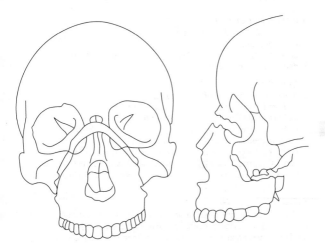

Fig. 1.13 Le Fort II fracture.

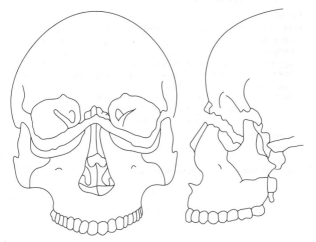

Fig. 1.14 Le Fort III fracture.

Indications for treatment
- Occlusal abnormality, e.g. anterior open bite.
- Mobility of maxilla.
- Lack of facial projection and width as a result of zygomatic arch deformity in Le Fort III fracture.

Surgical access
Dependant on the level of the fracture:
- **Le Fort I**: incision in the upper buccal sulcus.
- **Le Fort II**: the lower part of a Le Fort II fracture can be accessed via a Le Fort I incision, but the infraorbital part aspect of the fracture requires transcutaneous/transconjunctive access.
- **Le Fort III**: accessed via multiple cutaneous incisions or from above via a coronal approach (see ➜ Zygomatic fractures, p. 48). Full exposure of the zygomatic arch is essential in the presence of ↑ facial width and lack of facial projection.

Reduction
Le Fort fractures are often driven backwards along the skull base in an inferior and posterior direction, resulting in the classic open bite deformity. They often impact in this position and, therefore, initially may require disimpaction with Rowe's forceps. The problem of impaction can be compounded by the fact that sometimes fractures are incomplete. Under this circumstance, fractures should be completed at the Le Fort I fracture level to aid reduction of the occlusion.

Fixation
Fixation with internal wiring has been superseded with semi-rigid miniplate fixation. In order to restore facial proportions the fractures are repaired in the following sequence:
- Zygomatic arch reconstruction to restore facial projection and width.
- Stabilization of the fronto-zygomatic sutures to restore orbital height.
- Stabilization of the inferior orbital rims.
- Restoration of the vertical buttresses of the maxilla:
  - anterior buttress, namely the lateral piriform apertures;
  - middle buttress, namely the zygomatic buttresses.

Complications
- 'Dish face' deformity (inadequate reduction).
- Infection.
- Occlusal changes (inadequate reduction).

Zygomatic fractures

Zygomatic fractures often occur secondary to blunt trauma to the periorbital area (Fig. 1.15).

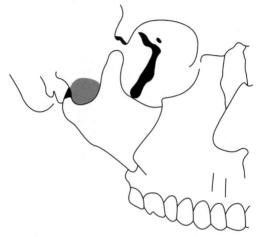

Fig. 1.15 Fracture sites of zygomatic complex.

Indications for treatment

Zygomatic fractures can be undisplaced, in which case they are managed conservatively. All displaced fractures need assessment for potential correction (Fig. 1.16 and Fig. 1.17).

Indications for correction include:
- Asymmetry of the malar prominence.
- Unresolving diplopia.
- Orbital deformity: can be clinically underestimated in the presence of facial swelling. Complex comminuted fractures may require CT scanning.
- Restricted mouth opening due to impingement on the coronoid process.
- There is no firm evidence that reduction improves infraorbital nerve sensation/dysaesthesia.

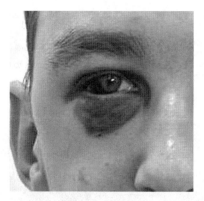

Fig. 1.16 Clinical appearance of fractured right zygoma.

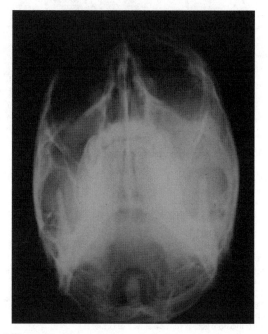

Fig. 1.17 OM view of fractured right zygomatic complex.

Surgical access

Closed

- Gillie's approach (Fig. 1.18):
  - temporal cutaneous incision;
  - incision through temporalis fascia allows instrument to be passed under zygoma.
- Intraoral.
- Extraoral with Poswillo hook.

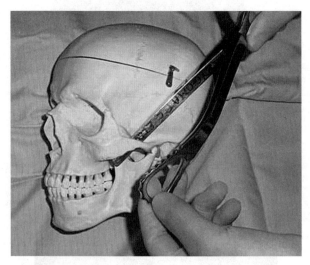

Fig. **1.18** Gillie's approach to fractured zygoma.

Open

- Through pre-existing laceration.
- **Fronto-zygomatic suture:**
  - upper lateral blepharoplasty;
  - crow's foot;
  - lateral eyebrow;
  - lower lid transconjunctival with lateral canthotomy.
- **Inferior orbital rim:**
  - transcutaneous—subcilary, blepharoplasty, midtarsal, infraorbital;
  - transconjunctival.
- **Zygomatic buttress:** infraorbital buccal sulcus.
- **Zygomatic arch:** coronal flap incision or temporomandibular joint (TMJ) approach.
- **Lynch incision:** access to medial wall of orbit.
- **Coronal:** complex/comminuted fractures.

Points of note regarding open access
- Motor nerve supply of orbicularis oculi muscle in lower lid enters on deep surface.
- Risk of ectropion reduced by stepped approach and low incision.
- Risk of ectropion highest with subciliary incision.
- Transconjunctival access can be improved by incorporation of:
  - canthotomy (lateral wall of orbit);
  - transcaruncular approach (medial wall of orbit).
- Coronal incision:
  - provides access to frontal bones, frontal sinuses, orbital rim, zygomatic arches, naso-ethmoidal complex;
  - consider stealth incision;
  - subgaleal approach initially;
  - frontal branch of facial nerve protected by reflecting superficial layer of temporalis fascia;
  - supraorbital bundles may need to be released with osteotomy.

Reduction
The zygoma has an axis of rotation around a line drawn from the fronto-zygomatic suture to the zygomatic buttress. Broadly, two types of deformity occur:
- **Rotation around the axis:**
  - external rotation results in out-fracture of the infraorbital rim and in-fracture of the zygomatic arch;
  - internal rotation results in out-fracture or bowing of the zygomatic arch and in-fracture of the infraorbital rim.
- **Shift of the entire axis:** cardinal sign of this is displacement at the fronto-zygomatic suture or the maxillary buttress.

Fixation
- None.
- Miniplate fixation at one or more sites.

Medial process of maxilla
- Palpable/radiographical evidence of infraorbital step; can be misdiagnosed as zygomatic fracture.
- Can be associated nasal bone fracture.
- No clinical or radiographic signs of zygomatic fracture.

Complications
- Loss of vision (all orbital surgery including zygoma surgery caries a remote risk of visual loss).
- Retrobulbar haemorrhage (see Initial management of ocular injuries, p. 16).
- Flat zygoma (inadequate reduction).
- Bowed zygomatic arch (usually due to inadequate anterior positioning of zygoma, can be due to over-reduction of the arch).
- Infraorbital anaesthesia.
- Worsening of diplopia due to iatrogenic damage to the extraocular muscles.
- Ectropion from cutaneous lower lid incisions.

Orbital fractures

The orbit consists of an outer and inner frame.

- Outer frame:
  - *inferior*—laterally zygoma, medially maxilla;
  - *superior*—frontal bone.
- Inner frame:
  - *floor*—roof of the maxillary sinus and orbital plate of palatine bone;
  - *medial wall*—ethmoidal and lacrimal bones anteriorly, lesser wing of sphenoid with optic canal posteriorly;
  - *lateral wall*—zygoma and greater wing of sphenoid;
  - *roof*—frontal bone.

Any part of the orbit both internal and external can be fractured. The most common areas of fracture are the zygoma and the inferomedial orbital wall. Isolated internal orbital injuries are termed *blow out* or *blow in* fractures.

Indications for treatment

- Enophthalmos.
- Non-resolving diplopia secondary to entrapment.

The following clinical guidelines can be applied:

- Entrapment more commonly results in diplopia looking upwards (Fig. 1.19).
- Muscle dysfunction usually results in diplopia looking downwards.
- Muscle dysfunction tends to get better with time, therefore delayed repair of orbital floor injuries is often employed.
- Orthoptic assessment is very useful in distinguishing muscle dysfunction from muscle entrapment.

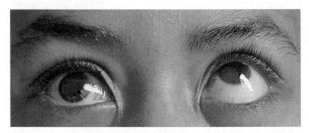

Fig. 1.19 Restricted upgaze right eye.

Paediatric orbital injuries

These fractures need treating *urgently* if there is entrapment present. Often a trap-door defect occurs, which can result in early necrosis of the trapped soft tissue the classic presentation is the so-called *'white eye blow out'*—a combination of an internal orbital fracture with an exaggerated oculocardiac reflex so that the child presents with diplopia and hypotension ± vomiting.

Enophthalmos

- Results from an increase in orbital volume.
- Normal orbital volume = 30mL, of which the globe occupies 6.5mL.
- Degree of orbital volume change is most marked if the orbit is fractured in its inferomedial portion, particularly in the area behind the globe. Displaced fractures in this area produce enophthalmos proportionate to increase in volume with 1mL of ↑ orbital volume producing around 1–2mm of enophthalmos.
- Enophthalmos may not be clinically apparent immediately following injury because of swelling of the orbital contents. True extent of enophthalmos is revealed at around 2–4 weeks following injury when this swelling has resolved.
- Enophthalmos clinically obvious to most patients when exceeds 2mm.

Surgical access

- Access is usually via a transcutaneous or transconjunctival approach (Fig. 1.20) (see ➲ Zygomatic fractures, p. 48), although endoscopically assisted approaches from the nasal cavity and maxillary sinus have been described.
- Avoid damage to the orbital contents and optic nerve.
- Optic canal sits 40mm posterior to a normally positioned inferior orbital.
- The orbital plate of the palatine bone is rarely fractured and, therefore, solid bone is usually encountered before reaching the optic foramen.

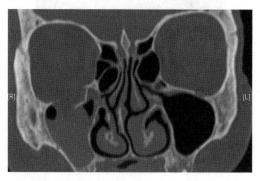

Fig. 1.20 CT right orbital floor fracture.

Isolated defect of floor causing entrapment

- Does not necessarily cause enophthalmos.
- Ensure thorough dissection at operation with freeing of soft tissue and identification of all bony defect edges.
- Checked intra-operatively with a forced duction test applied to the inferior rectus muscle.
- Reconstruct to prevent repeat herniation and entrapment of orbital contents.

Inferomedial wall defect with enophthalmos

One-third of orbital floor fractures have a medial wall component and associated enophthalmos. Additional exposure is sometimes required (Fig. 1.21) (see ➲ Zygomatic fractures, p. 48).

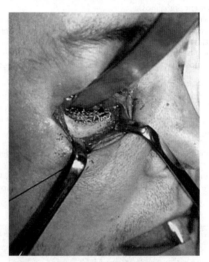

Fig. **1.21** Orbital floor exposure.

Reconstructive options for orbital defects

- Autologous bone:
  - maxillary antrum, outer table of skull or iliac crest;
  - well tolerated;
  - ultimately integrate with the surrounding orbit;
  - prone to resorption;
  - can be difficult to contour in three dimensions.

- **Alloplastic materials:**
  - titanium mesh ± polythene covering;
  - well tolerated;
  - rarely require removal;
  - easy to contour.

Complications
- Loss of vision (all orbital surgery including zygoma surgery caries a remote risk of visual loss).
- Retrobulbar haemorrhage (see ➲ Initial management of ocular injuries, p. 16).
- Worsening of diplopia due to iatrogenic damage to the extraocular muscles.
- Ectropion from cutaneous lower lid incisions.

Orbital roof

Orbital roof fractures are often associated with other fractures of the frontal bone ± dural tear and CSF leakage. Tend to be associated with exophthalmos due to a reduced orbital volume—this forms the main indication for treatment. If exophthalmos is present it may be pulsatile due to brain vascularity. This sign is most frequently seen in children and is an indication for repair. In some instances orbital roof fractures are best repaired in conjunction with a neurological surgeon as an intracranial approach may be required to reduce herniated brain.

Superior orbital fissure syndrome

- This is due to compression of:
  - abducens VI;
  - oculomotor (superior and inferior divisions) III;
  - trochlear IV;
  - frontal, lacrimal, and nasociary branches of ophthalmic nerve VI.
- Results in:
  - exophthalmos;
  - anaesthesia of the frontal branch of the trigeminal nerve;
  - ptosis;
  - ophthalmoplegia.

Superior orbital fissure syndrome can result from blunt facial trauma. It has a good prognosis if treated conservatively. Most cases make a full recovery within 3 months.

Orbital apex syndrome

- Superior orbital fissure syndrome associated with visual loss as a result of damage to the optic nerve.
- Patients with the superior orbital fissure syndrome or orbital apex syndrome should be assessed with CT scanning.
- Optic nerve injuries have a poor prognosis.
- Role of steroids controversial.
- Patients found to have bony fragments impinging on the optic nerve should be considered for surgical exploration.

Frontal bone fractures

Injuries to the supraorbital ridge produce fractures of two overlapping types:
- Frontal sinus.
- Naso-ethmoid.

Frontal sinus fractures

The frontal sinus is made up of an anterior wall, which forms part of the forehead, a posterior wall that is in contact with the brain, and a floor that is continuous with the naso-ethmoidal area. Management is dependent on the area fractured.

Classification
- Anterior wall.
- Posterior wall.
- Floor.
- Combinations.

Indications for treatment
- Cosmetic defect.
- Prevention of sequelae—meningitis, Potts puffy tumour, mucocoele.

Anterior wall injuries

Isolated fractures of the anterior wall are managed depending on the forehead deformity that they produce. Minimally displaced injuries producing no forehead deformity do not need treatment. Isolated displaced injuries tend to be associated with large frontal sinuses and are treated with:
- **Access:** coronal incision.
- **Reduction:** fragments are reduced to their anatomical position. This is sometimes easier if the fragments are removed, reconstructed on the bench and then replaced as a free bone graft.
- **Fixation:** titanium miniplate <1.5mm screw diameter.

Posterior wall injuries

Posterior wall injuries can be associated with brain injury and CSF leaks. Left untreated, there is a long-term risk of secondary infective meningitis. All posterior wall injuries should be discussed with a neurosurgeon. Treatment options:
- **Conservative:** if there is no CSF leak and the fracture is minimally displaced.
- **Open:** comminuted fractures can be treated with cranialization where the posterior wall of the sinus is removed and the brain allowed to herniate towards the reconstructed anterior wall. A pericranial flap can be interposed between the brain and the cranial vault to add an additional layer of protection against subsequent infection.

Floor injuries

Injuries of the floor of the frontal sinus are continuous with the naso-ethmoidal area and involve damage to the frontonasal duct. There is abundant literature on frontonasal management in relation to frontal sinus fractures. However, the realization that the duct is also damaged in naso-ethmoidal injury, which itself does not appear to lead to problems with frontal sinus drainage, has led most authors to realize that it has an immense capacity to spontaneously reform. No attempt should therefore be made to repair the frontonasal duct.

Naso-ethmoidal injury

Continuous with inferior wall of the frontal sinus is the naso-ethmoidal complex. Injuries to this area result from trauma across the bridge of the nose. The nasal and ethmoidal bones are delicate, and comminute easily. The clinical hallmarks of naso-ethmoidal injury include:

• Depression of nasal bridge.
• Upturned nasal tip.
• Telecanthus as a result of lateral displacement of the medial canthal ligament. This usually occurs because the bone that is attached to the medial canthal ligament is separated from surrounding fragments (Fig. 1.22).

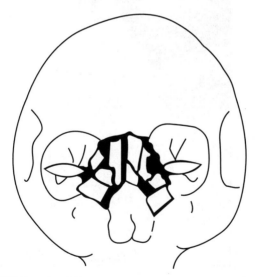

Fig. 1.22 Naso-ethmoidal fractures.

Indications for treatment
Significant nasal deformity or telecanthus should be treated in the primary setting since secondary correction of facial deformity in this area is notoriously difficult (Fig. 1.23 and Fig. 1.24).

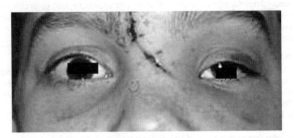

Fig. 1.23 Facial view of naso-ethmoidal fracture.

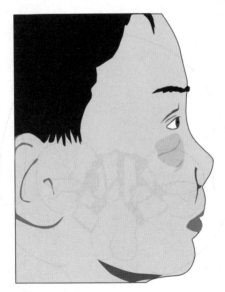

Fig. 1.24 Lateral facial view of naso-ethmoidal fracture.

Surgical access
As a rule, coronal access is required.

Reduction and fixation
Nasal reconstruction is accomplished by reducing the comminuted nasal fragments and fixing them in position to the frontal bone. Primary bone grafting is often required in this area. The key to successful treatment of naso-ethmoidal injury is accurate repositioning of the medial canthus. This is technically difficult as the bony fragment to which the medial canthus is attached is usually small, and has to be reattached posteriorly in order to regain normal appearance and lacrimal function.

Complications
- Inadequate repositioning of medial canthal ligament.
- Residual nasal deformity.
- Infection.

Pan-facial fractures

Pan-facial injuries are a combination of mandibular, maxillary, and orbital injuries. CT assessment is mandatory. Timing of treatment is often delayed as patients are likely to have other injuries that demand urgent assessment and treatment. The techniques for repairing the individual injuries are in general the same as those described for an isolated injury, the only difference being in the sequencing:
- Reconstruction of the zygomatic arches and frontal area to restore upper facial width and facial projection.
- Reconstruction of the orbits, orbital floors, and naso-ethmoidal area.
- Anatomical reconstruction of mandible, including condylar fractures, to restore lower facial width and projection.
- Repositioning of the maxilla at the Le Fort I level including reconstruction of the anterior and middle buttress of the maxilla (piriform aperture and maxillary buttress).

Isolated nasal fractures

- Isolated fractures of the nose are common.
- Easy to undertreat at primary surgery, but often requires revision because of inadequate treatment of the cartilaginous part of the nose.
- Treatment can be in the acute setting if there is little swelling.
- Reassess at 10 days if swelling on presentation.
- Radiology has no role in assessment.

Indications for treatment

- Nasal deviation/cosmesis.
- Nasal blockage.

Surgical access

These are often treated as closed injuries. Injuries to the nasal septum should be considered for primary open septoplasty via an intranasal incision.

Reduction

Since nasal bones are often impacted they may require disimpaction prior to repositioning under LA or GA.

Fixation

Fixation is achieved with a temporary nasal splint.

Complications

Inadequate reduction and therefore secondary rhinoplasty.

Dental injuries

Avulsed teeth

Avulsed primary dentition does not need any specific treatment. Avulsed adult teeth are most common in the 6–7-year age group and need re-implantation. Avulsed teeth are best managed as follows:

Pre-hospital care
- Ideally teeth are re-implanted as soon as possible.
- Extra-alveolar time (EAT) exceeding 15min has a significantly lower long-term success rate.
- After 1h most periodontal ligament cells are non-viable.
- If it is not possible to re-implant the tooth at the scene of the accident the tooth should be stored in milk (has been shown to preserve periodontal ligament cells for up to 3h).

Hospital care
- If grossly contaminated rinse off the root of the tooth.
- The tooth should be splinted to the adjacent teeth (wire, composite).
- Prescribe antibiotics.

Secondary care
- Follow-up with dentist.
- Splint removal at 10 days.
- Most avulsed teeth need root canal treatment (exception—open apex incisors with short EAT).

Complications
- Pulp necrosis.
- External root resorption.
- Ankylosis.

Dento-alveolar fractures
- Distinguish from basal bone fractures.
- Reduced (under LA or GA).
- Fixation with archbars to correct occlusion.
- Remove fixation at 4–6 weeks.
- Consider endodontic treatment in the long term.

Post-traumatic deformity

Post-traumatic facial deformity is a common problem since facial trauma can be complex to treat and the results are not always ideal. There are many procedures that can be used to improve the appearance and function of the face and jaws. A number of factors need to be taken into account.

Patient concerns

Only correct what the patient is actually concerned about.

Timing

Secondary procedures should be delayed until the primary surgery has healed, and time has taken place for maturation of the hard and soft tissues.

Soft tissues

Facial scars take up to 2 years to mature. Since soft tissue overlying under-reduced bone shrinks to fit, the reduced bony volume correction of long-standing mal-united fractures of the face may never look aesthetic unless there is simultaneous correction of the soft tissue drape. This may require augmentation with:

- Tissue expansion.
- Dermal fillers.
- Dermal grafts.
- Fat grafts.
- Free soft tissue transfer.

Hard tissues

Correction of hard tissue can usually be undertaken with standard orthognathic techniques, onlay grafts or, rarely, osteotomizing fracture sites.

Oral cavity and oropharyngeal cancer

Introduction

The management of oral and oropharyngeal cancer is a challenge to the head and neck surgeon. Whilst oral cancer presents in an environment that can be readily examined by patients and professionals alike, oropharyngeal tumours lie at the posterior aspect of what is visible and, as such, may often present late. Rarely, neglected tumours can cross both anatomical zones giving a unique spectrum of clinical presentations.

Cancer of the oral cavity and oropharynx is most frequently squamous cell carcinoma. Occasionally, rarer tumours can present at this site (lymphoma, salivary tumours) or tumours from deeper structures (e.g. deep lobe parotid tumours) can present in this anatomical region. This chapter will principally consider squamous carcinoma of the head and neck presenting in the oral cavity and oropharynx.

Anatomy

- The oral cavity commences at the vermillion of the lips and extends posteriorly to the oropharynx (Fig. 2.1). It contains the hard palate, tooth-bearing tissues, and anterior two-thirds of the tongue.
- The oropharynx is defined as that part of the upper aerodigestive tract that commences at the anterior pillar of the fauces, hard/soft palate junction, and the junction of the anterior two-thirds and the posterior one-third of the tongue. Comprises of soft palate, anterior and posterior tonsillar pillars, and tonsillar fossa, lateral and posterior walls, and the tongue base down to epiglottis (Fig. 2.2 and Fig. 2.3).
- The surface of both oral cavity and oropharynx is lined with stratified squamous epithelium from which the most frequently presenting tumour arises.
- Tissues at both sites have very rich lymphatic drainage, which has clinical significance in the loco-regional spread of malignant disease.
- Various sub-sites are considered to have differing prognostic significance in the context of carcinoma, e.g. tumours of the palatine arch (anterior pillar, soft palate, and uvula) are less aggressive than those of the other oral cavity and oropharynx sites.

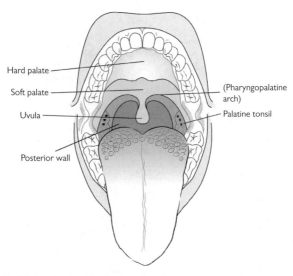

Hard palate

Soft palate

Uvula

Posterior wall

(Pharyngopalatine arch)

Palatine tonsil

Fig. 2.1 Anterior view of oral cavity and oropharynx.

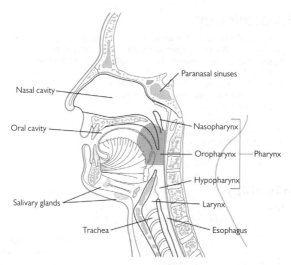

Fig. 2.2 Sagittal view of oral cavity and oropharynx.

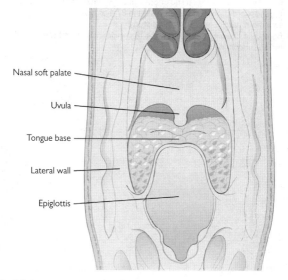

Fig. 2.3 Posterior view of oropharynx.

Epidemiology

- Around 7500 cases of all head and neck cancer types occur in the UK per annum, making it the 6th most common form of cancer.
- Approximately 2600 occur in the oral cavity and 900 in the oropharynx.
- In the USA, approximately 30,100 new diagnoses of oropharynx carcinomas are made and an estimated 7800 deaths occur.
- In India, oral cavity and oropharyngeal tumours comprise 40% of cancers.
- There is between 2 and 5 times greater incidence in men than women depending on site.
- Traditionally, it is most common in the 6th and 7th decades, although there is evidence that it is increasing in young adults.

Aetiology

- Smoking and consumption of alcohol are the two principal aetiological factors in this disease. These factors act separately but also synergistically in causing this form of cancer.
- Diet containing high proportions of vegetables and fruit might modulate carcinogenic effects and low body mass index (BMI) appears to increase the risk of oropharynx cancer.
- Human papilloma virus (HPV) is now recognized as an independent risk factor for oropharyngeal squamous cell carcinoma—HPV type 16 is the most prevalent genotype present in 87% of cases of oropharyngeal squamous carcinoma in one large study.
- Betel quid chewing is related to the high incidence of oral cancer in the Indian subcontinent.

Premalignant conditions

Conditions of definite premalignant potential

- Leukoplakia.
- Erythroplakia (Fig. 2.4).
- Chronic hyperplastic candidiasis.

Conditions associated with an increased risk of malignant transformation

- Lichen planus.
- Oral submucous fibrosis.
- Syphilitic glossitis.
- Sideropenic dysphagia.

These include conditions are that not themselves premalignant, but confer an ↑ rate of malignancy by the atrophy that they produce within the mucous membranes (see ➔ Lichen planus, p. 432, and ➔ Syphilis, p. 460).

Conditions erroneously considered to be premalignant

- Stomatitis nicotina.
- Habitual cheek biting.
- White sponge naevus.

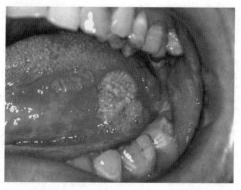

Fig. 2.4 Oral squamous cell carcinoma presenting in area of erythroplakia.

Diagnosis

This is made on the basis of clinical features and special investigations. Clinical features include symptoms and signs.

Symptoms

In early disease small tumours may produce very few or only specific symptoms, and are therefore difficult to detect. Presenting symptoms may include:

- Painless ulcer.
- Sore throat.
- Sensation of a foreign body in the throat.
- Change in voice, otalgia, or odynophagia (pain referred to the ear mediated via glossopharyngeal and vagus nerves).
- Lump in the neck.
- Weight loss.

With increasing tumour size, tongue movement may be impaired, affecting speech and swallowing. In late stage disease patients may complain of spontaneous bleeding and halitosis.

Signs

- Indurated ulcer (Fig. 2.5).
- Exophytic mass.
- Area of abnormal mucosa, e.g. red patch.
- Cervical lymphadenopathy: (Fig. 2.6) may be reactive or metastatic. A metastatic node will classically be:
  - hard;
  - non-tender;
  - may be fixed to surrounding structures.
- Alteration of voice.
- Cranial nerve lesions:
  - hypoglossal palsy (deviation towards affected side with wasting and fasciculation of ipsilateral side of tongue);
  - vagus nerve palsy (impaired movement of soft palate, ipsilateral vocal cord paralysis);
  - trigeminal nerve anaesthesia in territory supplied by lingual nerve and mental nerves.

Clinical examination must include a methodical examination of the oral cavity, as well as the anterior and posterior triangles of the neck. Fibre-optic naso-endoscopy must always be carried out when an oropharyngeal lesion is suspected. This can be carried out under topical anaesthesia.

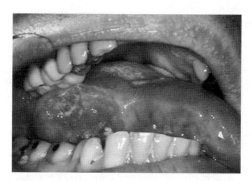

Fig. 2.5 Oral squamous cell carcinoma presenting as indurated ulcer.

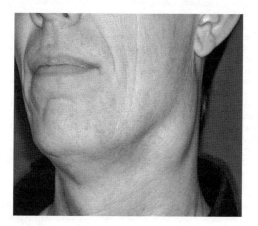

Fig. 2.6 Upper deep cervical lymph node enlargement from oral cavity primary.

Investigations

Plain radiography

Plain radiographs have a limited role to play in the diagnosis and pre-operative assessment of oropharyngeal tumours. Nonetheless, they are frequently performed as part of the diagnostic pathway, particularly in patients who present with non-specific symptoms.

The orthopantomogram

- Frequently undertaken as a screening investigation for patients presenting with facial pain.
- A rotational tomogram and, therefore, only of diagnostic value for those tissues that lie within the focal trough.
- Of little practical value in assessing soft tissue pathology.
- Bony pathology is only demonstrated where significant decalcification has occurred as a result of either pressure or direct invasion by a malignant process.
- Occasionally useful in diagnosing the much rarer osteosarcomas where characteristic features, including the 'sunray' appearance, are almost pathognomonic.
- Bone invasion by the more common squamous cell carcinomas is indicated by loss cortical outlines and irregular areas of radiolucency in either the mandible or maxilla (Fig. 2.7). Rarely resorption of dental roots can also be identified.
- Malignant transformation within pre-existing benign pathology cannot be excluded with plain radiology.
- Multiple lesions may occur with metastatic bony deposits, such as in myeloma or breast carcinoma.
- Main value of the OPG in patients with oropharyngeal malignancy is in aiding dental assessment prior to surgery or radiotherapy:
  - planning of mandibular resections or access osteotomies must take into account the position of the teeth in order to minimize functional disability;
  - extent of caries and periodontal disease can be determined in order to ensure that appropriate therapy including dental extractions are undertaken preferably at the examination under anaesthesia (EUA) stage, and certainly prior to the commencement of major therapeutic interventions.
- Finally, the OPG is used to confirm the appropriate reduction and fixation of access mandibulotomies and to ensure that, where mandibular reconstruction has been undertaken, bony contour, plate position, and accurate location of the condyle within the glenoid fossa have all been achieved.

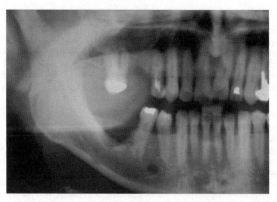

Fig. 2.7 Orthopantomogram demonstrating mandibular invasion in molar region.

Occipito-mental radiograph
- Seldom used in modern diagnostic practice outside the realms of facial trauma.
- Occasionally indicated in the investigation of facial pain thought to be of maxillary sinus origin.
- Opacity of maxillary sinus coupled with bony destruction is most likely to indicate a malignant process although long-standing chronic suppurative disease (e.g. aspergillosis) can give rise to similar appearances.

Chest radiograph (CXR)
The pre-operative CXR still has a number of important functions in the overall assessment of patients with oropharyngeal malignancy.
- Many patients present with cardiorespiratory co-morbidities and the CXR can form a valuable tool in supplementing clinical assessment of respiratory and cardiac function.
- Given the high incidence of post-treatment complications involving the cardiorespiratory system, a pre-treatment baseline CXR can provide invaluable information about the developing clinical picture.
- May demonstrate pulmonary metastases, although it is not as sensitive as other imaging modalities in the detection of smaller lesions. Nonetheless, a CXR that demonstrates widespread pulmonary metastases at the beginning of the diagnostic pathway may save a great deal of unnecessary time and investigation, and allows the patient to receive appropriate therapy at a much earlier stage.
- The role of CXR as part of the routine follow-up of patients following definitive therapy is less certain. In general, follow-up radiography is only recommended where symptoms dictate. Follow-up screening for pulmonary metastases or second primary malignancies is not recommended.

Contrast radiography

Sialography

Whilst sialography has no role to play in the planned assessment of a patient with known oropharyngeal malignancy, occasionally patients with such a malignancy may present with symptoms consistent with obstructive sialoadenitis. It is important to recognize that space-occupying lesions within the major salivary glands or extrinsic compression of the ducts may be identified on sialography.

Carotid angiography

High-resolution contrast MRI, duplex ultrasound scans (DUSS), and subtraction angiography have largely superseded the need for carotid angiography in the pre-operative assessment of oropharyngeal malignancy. Occasionally, however, where previous neck surgery or radiotherapy has been undertaken, angiography may be required in order to assess the patency and condition of the vascular tree in order to facilitate appropriate reconstructive choice. In highly vascular tumours embolization may be of value as an adjunct to surgery.

Barium swallow

This investigation can give useful information about tongue base lesions. It is of particular value when coupled with naso-endoscopy in the post-operative assessment of swallowing function.

Cross-sectional imaging

Computed tomography

- High-resolution CT scanning with and without contrast probably represents the best all-round imaging modality in the pre-operative assessment and staging of oropharyngeal malignancy.
- Details of bony anatomy and potential bone involvement by tumour are superior to MRI.
- Single CT scan of the head, neck, thorax, and upper abdomen allows a comprehensive staging scan to be undertaken rapidly at one sitting.
- In order to assess the para-nasal sinuses coronal scans can be undertaken or reformatted and give excellent detail regarding involvement of the orbit and cranial base. Sagittal scans can also be of value in the fronto-nasal area.
- CT is widely available and the criteria for determining the probability of nodal involvement are well developed.
- Main drawbacks of CT:
  - distortion of images caused by amalgam artefact;
  - limitations of imaging smaller lesions in mobile areas of the oropharynx.
- Whilst exposure doses have been significantly reduced with modern CT machines, this modality still has the disadvantage of subjecting patients to ionizing radiation.

- CT scan provides a high level of accuracy in assessing the involvement of lymph nodes in the neck (Fig. 2.8). The criteria for identifying positive neck nodes are:
  - increase in size (short axis >8–10mm);
  - central necrosis and rim contrast enhancement;
  - extra-capsular extension;
  - obliteration of surrounding fat planes.
- Surpasses plain radiography in diagnostic accuracy for determining the presence of pulmonary metastases or early primary lung tumours.
- Since image acquisition times with modern spiral scanners are short, there is little reason for not undertaking chest examination as part of a standard head and neck staging protocol.
- There remains the method of choice for radiotherapy treatment planning. However, an additional 'planning CT scan' is usually required with the patient positioned in the treatment position.

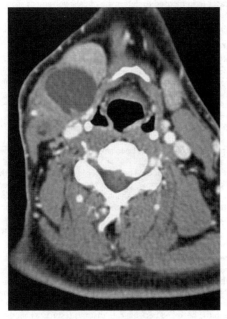

Fig. 2.8 Positive node identified on CT by imaging criteria.

Magnetic resonance imaging
- Superior to CT scanning for determining the depth and volume of primary soft tissue oropharyngeal tumours.
- Not susceptible to dental amalgam artefact.
- No exposure to ionizing radiation.
- Coupled with administration of gadolinium gives excellent information about potential proximity to vascular and neural structures.
- Acquisition times greater than for CT.
- Some patients find it unbearably claustrophobic and noisy.
- High false positive rate when assessing patients for recurrent tumour following therapeutic intervention.
- High-resolution MRI scans can be of particular benefit in identifying small naso-pharyngeal tumours and recurrence at the base of skull.
- Investigation of choice for assessing primary salivary gland malignancies and in particular is of value for identifying perineural spread.
- Gives almost equivalent accuracy to the CT for detecting cervical node metastases (criteria used to determine nodal involvement are similar to CT).
- Contraindicated in presence of ferrous implants.

Nuclear medicine

Bone scintigraphy
- Radioisotope scanning with technetium 99-labelled methylene diphosphonate (MDP) can be of benefit in determining whether early bony invasion exists.
- Computerized co-location on sectional anatomical images can be of benefit in identifying areas of bony invasion where no change is identified on either the CT or plain radiographs.
- Highly sensitive test and false positives may occur where there is active dental pathology, if there has been a recent biopsy, or where there is simply a periosteal reaction.
- Results of scintigraphy should be considered in the context of the clinical picture and other investigations. When positive, but where significant clinical doubt exists, an intra-operative periosteal strip should be performed before committing the patient to a segmental bone resection.
- Also of value in assessing the viability of microvascular free bone transfers in the post-operative period.

Positron emission tomography (PET)
- PET provides a functional assessment of tissue metabolism using radiolabelled fluoro-deoxy-glucose (FDG).
- Should give the maximum diagnostic information by distinguishing between the metabolic behaviour of cancer and normal tissues.
- Studies in the head and neck indicate that this test has a high diagnostic accuracy particularly for:
  - detecting primaries of unknown origin;
  - detecting tumour recurrence by distinguishing between active tumour and post-treatment scar tissue.

- Requires the use of radiolabelled products that only have a short half-life—therefore expensive.
- At present PET should be reserved for selected cases where a primary cannot be identified or where tumour recurrence is suspected, but cannot be detected by other methods, and patients should be considered for entry into ongoing clinical trials.
- It is important that no therapeutic intervention or biopsy has been recently undertaken in order to limit the false positive rate.

Ultrasonography

- Diagnostic ultrasound has become an important adjunct to the clinical assessment of neck masses—does not replace the requirement for either a CT or MRI scan since these give much more anatomical detail and permit staging of the neck, thorax, and abdomen.
- Accurate determination of the size and morphology of neck masses can be made, and in many cases normal and abnormal architecture of cervical lymph nodes can be assessed.
- When used in conjunction with fine needle aspiration cytology or biopsy (FNAC or FNAB) enhances diagnostic yields.
- DUSS of value in assessing the patency of the vascular tree and vascularity of the tumour.
- Does not expose the patient to ionizing radiation or strong magnetic fields.
- Simple to undertake.
- Highly operator dependent. Real-time imaging provides much more valuable information than can be conveyed in static images.
- Has a high diagnostic accuracy in the detection of salivary gland tumours; however, its ability to discriminate between benign and malignant tumours is less certain.
- If coupled with FNAC or FNAB, USS diagnostic accuracy for salivary neoplasms is improved, but high false positive and false negative rates for cytology still exist such that radical surgery cannot be justified on the basis of USS and cytology alone (however, demonstration of diffuse enlargement of gland may justify incisional biopsy to distinguish an inflammatory process from lymphoma). USS can be of benefit in monitoring patients with Sjögren's syndrome and assess whether a discrete lymphoma is developing within sialectatic salivary tissue (see ➲ Sjögren's syndrome, p. 186).

Fine needle aspiration for cytology or biopsy
FNAC

- Of benefit when abnormal squamous cells are identified from aspiration of a mass in the neck—triggers diagnostic pathway in search of a primary oropharyngeal malignancy. Where a metastasis from a mucosal malignancy is suspected, every attempt should be made to reach a sound diagnosis without resort to compromising the neck with open surgery.

- Where abnormal lymphocytes are identified suggesting lymphoreticular malignancy, cytology is rarely sufficient to determine the most appropriate therapy—next most appropriate diagnostic step is excision biopsy through a defensive neck incision (where the approach allow for a future neck dissection).
- Risk of seeding using FNAC is believed to be extremely remote—nonetheless, where there is unequivocal histological diagnosis of the primary tumour, and imaging of the neck demonstrates abnormal nodes on size or architectural criteria, any additional information obtained by FNAC is of questionable benefit as it is unlikely to influence therapeutic decisions.

FNAB

- Offers greater information regarding tumours because it provides not only evidence of abnormal cytology, but also information regarding the histology of the tissue.
- Occasionally will provide sufficient information regarding lymphomas to initiate treatment without resort to formal nodal excision biopsy.
- Theoretical risk of seeding using this technique, but there is no evidence to demonstrate a true risk.

Staging

Oropharynx cancer is staged using the TNM system (tumour, lymph nodes, distant metastases). Staging can be further classified as clinical, radiological (based on imaging), or pathological (based on the outcome of histopathological examination of excised tissue).

T stage

The primary tumour is staged on the basis of surface extent (Table 2.1).

Table 2.1 T stage

T stage	Tumour maximum surface diameter
Tx	Primary tumour cannot be assessed
T0	No primary tumour
Tis	Primary lesion contains *in situ* cancer only
T1	<2cm
T2	>2cm <4cm
T3	>4cm
T4a	Tumour invades larynx, deep/extrinsic muscles of tongue, medial pterygoid muscle, hard palate, or mandible
T4b	Tumour invades lateral pterygoid muscle, pterygoid plates, lateral nasopharynx or skull base, or encases carotid artery

N stage

The cervical lymph nodes are staged as shown in Table 2.2.

Table 2.2 N stage

N stage	Nodal status
Nx	Regional nodes cannot be assessed
N0	No regional lymph node metastasis
N1	Metastasis in a single ipsilateral node 3cm or smaller in maximum dimension
N2	Metastasis in a single ipsilateral node >3cm, but 6cm or less in greatest dimension, or in multiple ipsilateral nodes 6cm or less, or in bilateral or contralateral lymph nodes 6cm or smaller
N2a	Metastasis in a single ipsilateral lymph node >3cm, but <6cm
N2b	Metastases in multiple ipsilateral nodes 6cm or smaller
N2c	Metastases in bilateral or contralateral nodes 6cm or smaller
N3	Metastasis in a lymph node >6cm

When evaluating nodal metastases clinically the actual size of the mass is measured taking account of the intervening soft tissues. Most neck masses >3cm are not single nodes, but confluent nodes or tumours in soft tissues of the neck.

M stage

Distant metastases are staged as shown in Table 2.3.

Table 2.3 M stage

M stage	Distant metastasis
MX	Distant metastasis cannot be assessed
M0	No distant metastasis
M1	Distant metastasis

Disease stage

Taking the TNM status together for a tumour, the stage of disease is as shown in Table 2.4.

Table 2.4 Disease stage

Stage group	T Stage	N	M
0	Tis	0	0
I	T1	0	0
II	T2	0	0
III	T3	0	0
	T1	1	0
	T2	1	0
	T3	1	0
IVA	T4a	N0	0
	T4a	N1	0
	T1	N2	0
	T2	N2	0
	T3	N2	0
	T4a	N2	0
IVB	T4b	Any N	0
	Any T	N3	0
IVC	Any T	Any N	M1

Principles of treatment

Treatment intent—to cure or palliate?

- Having established a diagnosis of oropharyngeal malignancy, the histological type, and the stage of disease it is important to take account of the overall physical and mental state of the patient.
- The relative risks and benefits of the various treatment options should be identified and it should be ensured that the patient, and preferably also their relatives and carers, fully understand the implications of treatment and are in a position to make an informed choice.
- Where remediable factors exist in terms of general co-morbidities these should be addressed prior to treatment decision.
- Treatment involves three potential modalities:
  - surgery;
  - radiotherapy;
  - chemotherapy.
- Achieving loco-regional control is key and relates directly to overall survival.
- Management of the primary cancer can be either surgical or by radiotherapy, and remains controversial. Surgery is often combined with adjuvant radiotherapy based on histopathological outcomes of surgical resection.
- Ionizing radiation and chemotherapy are used increasingly for this patient group as a combined modality.
- Management of stage III and IV resectable oropharynx cancer—there has been only one prospective randomized controlled trial (RCT) comparing chemoradiotherapy with primary surgery plus adjuvant therapy.
- In early disease, surgery and primary radiotherapy are equally effective in eradicating primary disease.
- All surgical complications are well known to be far more prevalent and complex in the post-radiotherapy patient.
- Quality of life should be considered alongside the chances of survival.
- All members of the multidisciplinary team (MDT) should have the opportunity to express their views about treatment options from their own perspectives. A designated member of the team should take a lead role and ultimately be responsibility for the management of an individual patient's care.
- A head and neck MDT should comprise of:
  - oral and maxillofacial surgeons;
  - ear, nose, and throat (ENT) surgeons;
  - reconstructive surgeons (oral and maxillofacial surgery (OMFS), ENT, or plastic);
  - specialist anaesthetists;
  - clinical/medical oncologists;
  - specialist nurses;
  - speech and language therapists;
  - palliative care physicians;
  - specialist radiologists;

- specialist pathologists;
- dieticians;
- restorative dentists;
- dental hygienists;
- psychologists.

Having weighed the evidence and discussed all the treatment options with the patient it is vital that the intention of treatment is clearly understood by the whole team, patient, and carers. Where treatment is given with palliative intent it is important that this is targeted at the specific relief or prevention of symptoms, and that the treatment is designed to minimize side effects. Regular reassessment is required to ensure that therapeutic goals are being achieved and that the side effects of treatment are not outweighing the benefits. There must be a clear evidence-based stepwise strategy for managing common symptoms such as pain and nausea.

When appropriate, advance life directives should be discussed and an end of life resuscitation policy agreed with the patient and preferably carers.

Therapeutic options

The overwhelming majority of oropharyngeal cancers are mucosal squamous cell carcinomas. Most of the discussion regarding therapeutic options will be directed to the management of these relatively common tumours. There are three main treatment modalities to consider:

- Surgery.
- Radiotherapy.
- Systemic anti-cancer therapies (SACT).

These modalities can be used in isolation or combination. When used in combination surgical resection normally precedes adjuvant radiotherapy as post-irradiation surgical resection carries with it a much higher risk of complications. Primary chemoradiation may be indicated for certain tongue base and tonsillar tumours. However, the use of chemotherapy as a stand-alone primary modality or as adjuvant treatment with surgery is often only undertaken in the context of clinical trials. It is not possible to consider every permutation and combination, but the following factors all have a bearing on the choice of treatment:

- Site of primary tumour.
- Stage of disease.
- Proximity or involvement of bone.
- Treatment intent.
- Physical status of patient.
- Patient preference.

As far as the physical status of the patient is concerned a number of risk stratification models are available to assist the MDT in advising the patient. At the simplest level, the American Society of Anaesthesiologists (ASA) I–V scale gives a reasonable prediction of the risk of morbidity and mortality (see ➲ Anaesthesia, p. 376). Pre-operative risk stratification not only assists in choosing the modality of treatment and even the extent of surgery, but is also a prerequisite for meaningful comparative audit.

Surgery

There are a number of different options available under the banner of surgery:

- Conventional excision.
- Laser surgery.
- Thermal surgery.

The primary site

- Choice of primary modality treatment depends upon the tumour site and histological features, coupled with the stage of disease and ultimately patient choice.
- Size and location of tumour will determine whether a resection followed by primary closure or healing by secondary intention will be satisfactory, or whether reconstruction of the defect with a local or distant tissue will be necessary to restore form and function.
- In borderline cases there may have to be careful consideration of the trade-off between loss of function and the risks of the procedure.

Access to the primary tumour

Many tumours in the anterior part of the oral cavity can be accessed via the transoral route. This is ideal since the oral sphincter is maintained and no scars are produced above the jaw line. The cosmetic result is usually excellent. However, as tumours increase in size and as their position becomes more posterior it may not be feasible to undertake a safe resection via the transoral route. Three main alternatives exist to achieve access under these circumstances:

- Lip split and mandibulotomy (Fig. 2.9 and Fig. 2.10).
- A 'pull through' technique via the neck.
- For maxillary tumours, an upper lip and para-nasal incision (lateral infraorbital extension is rarely required and has a high complication rate).
- Transoral robotic surgery may be of benefit in performing ablative surgery, in otherwise inaccessible site. However this technique is still under evaluation and should be restricted to a small number of specialist centres.

There are several options for the lip skin incision. However, in most circumstances, some form of stepped incision is desirable both in the upper and lower lip. This disguises and lengthens the scar to prevent post-operative wound contraction, which otherwise distorts the vermilion border. After a lengthy operation the tissues can become oedematous by the time closure is undertaken and it is therefore advisable to mark the skin with methylene blue temporary tattoos prior to incision in order to ensure accurate apposition during closure. It is also important to ensure that the orbicularis muscles are correctly realigned in order to maintain an effective oral sphincter and prevent unsightly post-operative clefting of the lip.

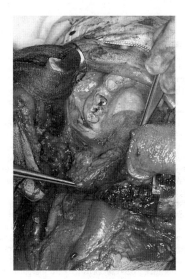

Fig. 2.9 Operative photograph of lip split and mandibulotomy.

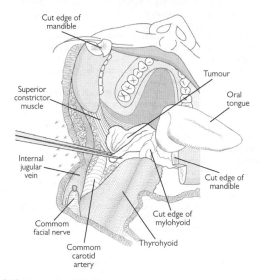

Fig. 2.10 Line diagram of Fig. 2.9.

Ablation

- Effective tumour ablation is achieved by ensuring that good visibility is maintained. This in turn results from appropriate access.
- In order to maximize the chances of achieving complete tumour resection with a clear margin of normal tissue the surgeon must employ both visual inspection and palpation.
- The method of cutting (cold steel, harmonic scalpel, laser, diathermy, or coblation) is, to some extent, a matter of personal preference. In many cases, a combination of techniques will be used.
- For some small and superficial lesions laser vaporization may be employed; however, this does not permit histological assessment of the adequacy of tumour resection. Similarly, lasers and thermal techniques, whilst reducing the amount of intra-operative bleeding, cause morphological distortion of tissues at the margins, which can lead to histological artefacts and some difficulty in assessing the adequacy of tumour resection.
- Coblation involves the generation of bipolar radiofrequency waves that generate tissue temperatures of around 60°C, much lower than temperatures generated by conventional diathermy. This is claimed to reduce post-operative pain, but the technique has been associated with ↑ levels of post-operative haemorrhage. It should therefore only be used by surgeons who have had specific training in its use.
- Use of intra-operative frozen sections to assist marginal clearance is controversial:
  - given that the primary aim is tumour resection with a clearance preferably with clinical margin of 1cm (vital structures permitting) if the surgeon believes that close or positive margins could be possible then a wider resection should be undertaken if feasible;
  - random frozen sections are unlikely to be able to identify positive margins;
  - they may give a false sense of security to the surgeon and invariably prolong the operative time.
- Intra-operative tumour tissue marking has been attempted (e.g. toluidine blue), but this has limited value at detecting mucosal margin clearance because of the high false positive rate. The technique is unsuitable for detecting deep margin clearance (area where resection is most likely to be inadequate).
- Where bony resection is required extent is largely based on the clinical and radiological findings:
  - extensive subcortical spread of tumour within the mandible is a relatively rare phenomenon, but will usually be suspected pre-operatively;
  - prior to bone resection, a titanium reconstruction plate is fashioned to restore the contour of the resected bone (plate extended well beyond planned resection site in order to provide adequate fixation of the bone graft).

- For posterior oropharyngeal tumours it is important to visualize the great vessels of the neck up to the skull base and ensure that these are lateralized prior to resection of the primary tumour in order to avoid inadvertent damage.
- In rare instances where there is true tumour invasion of the major vessels, carotid resection is seldom warranted as the complications are severe, and neither palliation nor survival is enhanced.
- Following resection and prior to reconstruction, it is of vital importance that meticulous haemostasis is achieved:
  - anaesthetist should be asked to restore the pre-operative blood pressure if hypotension has deliberately been employed;
  - patient should be tipped head down to enhance identification of potential bleeding.

Photodynamic therapy

- Advocated as a technique that causes selective tumour destruction by cell apoptosis with minimal scarring and preservation of uninvolved tissue (thereby minimizing functional deficit).
- Photosensitizing agents currently available are insufficiently selective to prevent normal tissue damage.
- Patients must be protected from exposure to sunlight for several days.
- Following tumour ablation, the wound sloughs and heals by secondary intention and scarring.
- There does not appear to be any benefit of this technique over the more traditional resection methods.

The neck

- Several classifications of neck dissection (ND) are in existence.
- The term radical neck dissection should only apply to the classical ND described by Crile, which involves resection of the lymph nodes in level I–V of the neck together with sacrifice of:
  - sternocleidomastoid muscle (SCM);
  - spinal accessory nerve (SAN);
  - internal jugular vein (IJV).
- All other neck dissections are selective and best described by the levels of lymph nodes resected, and which of the vital structures have been sacrificed, e.g. level I–IV with resection of IJV. This avoids confusion regarding the meaning of terms such as modified radical, functional, comprehensive, supra-omohyoid, and extended, which are all open to interpretation and lack clarity.
- Whether elective (staging ND in cN0) or therapeutic (ND in clinically or radiologically N+ disease) most neck dissections performed today preserve the vital structures of the neck to minimize functional deficit. The following structures are preserved unless they are directly invaded by tumour:
  - SCM;
  - carotid artery;
  - IJV;
  - SAN;
  - vagus;

- laryngeal nerves;
- sympathetic chain;
- phrenic nerve;
- cervical plexus;
- hypoglossal nerve;
- mandibular branch of the facial nerve.

Neck access

There are four main types of incision described to access the neck:
- Apron.
- Wine glass.
- 'H'.
- MacFee.

In most situations some form of the apron incision is the most appropriate. This should be raised in the sub-platysmal plane unless tumour invasion dictates otherwise. The subcutaneous blood supply is derived from a plexus of vessels with a vertical axis and therefore the MacFee (parallel transverse) incision, although preserving a bi-pedicle skin flap, does not make best use of the skin blood supply and produces poorer access to the neck. The 'H' and wine glass incision both give excellent access, but create points with reduced blood supply, which often lie over underlying vital structures. Where a previous incision has been made in the neck this should normally be excised and the neck incision planned around this.

Elective neck dissection (END)

- Where there is no clinical or radiological evidence of nodal involvement, END may be indicated because up to 30% of patients with tumours of the floor of mouth or tongue will have occult micrometastases.
- Access to the neck is also often required in order to facilitate microvascular reconstruction—under either of these circumstances a neck dissection will be indicated unless the patient is not fit enough for major surgery. When a simple local resection and 'watch and wait policy' can be employed.
- At present there is insufficient evidence to know whether any survival advantage is gained in performing END and what detriment in may have in terms of quality of life. However, it is hope that the ongoing UK-wide clinical trial 'selective elective neck dissection' (SEND) trial will address this issue. This is a prospective RCT comparing survival in patients who undergo either an END, or a 'watch and wait policy' for early carcinoma of the tongue. Study start date January 2007 with estimated primary completion in December 2015.
- Further benefit arising from END is accurate pathological staging of the neck that helps inform the need for adjuvant radiotherapy and increases prognostic accuracy.
- The extent of END determined by the site and size of the primary tumour, e.g. in anterior tumours:
  - neck dissection should harvest levels I–IV (accounts for the possibility of skip lesions in level IV—particular phenomenon associated with primary tumours of the tongue and floor of mouth);

- incidence of spread to level IIb (above the spinal accessory nerve) is very low—therefore only included in large, posterior tumours;
- incidence of spread to level V in N0 neck is very low (1–3%)—therefore, level V not usually removed because morbidity to shoulder arising from devascularization of the spinal accessory nerve is high.
- If metastases are detected pathologically in levels I–IV (more than one positive node or any positive node with extracapsular spotted) then post-operative adjuvant radiotherapy is usually employed to include level V.

Sentinel node biopsy
- Advocated by some for the N0 neck.
- Injection of radiolabelled dye 1 day pre-operatively of the primary tumour area with intra-operative blue dye injected at the time of surgery.
- This then drains to the lymph nodes in the same order that tumour would spread.
- Gamma camera then used to determine the pattern of lymph node drainage for that tumour.
- Small incision made in the neck and the dye-bearing node(s) with high gamma signal excised and submitted for histology.
- If metastasis subsequently detected pathologically, formal neck dissection is undertaken at a second operation.
- Application of technique to oropharyngeal malignancies still under evaluation.

Therapeutic neck dissection
- Where the neck is N+.
- Where there is extensive disease in the neck with invasion of the SCM, SAN, and IJV, a radical ND is justified. On occasion it is necessary to extend the dissection beyond the boundaries defined by Crile (extended radical neck dissection (RND)).
- In other N+ cases a selective ND is indicated with preservation of as many vital structures as possible. In the majority of cases clear tissue planes between the vital structures and involved nodes are preserved, which means that some preservation of function is feasible.
- Occasionally it is not possible to safely resect involved nodes from a vital structure and, at that point, the ND should include the involved structure. This should be tailored to each individual patient. Whilst pre-operative imaging may give some idea about the likelihood of involvement, it is not infallible and often the decision will have to be made at operation.
- If this inclusion involves SCM, IJV, and SAN, and levels I–V, the ND is said to be 'radicalized'.
- Care should be taken when undertaking the neck dissection to avoid unnecessary sacrifice of vessels that may have potential value for reconstruction—this should never take precedence, risking compromise of tumour resection.

Tracheostomy

The majority of patients who undergo resection of oropharyngeal tumours and ND do not require an elective tracheostomy provided that a level 3 critical care facility is available for the management of the patient in the immediate post-operative period. Where there has been a large oropharyngeal resection it is prudent to undertake a naso-endoscopic assessment of the airway prior to extubation. Occasionally, where the anaesthetist has assessed the intubation as difficult, it may be prudent to undertake an elective tracheostomy. Some units undertake elective tracheostomy where a bilateral ND or a large posterior resection has been carried out.

Where patients are taken back to theatre for re-exploration of the neck for flap insufficiency or bleeding it is usually wise to undertake a tracheostomy at that stage as swelling is likely to be much more significant (see ➔ Anaesthesia, p. 376).

Reconstruction

There have been major advances in this area over the last 3 decades. Previously, techniques available to repair defects following cancer ablation were limited. Patients were left deformed with little function. The use of free tissue transfer had transformed cancer treatment by extending what can be safely resected and with the resulting reconstruction, improved quality of life.

The oral cavity and oropharynx has many important functional roles. Resection of any tumour in this region may impact on function. The key functions to preserve with reconstruction of oropharyngeal cancer defects include:

- Speech.
- Swallowing.
- Eating.
- Chewing.
- Sensation.
- Cosmesis.

Reconstruction: issues to consider

The choice of reconstruction technique will depend on:

- Defect: site and size.
- Type(s) of tissue required.
- Patient factors:
  - general fitness;
  - existing medical problems;
  - suitability of donor site;
  - patient's preference.
- Resources available.

General principles of reconstruction

- Replace like with like.
- Keep it simple.
- Immediate reconstruction is better than delayed.
- Minimize donor site morbidity.
- Resection to achieve clear margins must not be compromised to enable easier reconstruction.

Reconstructive ladder

The techniques available for repair are usually described as a reconstructive ladder, with simple techniques at the bottom rung (less effort/expertise) and more complex ones higher up. The success of reconstruction may be compromised by bleeding, haematoma, breakdown of wound, and infection. A more complex treatment, such as free tissue transfer, is an all or none phenomenon—its failure will result in a persisting defect, donor site morbidity, and a weaker patient.

Reconstructive techniques

The techniques available are described from a simple to more complex order.

Open wound

A laser bed wound is left open and heals with good mucosa coverage and minimal contracture. Conventional non-laser wounds, if left open, will heal slowly, with a combination of contracture and re-epithelization. The resultant scar is poor, deformed, and may have a deleterious affect function.

Primary closure

- Ideal for small defects where the edges of the wound can be advanced for closure, enabling healing by primary intention.
- No donor site morbidity with maximal preservation of function and cosmesis.
- Use limited to small defects with lax adjacent tissues to advance for closure. Excessive tension to achieve primary closure may result in distortion, dehiscence and widened scar.

Graft

This involves using a piece of tissue (e.g. mucosa, skin graft, or bone) removed from its original donor site and transferred to a recipient site where it gains a new blood supply from the wound bed. The graft is usually harvested from the same individual (*autograft*), but may be from another individual of same species (*allograft*) or even different species (*xenograft*). A graft cannot be used if the recipient bed is absent (through and through defect) or hostile (no prospect of revascularization).

- Mucosal grafts:
  - can be harvested from buccal mucosa (primary closure) or hard palate (allowed to re-epithelialize);
  - good match for mucosal repair;
  - easy to harvest;
  - healing of donor site may cause further distortion of the oral cavity.
- Split-thickness skin graft:
  - epidermis and part of dermis taken with a manual or electric dermatome knife;
  - donor site left to re-epithelialize;
  - high success rate as little tissue thickness is required for re-vascularization, but has minimal intrinsic features and may contract;
  - donor site (e.g. thigh, upper arm) can be sore, requires dressing for several weeks, and has a paler appearance in the long term.
- Full-thickness skin graft:
  - Reliable, but the success rate is slightly less than partial thickness counterpart;
  - better appearance than partial-thickness graft;
  - donor site (pre- or post-auricular, supraclavicular, abdomen) closed primarily.

- Bone:
  - cancellous blocks (rich in osteogenic material), cortico-cancellous blocks, or cortical pieces;
  - long-established technique that provides rigid scaffolding (osteoconductive), whereby the bony structure is gradually replaced by new bone formation;
  - variety of donor sites, e.g. mandible, iliac crest, rib, tibia, or calvarium;
  - can be used for repairing bony defects, and to augment or reconstruct discontinuity;
  - as non-vascularized requires immobilization and a healthy vascular bed to take (radiotherapy will result in subsequent loss);
  - in addition to generic operative side effects/possible complications (bleeding, haematoma, dehiscence, infection, and scarring), each donor site will have some specific morbidity, e.g. anterior iliac crest (numbness side of leg and groin, aching, and deformity).
- Cartilage grafts:
  - used in reconstruction of composite ear or nose defects;
  - usually harvested from the patient and has a good success rate if covered due to its low metabolic requirements;
  - can be harvested from nose, ear, and rib as a composite graft with skin/mucosa.
- Nerve and vein grafts:
  - occasionally required and often taken locally, e.g. as part of flap harvest, great auricular nerve, or external jugular vein;
  - fascial grafts provide a band of firm tissue (from temporalis area or fascial lata of thigh) for use as slings or craniofacial dural repair.

Flaps

A flap is a piece of tissue retaining its attached vascular supply transferred to repair a defect within reach. Unlike a graft it is not dependent on initial re-vascularization since its blood supply is maintained. This also enables a more substantial bulk of tissue to be used, providing structure form and volume.

The vascular supply of a flap can be random or axial in pattern. The random pattern flap relies on subcutaneous vasculature. This limits the design on the length of flap before distal necrosis occurs (usually base width equal to length, but can be longer with the rich blood supply in the head and neck region). An axial pattern with specific associated vessels means a larger and longer flap can be raised safely.

- Local flaps: there are many local flaps that can be used for defects around the face, oral cavity, and pharynx, as well as neck. Examples include:
  - *local intra-oral options*—buccal mucosal advancement/rotational flaps, tongue flap, palatal mucosal flap, and buccal fat pad flap. Suitable for small adjacent defects. Ease of harvest of a local flap and its matching tissue characteristics is offset by its limitation of size. Too large a harvest can distort anatomy and compromise function;

- *naso-labial flap*—random finger of skin taken from the naso-labial fold (primary closure of donor site with good resultant cosmesis) is turned into the oral cavity through a created opening in the cheek and buccal mucosa. Can be used to repair small defects (buccal, alveolus, and floor of mouth). The inferiorly based pedicle is divided 2–3 weeks after gaining co-lateral vascularization from the bed of the defect. When used bilaterally can repair anterior floor of mouth while retaining good function of the tongue;
- *Karapandzic flaps*—this sensate flap closes lower lip defects of up to 60% by advancing adjacent tissue, while preserving the peri-oral vascular ring and nerves (blunt muscular dissection technique). Microstomia can be a problem. There are numerous other rotational/advancement flaps for lip defects.
- **Regional flaps:** temporalis flap—muscle flap based on deep temporal vessels, reflected over the zygomatic arch to reconstruct small defects in the upper cheek, pharynx, and palate. Limited by its arc of rotation. Has a role in facial reanimation.
- **Distant flaps:**
  - *pectoralis major myocutaneous flap (PMMF)*—workhorse, pedicled non-microvascular option in reconstruction of medium to large oral defects. Provides large muscle and associated chest wall skin based on the pectoral branch of thoraco-acromial artery. Often raised as a myocutaneous (muscle and skin) or muscle-only flap, reflected over the clavicle into the neck, and can reach up to the zygomatic arch. Donor site is primarily closed. Reliable and can be raised without need to change position of patient on table for oral cancer ablation. Its bulk is both advantageous (protect neck vessels, good for big defects) and disadvantageous (too rigid for defects requiring a more pliable repair). The shoulder function can be impaired when combined with radical ND;
  - *delto-pectoral flap*—two-stage fasciocutaneous flap medially based on 2–3 perforating branches of the internal mammary artery. Limited by its reach into only the lower half of oral cavity and face. When collateral vascularization is achieved at 2–3 weeks, the tubed pedicle is divided and repositioned. The donor site defect is skin grafted (split-thickness). Superseded by other options but worth considering as a fall back in rare circumstances.
- **Free flap:** involves harvesting a flap of soft tissue or bone with its associated vascular supply, detaching it and re-anastomosing with donor vessels in the neck using microsurgical techniques (loupes or microscope). Surgery is complex and technically challenging. However, the type of tissue available for repair is no longer restricted by its ability to reach the defect. Success rate is high (around 95%) in specialized units. Post-operative monitoring is essential as a haematoma or venous thrombosis can threaten the viability of the flap.

There are many flaps suitable for oral and oropharyngeal defects following cancer ablation.

Four common free flaps used

Radial forearm flap

This is a distal skin paddle of the forearm based on a pedicle of the radial artery, vena commitantes, and/or superficial subcutaneous vein (Fig. 2.11). The soft pliable skin paddle provides a good reconstruction for small to medium oropharyngeal defects, enabling the residual tissue (e.g. tongue, floor of mouth) to function. The skin paddle is usually taken from the volar surface.

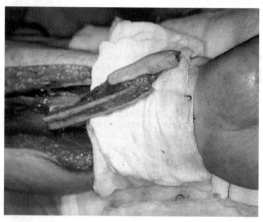

Fig. 2.11 Composite radial forearm free flap.

- Indications and strengths:
  - workhorse for oral soft tissue defects;
  - provides thin, pliable skin paddle with reliable long vascular pedicle;
  - good size vessels;
  - easy to raise;
  - permits two-team operating.
- Modifications:
  - can include vascularized bone (part of radius, risk of fracture in 1/5 cases, but can reduce with prophylactic plating);
  - nerve (innervation);
  - tendon (sling effect with palmaris longus);
  - usually fasciocutaneous—can be suprafascial or fascia only.
- Pre-operative assessment:
  - use non-dominant forearm;
  - check no previous surgery/injury or Raynaud's disease;
  - ensure normal (negative) Allen's test for patency of radial artery, ulnar artery, and collateral palmar arch;
  - if doubt use Doppler duplex assessment to investigate further, another limb or another flap;
  - ensure no venepuncture made in the donor arm.

- Positioning:
  - supine with arm extended on side support board (<90°);
  - tourniquet applied to arm (above elbow), but **do not** inflate until flap is marked and ready to start harvesting.
- Preparation:
  - radial artery is palpated and skin paddle is marked out;
  - forearm is elevated and the tourniquet inflated to twice the blood systolic pressure (usually 200–250mmHg).
- Procedure:
  - dissection of skin paddle commenced on ulnar border of flap;
  - incise skin, fat, and fascia to underlying muscle (watch for superficial ulnar vessels ~2%);
  - haemostasis achieved with bipolar diathermy or ligation;
  - para-tenon left intact to maximize skin graft take;
  - dissection continued until the condensation of the inter-muscular septum between brachioradialis and flexor carpi radialis is reached (median nerve sits deep to the flexor muscles);
  - flap must be raised with care to preserve the connection between radial pedicle and skin flap;
  - distal and radial side of skin flap is raised;
  - brachoradialis tendon is used to guide dissection on radial side of flap/pedicle;
  - radial artery and venae commitantes at the distal end of the skin paddle are ligated and divided;
  - the skin paddle and associated radial pedicle is then elevated proximally, preserving the cephalic venous system if required;
  - preserve superficial radial nerve if possible;
  - perforators from the radial pedicle run into the adjacent muscles at regular intervals—they should be controlled with bipolar diathermy or ligation well away from the pedicle at the muscle surface;
  - once the flap is raised to an adequate length, the tourniquet is released, any bleeding controlled and the flap left to perfuse for at least 20min;
  - adequate residual circulation to the hand should be ensured at this stage; when ready for transfer the pedicle is divided.
- Closure:
  - donor site is closed primarily apart from the distal end;
  - skin paddle site is repaired with a full-thickness skin graft (VY skin graft or abdominal skin graft), split-thickness skin graft, or local (ulnar) transposition flap;
  - the skin graft is pressure dressed;
  - a backslab can be applied to improve skin graft take.
- Post-operative care:
  - elevate limb in Bradford sling for 2 days with regular checks on hand viability;
  - the transferred flap is also monitored regularly (Fig. 2.12);
  - forearm dressing is changed at 9–10 days and at weekly intervals thereafter. If heals uneventfully dress forearm for about 4–5 weeks;
  - function of the hand following harvest is usually normal unless complicated by skin graft loss or fractured radius (composite flap) (Fig. 2.13).

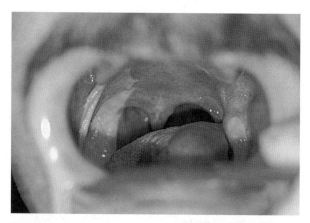

Fig. 2.12 Oropharyngeal reconstruction with radial forearm free flap.

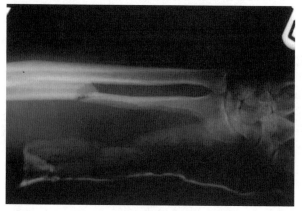

Fig. 2.13 Fracture of residual radius following composite harvest.

- Complications (donor site):
  - bleeding (rare);
  - excess exudate can soak dressing and will require changing;
  - wound infection or skin graft loss with tendon exposure can occur; exposed tendon usually heals after lengthy regular dressings;
  - paraesthesia at root of thumb is common;
  - power and range of movements in hand not usually impaired;
  - scarring problematic in younger patients—camouflage can be offered.

Anterolateral thigh flap
- Indications and strengths:
  - as per radial forearm soft tissue flap;
  - larger area can be harvested;
  - donor site morbidity is very low.
- Anatomy and procedure:
  - a fasciocutaneous flap based on the septocutaneous or musculocutaneous perforators of the descending branch of the lateral circumflex femoral artery. A satisfactory perforator is generally found within 3cm of the midpoint of a line connecting the anterior superior iliac spine with the superolateral border of the patella. More than half of perforators traverse the substance of the vastus lateralis muscle. The descending branch of the lateral circumflex femoral artery, and its vena comitans, lies between the vastus lateralis and rectus femoris muscles, along with the nerve to the vastus lateralis. The descending branch can usually be safely dissected proximally to its major branch to the rectus femoris, which should be preserved during flap harvest;
  - skin paddles can be 20cm in length;
  - vascular pedicle can be up to 20cm;
  - primary closure is possible for paddles 8–9 cm in width;
  - in most cases, the fascia lata represents the deep aspect of the harvested flap, but suprafascial harvest is possible. Portions of vastus lateralis muscle can be harvested with the flap if necessary;
  - the position of the nerve to vastus lateralis is variable with respect to the vascular pedicle, and the nerve cannot always be left intact during harvest. It is likely that nerve division will result in morbidity.

Fibula flap
Up to 25cm of fibula bone ± skin paddle on lateral leg can be harvested based on the peroneal artery and veins. The bone is osteotomized to match mandible or maxillary alveolus. The skin paddle provides a good soft tissue reconstruction with the bone readily accepting implants, but does not match the height of a dentate mandible. Provided 6cm of bone is preserved at both ends of the donor site there is no significant impact on joint function or weight bearing. The donor site skin is closed primarily or with a split-thickness skin graft for larger defects.
- Modifications:
  - bone and muscle cuff only;
  - lateral sural cutaneous nerve can be included to provide for sensate flap;
  - bone can be 'double barrelled' at the recipient site to increase the height of the neo-alveolus (Fig. 2.14).

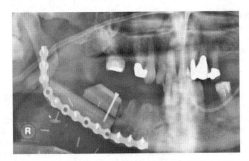

Fig. 2.14 Post-operative view of double-barrelled fibula flap.

- **Pre-operative assessment:**
  - exclude previous trauma, surgery, or peripheral vascular disease;
  - mandatory investigation to ensure all three vessels in leg are patent and healthy (DUSS, conventional angiograms, or MRA are common options).
- **Positioning:** supine position with the leg partly flexed and internally rotated to allow access to dissect the posterior part of skin paddle.
- **Preparation:**
  - leg is prepped and landmarks marked (line from fibula head to lateral epicondyle of ankle inferiorly);
  - skin paddle is fusiform in shape, and includes the junction of the upper two-thirds and the lower third of the above line to capture a dominant septocutaneous or musculocutaneous perforators to the skin;
  - tourniquet is inflated to twice the systolic blood pressure.
- **Procedure** (Fig. 2.15):
  - skin paddle is incised anteriorly through skin and subcutaneous tissue to the peroneus muscles;
  - dissection is continued backwards in a subfascial plane towards the intermuscular septum;
  - peroneus longus and brevis are dissected anteriorly off the fibula in a supra-periosteal plane;
  - when the anterior aspect of the fibula is reached, care is taken to keep close to bone to avoid injuring the anterior tibial vessels and deep peroneal nerve in the anterior compartment;
  - extensor hallucis longus is dissected off the fibula to expose the interosseous membrane;
  - after osteotomies of the distal and proximal ends of the fibula with saws (at least 6cm length preserved both ends to maintain integrity of joints) with protection of the tissue deep to bone, the distal ends of the peroneal vessels are identified, ligated, and transected;
  - interosseous membrane is then divided after external rotation of the osteotomized fibula for easier access;

- chevron-orientated muscle fibres of the tibialis posterior are visualized to identify the fascial plane superficial to the peroneal vessels. Dissection along this plane enables continuous visualization of the peroneal vessels. The entire length is dissected to the bifurcation of the posterior tibial vessels;
- posterior aspect of the skin paddle is dissected including a muscle cuff of flexor hallucis longus and soleus to preserve the musculocutaneous perforators to the skin paddle. The flexor hallucis longus is transected before the pedicle is freed;
- tourniquet is deflated and haemostasis achieved. The fibula composite flap is hinged on the pedicle ready for transfer.
- Closure:
  - primary closure possible with small fusiform skin paddle design;
  - larger defects need split-thickness skin grafting;
  - drain is employed as can be a catheter for long-acting LA infusion.
- Post-operative care:
  - elevate foot with pillow;
  - viability of the foot must be checked regularly;
  - leg dressing is changed at 10 days;
  - patient is gradually mobilized with physiotherapy input and walking aids.
- Complications:
  - muscular pain;
  - oedema;
  - paraesthesia—anterior and lateral side of leg and dorsum of foot;
  - weakness of dorsiflexion of the great toe;
  - ischaemia to foot.

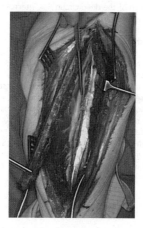

Fig. 2.15 Intra-operative view of right fibular harvest.

Deep circumflex iliac artery flap

This is another common hard tissue flap used for oropharyngeal bony defects reconstruction. Bone from the anterior iliac crest ± internal oblique muscle (or thicker skin adjacent to bone) is harvested based on the deep circumflex iliac artery (DCIA) and veins. The pedicle is relatively short. The donor site muscle defect may need a mesh closure. Any skin defect is closed primarily.

- **Pre-operative assessment:** clinical exclusion of previous abdominal injury/surgery.
- **Positioning:**
  - supine position;
  - a sandbag can be used to improve access to more posterior part of the iliac crest to achieve a longer pedicle.
- **Preparation:**
  - exposure from lower chest wall down to groin;
  - include midline medially.
- **Procedure (DCIA and internal oblique muscle flap):**
  - skin incision runs obliquely from the pubic crest 2cm medial to the iliac crest in a supero-lateral direction to just below the costal margin;
  - dissection continues on a wide front down to the external oblique muscle which is then incised to expose the internal oblique muscle (fibres run in different plane);
  - internal oblique muscle is initially divided at its cephalad extent, the plane between the internal oblique, and transversus being revealed by a white fascial flash;
  - internal oblique muscle is dissected from cephalad to caudal leaving it hinged on the iliac crest;
  - ascending branch of the deep circumflex internal artery (and vein) runs on the deep surface of the internal oblique muscle and is used to identify the main DCIA pedicle;
  - DCIA is traced to the external iliac vessels;
  - lateral portion of the transversus abdominus is then transected about 2cm from the inner table of the iliac crest;
  - DCIA runs between the iliacus and transversus abdominus along the inner table of the iliac crest and the iliacus is transected (with 2cm cuff) to expose the inner table of iliac crest (Fig. 2.16);
  - lateral dissection is carried out next lifting the muscles of the lateral aspect of iliac crest;
  - pedicle is protected and a segment of iliac crest osteotomized according to the desired shape, and the anterior superior iliac spine is preserved with the inguinal ligament attachment;
  - the harvested flap is then ready for transfer (Fig. 2.17) and insertion (Fig. 2.18).

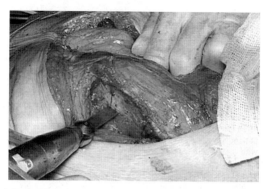

Fig. 2.16 Medial bone cut during DCIA harvest.

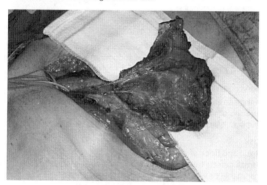

Fig. 2.17 DCIA harvest completed prior to division of pedicle.

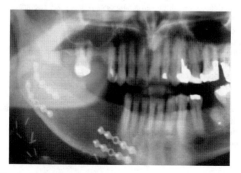

Fig. 2.18 Mandibular reconstruction with DCIA (post-operative image of Fig. 2.7).

- Closure:
  - meticulous closure is necessary to prevent hernia formation;
  - transversus muscle is approximated to iliacus. If a significant part of internal oblique muscle has been removed a mesh is used to repair the ensuing defect. The external oblique aponeurosis is then approximated to the tensor fascia lata and gluteus medius;
  - in addition to a drain, an infusion catheter is placed in the wound to permit the use of long-acting LAs to supplement pain control;
  - remaining subcutaneous tissues and skin are closed conventionally.
- Post-operative care:
  - listen for bowel sounds to ensure no ileus;
  - patient is gradually mobilized from day 2 to 3. Physiotherapy input with walking aids is required.
- Complications:
  - muscular pain;
  - weakening and bulging of abdominal wall;
  - hernia formation;
  - femoral nerve injury;
  - damage to intraperitoneal contents;
  - paraesthesia—lateral aspect of thigh.

There are many other flaps that include the anterolateral thigh, latissimus dorsi, lateral arm, scapula, and rectus abdominus. (For detailed descriptions please see ➲ Further reading, p. 147.)

Reconstructive options and common defects

A common strategy is to use two-team operating, one to perform the ablation and the other reconstruction. Harvesting of a free flap should be carried out simultaneously, if at all possible, to reduce overall operating time.

Defects

- **Tongue and floor of mouth:**
  - small defects may be left to re-epithelialized (laser) or closed primarily or with a local flap (e.g. naso-labial flap);
  - medium size defects require a pliable flap to allow residual tissue function (e.g. radial forearm flap, antero-lateral thigh flap);
  - large defects with little remaining organ/tissue will require bulkier flaps, such as pectoralis major, latissimus dorsi, or rectus abdominus flaps.
- **Buccal:**
  - superficial tumours can be removed with a laser or skin grafted;
  - small defects can be closed with local flaps;
  - larger defects can be reconstructed with radial forearm flaps;
  - through and through defects will require a bi-paddled radial forearm flap or larger soft tissue flap such as the antero-lateral thigh.
- **Mandible:** where mandibular invasion necessitates a segmental resection (full-thickness mandible producing discontinuity) vascularized bone is preferable due to the high rate of post-operative radiotherapy. Common flaps used include fibula, DCIA or scapular.

- **Maxilla:** a low-level defect can be obturated with excellent oro-nasal seal, function, and cosmesis. Larger or more complex defects require free tissue transfer options such as fibula, scapula, or DCIA flaps.
- **Lip:** this is a difficult area when the defect is too big for primary closure or local flaps. Free tissue transfer is often suboptimal in terms of colour match, oral seal, and function, even though tendon modification can be incorporated.
- **Pharynx:** partial defects can be reconstructed with a pectoralis major flap or soft tissue flap, such as radial forearm flap. The latter can be tubed for full circumferential defects. Alternatives include antero-lateral thigh or jejunal flaps.

Developments

Recent and ongoing developments include modification to the planned flap site (e.g. tissue expansion), tissue engineering (i.e. prelamination or pre-fabrication of flaps), and transplantation. These techniques currently have limited roles in cancer patients as they require time for the modification. Immunosuppression is also best avoided with cancer patients.

Technology advances in medical modelling with 3D printers now enable surgeons to prefabricate accurate reconstruction plates for difficult composite defects (e.g. large tumours or pathological fractures) and produce templates to achieve optimal bony osteotomies. Operating times will also be shortened.

Perforator flaps may reduce donor site morbidity and improve reconstructive options for the defect.

Implants

This is a useful adjunct for reconstructed bony defects involving tooth-bearing segments. Retention of prostheses can be improved with the aid of implant placement. Chewing, and consequently quality of life, has been demonstrated to be significantly improved. Bone flaps suitable for implant insertion are favoured with this rehabilitation in mind during treatment planning.

Prosthetic rehabilitation

This well-established technique for small maxillary defects requires pre-operative planning with a maxillofacial technician. When chosen for the appropriate defect it provides an effective and well-accepted reconstructive option. An impression of the jaw is taken before surgery to make a dressing plate. The maxillary defect after resection is dressed with a suitable obturation material and plate to seal the oral cavity from the nasal and antral cavities. The raw inner surfaces are skin grafted to facilitate prompt healing. A dressing change is performed 2 weeks later to allow further accurate impressions or the fitting of a temporary hollow obturator. A more permanent obturator with teeth is fitted later. More complex defects can be filled with a multipieced prostheses or further retention gained with the aid of implants.

Surgical complications

A surgical complication is a development that is generally to the patient's detriment arising at the time of the operation or within the post-operative period. Overall, complication rates as high as 60% have been reported in some surgical series treating oral cancer.

Risk factors in oral cancer patients

The factors influencing complications are often multifactorial. They include:

Patient factors
- Age: usually older patients.
- Poor performance status.
- Medical co-morbidities, e.g. ischaemic heart disease, respiratory disease.
- Excess alcohol and smoking.
- Poor nutritional status.

Tumour factors
- Advanced stage tumours are a common presentation.
- Aggressive tumours.

Treatment factors
- Complex surgery, i.e. lengthy operation.
- Need for reconstruction.
- Previous surgical treatment.
- Previous treatment modalities, e.g. radiotherapy.

Consequence of complications
- Major complications (~20%):
  - can be life threatening (up to 4% mortality reported);
  - increase length of stay;
  - cause further suffering with adverse effect on quality of life;
  - require further treatment;
  - incur ↑ cost;
  - delay adjuvant treatment;
  - all may result in poorer outcomes.
- Minor complications: may not be life threatening, but can require further surgery or prolong inpatient stay. Nevertheless, they adversely affect patients and may contribute towards the development of major problems.

Prevention

Predisposing factors should be identified as part of pre-assessment and appropriate interventions used to optimize the patient's status. The quantification of risk is also useful for formulating treatment plans, consent, and rehabilitation. With effective pre-assessment and optimization of any pre-existing conditions, careful surgery with advanced intra-operative monitoring and vigilant post-operative care, complications can be prevented or at least kept to a minimum.

Complications associated with oral cancer treatment

General anaesthetic and positioning complications

- Nerve compression injury, e.g. ulnar.
- Soft tissue problems, e.g. precipitation of pressure sores.

General medical problems or arising from existing co-morbidities

- Pulmonary (atelectasis, pneumonia, acute respiratory distress syndrome (ARDS), respiratory failure).
- Cardiovascular (myocardial infarction (MI), tachyarrhythmias, heart failure).
- Neurological (cardiovascular accident (CVA), delirium).
- Deep vein thrombosis (DVT) and pulmonary embolism.
- Urinary tract infection.
- Renal failure.
- Alcohol withdrawal.

(See main surgical textbooks for specific diagnosis and management.)

The diagnosis and management of these conditions are dealt with in the conventional manner. Of these potential complications respiratory (up to 20%) and cardiovascular (~10%) make up a significant proportion of medical problems encountered following head and neck cancer surgery. Wound infections are next most common.

Specific surgical problems

Peri-operative complications

- **Carotid sinus sensitivity:** manipulation or pressure of the carotid bulb (baroreceptors) during surgery may cause asystole/marked bradycardia and hypotension. Avoiding further pressure or, if continued manipulation is required due to tumour dissection, topical or injected lignocaine may be beneficial. Post-operative sensitivity may be due to scarring around the bulb.
- **Increased intra-cranial pressure (ICP):** ligation of the IJV will cause a transient rise in ICP. This seldom causes overt symptoms, but may contribute to post-operative delirium or facial oedema and cyanosis. Simultaneous bilateral IJV ligations (rare nowadays) will give rise to spectacular acute facial swelling.

Immediate/early complications

Bleeding

Any bleeding immediately after oral cancer surgery usually declares itself quickly and is detected before vital signs deteriorate. Basic principles of controlling bleeding include:

- Application of pressure.
- Summoning of assistance.
- Resuscitation.
- Urgent return to theatre to identify and treat the cause and protection of airway (crucial).

Many major oral cancer ablation and reconstruction patients may have temporary tracheostomies. The cuffed tube will secure the airway and enable rapid return to theatre safely. Sources of bleeding include major vessels and their branches (usually slippage of ligation), suture lines, or from the undersurface of flaps (may be due to coagulated vessels reopening during hypertensive episodes). Any haematoma must be dealt with promptly as it can threaten free tissue transfer anastomoses, compress the airway, and subsequently promote infected.

Airway obstruction and tracheostomy problems

Surgery for oropharyngeal cancer has a significant risk of obstructing the airway through bleeding, soft tissue oedema, and haematoma in the neck.

- Where the airway is felt to be at risk an elective temporary tracheostomy should be carried out. An emergency re-intubation for a compromised airway post-operatively is best avoided.
- A patient with an in-dwelling tracheostomy tube can still be at risk of airway obstruction through a displaced or blocked tube.
- Prevent blockage with meticulous nursing care, regular clearing of secretions, humidification, inner tube hygiene, and appropriate tube change.
- Pressure of the inflatable cuff must not be excessive.
- Breathing exercises should be encouraged and the tube adequately secured.
- Decannulation should be attempted when the airway is no longer compromised (maintain self-ventilation), minimal suction is required for secretions, and the patient able to protect his or her airway through effective coughing.

Chylous leakage

~2% risk in neck dissections. Caused by damage to thoracic duct (left side) or lymphatic duct (right side). Diagnosed during surgery by the presence, pooling, or discharge of clear fluid. Promptly diagnose, and treat by ligating or over-sewing the affected vessels. Bipolar diathermy is not effective. If undetected at surgery a chylous leak will declare itself as a collection in the neck or excess fluid in drain. The fluid will be clear (if patient starved) or milky (if feeding due to fat content—biochemistry reveals high triglycerides). Management depends on volume of output:

- High chylous output (>600mL/24h) will need surgical exploration with ligation of affected vessel/tissue. Can affect the patient's fluid balance, deplete protein levels, produce immunocompromise, and prevent the neck from healing. Over-sewing, application of tissue glue, and pressure dressings are methods adopted to control the leakage.
- Low chylous output can be treated non-surgically with medium-chain triglyceride enteral feeding, supraclavicular pressure dressings, and careful attention to the fluid and electrolyte balance. If persistent, total parenteral feeding may be necessary.

Seroma and salivary collection

- A collection of fluid may form soon after removal or blockage of neck drains. It can result in separation of the skin flap from the underlying tissue bed and is usually gravity dependent at the base of the neck.
- The tail of the parotid may have been transected during neck dissection resulting in a salivary collection.
- The swelling is softer and more fluctuant than a haematoma.
- Usually managed by repeated aspiration to allow healing—safeguard the anastomoses where present and prevent infection.
- A sialocoele can be confirmed with high amylase content on analysis. Exclude an orocervical communication. If a sialocoele reforms regularly anti-sialogogues may be required.

Infection

Wound infections following oral cancer surgery (oral cavity—clean contaminated surgery category) is not uncommon. The incidence of wound infection is ~20% in most series. It is often multifactorial. The causative pathogens are often polymicrobial, with well-known pathogens including anaerobes. Risk factors for infection:

- Advanced disease.
- Existing co-morbidities.
- Longer duration of surgery.
- Previous treatment (chemotherapy and radiotherapy).
- Smoking.
- Excess alcohol intake.
- Presence of tracheostomy tube.
- Use of blood transfusions, often multifactorial. The causative pathogens are often polymicrobial, with well-known pathogens including anaerobes.
- Antibiotic prophylaxis for clean contaminated surgery is warranted and should be broad spectrum, covering common pathogens and anaerobes. Shorter courses of antibiotics/perioperative prophylaxis have been shown to have similar infection rates to longer courses (see ⊃ General surgical principles, p. 374).
- Management of wound infection: drainage of pus, debridement, systemic antibiotics for systemic/severe local signs, with best-guess antibiotics followed by adjustment after microbiology results.

Dehiscence/failure of wound healing/fistula

- Minor dehiscence or wound breakdown is not uncommon, and often has little impact on outcome.
- Ideally, prevention with meticulous techniques, antibiotic prophylaxis, and good nutritional support is best.
- Oral dehiscence is often associated with salivary collection/leakage through the neck, requiring nil by mouth (NBM) + enteral feeding approach.

- There is a risk of neck vessels becoming exposed with danger of major secondary bleeding.
- Larger wounds can be managed with the over-sewing of pack.
- More significant defects will need further surgery to cover and seal the oral cavity.

Nerve injuries
- Phrenic nerve injury: raised (ipsilateral) diaphragm may lead to impaired pulmonary function with ↑ risk of infection.
- Sympathetic chain injury: Horner's syndrome.
- Accessory/cervical plexus injury (see Shoulder and neck problems in ➲ Late complications, p. 113).
- Marginal mandibular branch of facial nerve: weak lower lip (transient or permanent), usually of cosmetic, rather than functional impact.
- Superior laryngeal nerve injury: weaker voice. Not a common problem declared by patients following neck dissection.
- Paraesthesia of neck skin, resection bed and peri-auricular region (associated cutaneous nerves from neck dissection or direct nerve resection during tumour ablation).

Flap failure
All flaps should be monitored frequently in the immediate post-operative phase so that circulatory problems can be detected early with a view to successful salvage:
- Local flaps in the head and neck are usually robust due to the profuse vascular supply.
- Pedicled flaps such as the PMMF may become compromised due to constriction of the pedicle as it is reflected over the clavicle or beneath a tight skin tunnel in the neck. The constriction may be exacerbated by post-operative oedema. Judicious removal of sutures may be enough to reverse the problem.
- Free flaps demand close monitoring for the first 48h when problems such as venous engorgement (flap becomes blue and mottled) or arterial occlusion (pale, white flap) are most likely to occur. The latter can be difficult to diagnose, but a reduced or absent pulse can be detected by hand-held Doppler probe. Flap monitoring devices may provide earlier warning for successful salvage. Examples include in implantable Doppler probes and microdialysis. In addition to anastomotic problems external compression (neck haematoma) or systemic disturbance (e.g. hypotension, arrhythmias) may also threaten the flap.
- Management of flap compromise includes resuscitation if required followed by urgent exploration to identify the cause of the circulatory insufficiency. Where surgical interventions have been exhausted or are not feasible (local flap), venous engorgement may be relieved with leeches, while waiting for collateral circulation to be established (7–10 days). In such circumstances antibiotic prophylaxis is required with attention to haemoglobin levels/fluid and electrolyte balance.

Donor site morbidity (see ➲ Reconstruction, p. 94).

Late complications
- **Recurrence:**
  - can be local, regional (neck, including contralateral side), or distant (usually lung);
  - risk of recurrence depends on tumour margins, stage of the disease, tumour behaviour, and treatment modality employed; the risk is highest for large tumours;
  - in general, salvage rates are poor, in particular for high-staged tumours and previous combined modality treatment.
- **Altered sensation:** in addition to being unpleasant (cold draught, shaving) swallowing can be affected (no oropharyngeal sensory feedback). Most patients adjust to numbness of the skin.
- **Shoulder and neck problems:**
  - incidence—up to 80% in radical neck dissections and 50% in selective neck dissections;
  - neck may ache and there is limitation in range of movements;
  - shoulder may be painful (at rest and in motion) with limitation of abduction and flexion;
  - patient may have problems with raising the shoulder and so may be unable to carry out activities of daily living (e.g. combing hair, putting on clothes);
  - shoulder is affected by RND, MRND, and SND in descending order of proportion, as well as severity (quality of life measurements);
  - spinal accessory nerve and cervical plexus may be damaged during surgery (or sacrificed in radical neck dissection), and adhesive capsulitis of the shoulder joint may be a contributory factor;
  - affected shoulder will have an atrophied trapezius muscles, the shoulder girdle will take up an inferior position compared to the contralateral side and there may be hypertrophy of the sternoclavicular joint (shoulder syndrome);
  - management is mainly preventative with careful surgery to preserve the nerves and relevant plexus; progressive resistance exercise training have been shown to reduce shoulder pain and disability;
  - chronic shoulder pain can be debilitating—consider referral to chronic pain specialist to review medications/pain control measures and consideration of nerve/ganglion blocks.
- **Hypertrophic scars:** lip split incisions and neck scars are designed to heal well. Most oral cancer patients tend to not worry about their scars (although with decreasing age incidence this may not always be the case). Occasionally, a scar may become hypertrophied particularly with infection or in young patients. Topical silicone gel may help and camouflage referrals should be considered.

- Lymphoedema:
  - neck and face may be swollen in the early post-operative phase, but tends to settle with time;
  - oedema can affect the face and eyes—tends to be worse in the morning and lessen over the day with gravity-aided drainage;
  - manual lymphatic massage may be useful.
- Fatigue:
  - common following major surgery (forewarn patient);
  - eliminate organic causes, e.g. anaemia, hypothyroidism;
  - develop a rehabilitation programme where gradual goals are set to build up patients' confidence and improve their exercise tolerance.
- **Depression**: the diagnosis and subsequent treatment of cancer is a major life event. Support from family and close friends will help. The clinical nurse specialist's input is vital in this area. In some cases medical treatment may be necessary (see ➔ Psychosocial aspects, p. 136).

Combined treatment modalities

Usually necessary to improve control of advanced disease and where surgical treatment alone is insufficient (close/positive margins, neck disease, aggressive tumour parameters). Side effects and complication rates will be predictably higher.

Prediction of complications

Identifying those at higher risk of complications, optimizing their pre-existing medical co-morbidities, meticulous surgery, followed by vigilance at an early stage in the post-treatment pathway should reduce the incidence of complications. The use of objective measurements such as ACE-27, ASA may also be beneficial.

Other head and neck cancers

Maxillary sinus tumours

Epidemiology
- <1% of all tumours.
- 3% of head and neck malignancies.
- ♂ > ♀.
- Most prevalent in 5th decade.
- Commonly presents late (T3/4 disease).

Risk factors
- Tobacco.
- Alcohol.
- Occupation, e.g. hard wood dust, nickel, benzene.
- Ionizing radiation.
- Oncocytic papilloma.
- HPV.

Classification
Based on site or pathology.

Pathology
- Benign:
  - osteoma;
  - fibroma.
- Malignant:
  - epithelial—squamous cell carcinoma (SCC), adenocarcinoma (more common in occupational disease), adenoid cystic carcinoma (ACC), small cell carcinoma, malignant melanoma (MM);
  - osseous—osteogenic sarcoma, Ewing's sarcoma;
  - connective tissue—chondrosarcoma, fibrosarcoma.

Presentation
- Nasal symptoms:
  - epistaxis;
  - rhinorrhoea;
  - obstruction.
- Oral symptoms:
  - pain;
  - palatal swelling;
  - tooth mobility;
  - ulceration.
- Eye symptoms:
  - epiphora;
  - diplopia;
  - proptosis;
  - ↓ acuity.
- Cutaneous symptoms:
  - swelling;
  - sensory change (distribution of infraorbital nerve);
  - fixation;
  - erythema.

Investigations
- OPG.
- CT (posterior wall/pterygoid involvement).
- MRI (more sensitive for orbital soft tissue involvement).

Presentation
- **T1**: tumour confined to sinus mucosa.
- **T2**: tumour invading bone but not posterior wall.
- **T3**: tumour invading:
  - posterior wall;
  - pterygoid plates;
  - subcutaneous tissues;
  - orbital floor;
  - infra-temporal fossa;
  - ethmoid sinus.
- **T4**: tumour invading:
  - orbital contents beyond floor;
  - naso-pharynx;
  - dura.

Management
- Surgery followed by radiotherapy if resectable.
- Consider orbital exenteration (if ocular involvement or post-radiotherapy ocular morbidity predicted to be high).
- Reconstructive options:
  - obturation;
  - free tissue transfer;
  - implant-retained ocular prosthesis.

Prognosis
- Local recurrence around 45% (mostly in first year).
- At presentation:
  - 20% nodal disease;
  - 20% distant metastasis.
- 40% 5-year survival.

Nasal cavity tumours

Clinical features
- Epistaxis.
- Congestion.
- Obstruction.
- Swelling.
- Rhinorrhoea.

Differential diagnosis
- Benign nasal polyps.
- Rhinitis.

Treatment
- Surgery ± radiotherapy.
- Radiotherapy alone if there are cosmetic concerns.
- Prognosis.
- 15% of patients develop second primary—40% in head and neck, 60% subcapital.

Radiotherapy

- Normally administered as external beam radiotherapy for oropharyngeal tumours in the UK.
- In parts of Europe interstitial radiotherapy (brachytherapy) is more commonly employed:
  - insertion of iridium wires into the tumour in order to deliver a highly targeted dose of radiotherapy whilst minimizing dose to adjacent normal tissues;
  - in UK practice this technique is usually reserved for those patients who have received a full previous dose of external beam radiotherapy and where all other options have been exhausted.
- Radiotherapy may be used as the primary modality to treat either the primary site, or the neck, or both. The fields covered and the dose delivered depend upon a complex number of factors, which involve careful planning and calculation. It is also important to decide whether treatment is being given with curative intent (radical) or in order to minimize or prevent symptoms (palliative).
- Ideally, planning is undertaken on a CT scan that is performed with the patient in the treatment position.
- A rigid facemask (constructed from moulds) is used to ensure that the head is always placed in exactly the same position in order that treatment is delivered accurately to the prescribed fields.
- Conventional external beam radiotherapy using mega-voltage photons from a linear accelerator is administered in 2G fractions over each weekday until the prescribed dose is achieved.
- There is some evidence to suggest that hyper-fractionating the dose to give three fractions per day, rather than one, and accelerating the time over which the total dose is delivered from 6 weeks to 12 days is beneficial.
- Intensity-modulated radiotherapy (IMRT) utilizes enhanced computerized technology to improve the precision of delivering the radiation dose to the tumour and decreases the dosage to surrounding normal tissues—of particular benefit when delivering radiotherapy to the complex area of the head and neck (Fig. 2.19).
- Electrons are occasionally used to treat superficial skin metastases or small lip tumours where minimal tissue penetration is required.

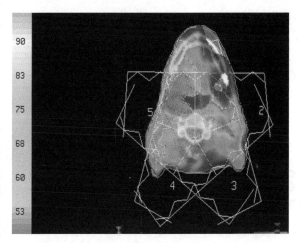

Fig. 2.19 Intensity-modulated radiotherapy plan.

Primary treatment

- As a general rule, most sites in the oral cavity and oropharynx are best managed with primary surgery, with or without adjuvant radiotherapy.
- For small tumours of the soft palate, tongue base, and tonsil, where the morbidity of the surgery is significant and the cure rates of radiotherapy are high, radiotherapy may be indicated.
- Where there is evidence of close proximity of the tumour to bone, radiotherapy is contraindicated as it is relatively ineffective and can give rise to osteoradionecrosis.
- Adenocarcinomas of salivary gland origin are relatively radio-insensitive and should be managed with primary surgery.
- Radiotherapy may also be indicated outside these criteria when the patient's physical status contraindicates surgery or where the patient will not consent to surgery.
- In the clinically N0 neck elective radiotherapy may be indicated to the neck where the primary site has a high incidence of occult metastasis, e.g. tongue and floor of mouth.
- Where high-risk primary tumours cross the midline consideration should be given to treating bilateral neck fields.
- Where there is clinical evidence of neck node metastasis, small volume disease without evidence of tumour necrosis may be managed by radiotherapy. However, for large volume disease or where there is tumour necrosis, a neck dissection should be performed prior to adjuvant radiotherapy.
- Where the primary site might be best managed by radiotherapy due to the morbidity of primary surgery, but where there is bulky neck disease, it is often best to undertake a neck dissection followed by primary radiotherapy to the primary tumour and adjuvant radiotherapy to the neck.

Adjuvant treatment

- Radiotherapy, in combination with surgery, has been demonstrated to deliver the best chance of cure for most oral cavity and oropharyngeal sites of advanced stage disease. When used in combination with surgery complications are minimized if surgery precedes radiotherapy.
- Indications for adjuvant radiotherapy following surgery include:
  - close (<5mm) or involved margins at the primary site and where further excision is impracticable;
  - peri-neural or peri-vascular spread;
  - large tumours;
  - poorly differentiated tumours;
  - >1 lymph node involved;
  - extra-capsular spread in a lymph node.

Complications and side effects of radiotherapy

Acute effects

- Mucositis.
- Skin erythema or ulceration (Fig. 2.20).
- Loss of taste.
- Impaired nutrition and weight loss.
- Bleeding.
- Infection.
- Lymphoedema.

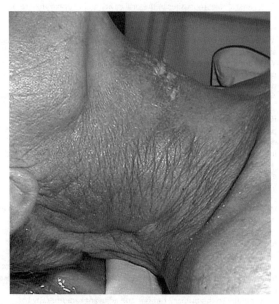

Fig. 2.20 Acute skin reaction during radiotherapy.

Late complications
- Fistula.
- Impaired healing.
- Osteoradionecrosis.
- Impaired swallowing.
- Impaired speech.
- Impaired taste.
- Xerostomia and radiation caries.
- Susceptibility to dental caries and periodontal disease.
- Loss of hair.
- Skin atrophy, telangiectasia, and colour changes (e.g. hypopigmentation).
- Radiation-induced tumours.
- Neuropathies.
- Lens cataracts.
- Hypothyroidism, e.g. bilateral neck dissections and adjuvant radiotherapy.
- Fibrosis.

Supportive care during radiotherapy

Nutritional support
Throughout the period of treatment many patients require nutritional support. Whilst, at one end of the scale, some patients will simply require careful dietary advice and possibly oral supplementation, others will require prolonged supplemental feeding with nasogastric tubes (NGTs) or feeding gastrostomies.

Mouth care
During active treatment and beyond, many patients have difficulty maintaining an adequate level of oral hygiene. Specialist hygienists should be available to provide dental hygiene instruction, support patients with fluoride treatments, and provide devices where manual dexterity is poor. A restorative dentist may be required to give expert advice regarding complex dental restorations or support the general dental practitioner in providing appropriate ongoing dental care. Those patients who have undergone radiotherapy require special attention as they are at high risk from dental caries and periodontal disease. If such problems can be minimized and anticipated then the incidence of osteoradionecrosis will be reduced.

Systemic anti-cancer therapies

Chemotherapy

The role of chemotherapy in oropharyngeal malignancy remains controversial. Most regimens rely on a combination of platinum-based drugs, fluorouracil, methotrexate, or the newer taxanes, and in some cases monoclonal antibody therapies, such as cetuximab (epidermal growth factor receptor inhibitor) There is no evidence that any existing regimens are as effective as a standalone curative treatment.

The timing of administration of chemotherapy can be:

- **Neoadjuvant/induction:** given prior to radiotherapy or surgery with the intention of improving organ preservation. Little evidence for this and no evidence of survival advantage.
- **Concurrent:** administered during the radiotherapy treatment schedule. When used as a primary modality treatment for tonsil, tongue base, and naso-pharynx, appears to offer an 8% survival advantage. Complication rates are high with many patients suffering severe toxicity reactions.
- **Adjuvant:** given after radiotherapy or surgery. Survival benefit when used as an adjuvant to surgery is less certain, but when given with radiotherapy as a post-operative adjunct toxicity rates are very high. This should only be used in the context of clinical trials.

Complications of chemotherapy

Acute effects

- Severe mucositis.
- Nausea and vomiting.
- Impaired nutrition.
- Weight loss.
- Diarrhoea.
- Soft tissue necrosis.
- Bleeding.
- Hair loss.
- Neurotoxicity.
- Immunosuppression.
- Septicaemia.
- Neutropenia.
- Thrombocytopaenia.
- Multi-organ failure.
- Neutropenic sepsis is a medical emergency, which requires rapid assessment, and the administration of appropriate IV antibiotics within 1h of presentation. Appropriate protocols must be in place so that these patients receive prompt care wherever they present, which is often not to the oncology treatment centre.

Late complications
- Nephropathy.
- Cardiomyopathy.
- Pulmonary fibrosis.
- Ototoxicity.
- Peripheral neuropathy.

Gene therapy

Clinical trials investigating the value of genetically modified viruses that selectively infect and kill tumour cells, are presently being undertaken, but at this stage it is too early to anticipate whether this technology may be of benefit in the management of head and neck cancers.

Prevention

Reduction in population tobacco usage is likely to reduce the incidence of new cases of oral cavity and oropharynx cancer. Recent measures, such as banning tobacco smoking in public places are beginning to show reductions in smoking rates in the population. However, the inherent lead-time of carcinogenesis means that these effects will take many years to manifest. This disease can also be prevented by modification of alcohol consumption. One intriguing new area is vaccination against HPV-16. Given the current vaccination policy in the UK to vaccinate females only, there is a case–control (if sex biased) study in progress in the population already.

Nutritional support

It is well documented that malnourished patients perform less well following surgery than their nourished counterparts. They take longer to recover and suffer more complications. Over 25% of hospital patients are malnourished due to a variety of reasons. Identification of such patients is not always easy. Prevention of malnourishment is paramount.

Caloric needs

Most patients require 2000–2500kCal (20–40kCal/kg) and 7–14g of nitrogen every 24h. It is rare for even catabolic patients to exceed these requirements. Very high caloric diets can lead to fatty liver. Dietetic input is a must.

Nutritional support for oral cancer patients

- Over 50% of head and neck cancer patients are malnourished because of the disease itself (e.g. pain, poor appetite, dysphagia), their pre-morbid lifestyle (e.g. excess alcohol and smoking, poor diet, poor social support) and co-morbidities, which affect their well-being and nutrition.
- Cancer-related malnutrition is likely to be multifactorial and has a negative prognosis.
- Side effects from cancer treatment (e.g. mucositis) will further exacerbate the problem.
- A vicious cycle of deficient nutrition with gastrointestinal consequences may develop. The immune system may also become depleted, making the patient more susceptible to infections.
- Malnourishment may be due to nutritional and/or swallowing difficulties.
- Management of patients should be multidisciplinary, with dietetic and speech and language therapy (SALT) input.

Problems specific to oral cancer

- The cancer itself: pain, restricted mouth opening, difficulties with mastication and swallowing.
- Surgical treatment: further exacerbation of the aforementioned functions with ablation (severity depends on site, extent of resection, and reconstruction employed), scarring, altered sensation, and loss of teeth.
- Radiotherapy or chemoradiation: mucositis, loss of taste, xerostomia, fibrosis, abnormality in motility and function of pharynx and oesophagus.
- Combined treatment regimens will compound side effects.

Assessment

- Detailed history and clinical assessment:
  - food intake;
  - weight change;
  - appetite;
  - ability to eat;

- presence of nausea, vomiting, or diarrhoea;
- psychological state;
- risk factors associated with disease or likely treatment.
- Look for dehydration and signs of malnourishment, e.g. loss of fat in skin folds, rough wiry hair.
- Measure body mass index (BMI) = weight (kg)/height (m²). Normally 20–25. If <19 consider malnourishment.

Other investigations

Include:
- Serum albumin.
- Total lymphocyte count.
- Body fat—generally unhelpful in routine practice.

Swallowing assessment

Dysphagia is assessed clinically and with the aid of special investigations such as videofluoroscopy and fibre-optic endoscope examination (see ➲ Swallowing in oral cancer, p. 132).

Nutritional support

Nutritional interventions and advice can positively influence outcomes. Three levels of nutritional support exist:
- **Meal fortification:** after assessing the patient's current intake and nutritional requirement, oral intake can be improved with advice and support, e.g. prescription of type, amount, and frequency of diet, and alleviation of symptoms affecting swallowing.
- **Oral nutritional supplements:** indicated if a patient fails to meet nutritional requirements in spite of advice and support. There are a variety of liquid and powdered preparations high in energy, protein, vitamins, and minerals. They can be used as adjuncts or in isolation. Their often bland consistency and monotonous nature can result in taste fatigue and negatively affect compliance.
- **Non-oral feeding:** whenever possible the oral route should be employed. If the swallow is not safe, try thickeners first (with SALT input) before using non-oral routes.

Enteral feeding

Nutrition administered by the stomach or jejunum via a tube. This route should be considered if the oral intake is inadequate (usually short term). It is ideal as oral cancer patients tend to have normal gut function. Enteral feeding includes:
- NGT feeding:
  - usually via a fine-bore tube for comfort;
  - short-term option;
  - narrow tube diameter is reflected in longer feeding times;
  - complications include incorrect site placement, risk of aspiration, tube blockage, infections, and obvious visibility on the face.
- Gastrostomy tube feeding:
  - placement of a tube from the abdominal surface into the stomach for feeding;
  - appropriate for longer-term use;

- associated with reduced risk of displacement and blockage compared with NGT;
- can be easily concealed beneath clothes;
- complications include bleeding, wound infection, separation of stomach from abdominal wall with resulting leakage and peritonitis.

Types of gastrostomy tube

- **Percutaneous endoscopic gastrostomy (PEG)**: placed under local anaesthetic and sedation with the assistance of an endoscope. Its use before treatment of oral or pharyngeal cancer has rarely been associated with implantation of oral tumour into the abdominal wall if the pull-through technique is adopted.
- **Radiological-inserted gastrostomy (RIG)**: alternative technique that requires the stomach to be inflated via an NGT and external puncture with aid of radiological imaging. The technique avoids disturbing the oropharyngeal region (cancer, recent reconstruction, restricted mouth opening).

Parenteral feeding

Intravenous feeding has significant risks. In oral cancer the gut is usually functioning and parenteral feeding is rarely required.

Placement of NGT

Check NGT feeding is right decision for patient, right time to place with appropriate equipment available and sufficient knowledge or expertise available to make sure it is safe.

- **Preparation:**
  - explain procedure to patient;
  - use an aseptic technique;
  - position patient almost upright (50–60°) with neck in neutral position;
  - apply topical LA to the nose (optional);
  - measure the radio-opaque fine-bore tube to know when to stop passing (reach stomach) by measuring the end from the xiphisternum to tragus of ear and the across the cheek to the alar rim.
- **Procedure:**
  - pass lubricated (with aqueous gel) tube along the floor of the nose until its tip reach the naso-pharyngeal wall (encounter resistance);
  - ask patient to swallow and with gentle pressure the tube should pass downwards into the pharynx;
  - do not allow the patient to tilt their head back as this may encourage the tube to go into the trachea instead (a pillow to prop the head can help);
  - encourage the patient to swallow as the tube will pass more easily with the peristalsis;
  - once the desired length is reached the tube is secured with taping and record the external tube length in the appropriate notes.

- **Check position:**
  - previous guide wire should be left *in situ* for radiological confirmation of tip beneath the diaphragm. A radio-opaque tube will be visible on the CXR;
  - pH testing is the first-line test method to confirm the NGT is in correct position (safe range pH between 1 and 5.5). Record whether aspirate obtained, its pH, and who checked and confirmed safe to administer feed/medication;
  - do not use litmus paper or air insufflation & auscultation of air turbulence method (National Patient Safety Agency);
  - CXR confirmation is second-line test method.
- **Caution:** if patient complains of a sharp pain in chest during the procedure, stop, and withdraw as the tube may have passed down a bronchus.
- **Side effects:** include nausea, vomiting, osmotic diarrhoea, tube blockage, or displacement.
- **Use:** the feed is started with water before gradual building up to liquid low-residue food. A pump can be used for the feed. Check local policy for monitoring. Repeat checks will be made before each feed, administration of medication, and at least once daily as well as any signs or symptoms of suspected displacement.

Speech and language therapy

Role of oral cavity and pharynx in speech

Voice production is dependent on a steady flow of expired air from the lungs. The passage of air through the vocal folds causes a wave-like motion of the cords. The consequent air molecules vibrate creating sound (phonation).

Speech is formed by the active movement of the articulators (soft palate, tongue, and lips) that modifies the shape of the vocal tract. These changes in vocal tract shape cause the acoustic waveform to form into vowels and consonants. In order to produce clear articulation and smooth speech, the structure and function of the vocal tract must be intact.

Articulation of consonants

Consonants are produced by creating an obstruction of the air stream through the vocal tract. They are classified according to the place of articulation and manner of obstruction. They can be voiced or voiceless (no vibration when passed through vocal folds). The consonants may be oral or nasal (depend on position of soft palate and amount of nasal airflow).

In the English language, places of articulation are *bi-labial* (between lips, e.g. p, b, m), *labiodental* (lower lip to upper front teeth, e.g. f, v), *dental* (tongue tip to front teeth, e.g. th), *alveolar* (tongue tip to behind front teeth and alveolus, e.g. t, d), *palatal* (front of tongue and hard palate, e.g. ch, j) and *velar* (back of tongue and hard palate, e.g. k, g).

Three common manners of articulation exist:
- **Plosives:** complete closure of articulators, e.g. p, t, k, b, d, g, m, n, ng.
- **Fricatives:** closed approximation of articulators causing turbulence, e.g. s, sh, f.
- **Approximants:** approximation of articulators, but no turbulence, e.g. r, j.

Articulation of vowels

Vowels are specified according to the position of the highest point of the tongue in the vocal tract, degree of lip rounding, or spread causing changes in the resonance of the vocal tract.

Effect of oral cancer and its treatment on speech

- Any alteration of the physiology and anatomy of the system due to oral cancer and its subsequent treatment can give rise to:
  - dysphonia (impaired voice production); or
  - dysarthria (any weakness, slowness, or inco-ordination of speech production).
- Speech, like swallowing, will be affected and cause problems with communication, psychosocial interaction, and impaired quality of life.
- Common sites affected by oral cancer are the tongue, floor of mouth, mandibular alveolus, tongue base, and palate.
- Speech will be affected depending on the site and size of the index tumour, mobility of the residual tongue or oral structures, presence or absence of teeth, and type of reconstruction. Other factors include age, hearing, pre-existing co-morbidities, and motivation.

- Poorer speech outcome is more likely with large tumours, restricted or absent residual tongue movements, poor oral seal, or absent teeth, all of which will produce difficulties in articulation.
- Tumours of the tongue base or soft palate can produce hypernasality, solid or liquid escape through the nose, and difficulty with oral plosives.
- Maxillectomy patients often have hearing problems, with Eustachian tube dysfunction causing middle ear effusions.
- Radiotherapy may contribute to speech problems as a result of xerostomia. Hearing defects can also occur from auditory canal inflammation, wax build-up, otitis media, fibrosis, and neuromuscular dysfunction.
- Chemoradiation causes much higher acute toxicities compared to radiotherapy. When used to treat non-laryngeal head and neck cancer, its effect on voice and speech can be long term.

The role of speech and language therapist

Involvement of SALT on the patient journey is well proven to have better speech and swallowing outcomes:
- Pre-operatively:
  - review what the patient understands and expects;
  - assess pre-operative communication;
  - prepare for the subsequent effects for treatment;
  - co-ordinate a rehabilitation plan.
- Post-operatively:
  - reinforce pre-operative information;
  - assess communication impairment;
  - provide exercises and support;
  - liaise with clinicians including prosthetic rehabilitation and audiology referral.

The aim is to maximize residual function, develop compensatory mechanisms, suggest substitutes for sounds that are impossible to achieve, and provide appropriate communication aids or strategies. As impaired communication can be devastating on a psychosocial basis, support is important. Liaison with other specialities, such as otolaryngology, audiology, and prosthetic/restorative dentistry may be necessary.

Swallowing in oral cancer

Normal process of swallowing

An anatomically intact and physiologically functioning oral cavity and pharynx is necessary for swallowing to take place normally. Swallowing is a complex process where food is carried from the oral cavity through the pharynx into the oesophagus and stomach. Once initiated it becomes an involuntary, reflex process.

- Oral stage:
  - this voluntary phase begins with entry of food or fluid into the oral cavity, and ends with start of the pharyngeal phase;
  - food is mixed with saliva to turn it into a consistency suitable for swallowing. For this process to occur normally it requires a competent lip seal and ability to manipulate food with saliva using oral cavity structures (jaws, teeth, tongue, floor of mouth, cheeks, and palate);
  - the mobile oral tongue is important in moving the food bolus around and propelling it backwards into the pharynx.
- Pharyngeal stage:
  - arrival of a food bolus into the pharynx triggers an involuntary process where the airway inlet is closed with a temporary cessation in breathing to prevent food entering the lungs (larynx is raised, epiglottis displaced backwards and glottis closed);
  - soft palate elevates with pharyngeal wall contraction to seal off the nose (velopharyngeal seal);
  - tongue base contracts and with the pharyngeal constrictor muscles produces a peristaltic wave that pushes the bolus down into the oesophagus;
  - cricopharyngeus muscle relaxes to allow entry into the oesophagus.
- Oesophageal stage: food bolus is propelled down the length of the oesophagus into the stomach as part of an involuntary process.

Impact of oral and oropharyngeal cancer

A large proportion of patients with oral and pharyngeal cancer will have swallowing problems. These problems may have significant impact on their recovery, physical, and emotional well-being, as well as psychosocial interactions. The standard curative treatment for early oral cancer is to try and embody one treatment modality only. The choice of that treatment modality will depend on site of tumour, and to some extent preference of MDT or patient. More advanced disease is usually treated with surgery and reconstruction followed by adjuvant radiotherapy. There is a trend towards chemoradiotherapy in the desire for organ preservation in oropharyngeal cancer. However, organ preservation may not be synonymous with preservation of function. All current treatment modalities have significant impact on swallowing.

Effect of cancer on swallowing

Oropharyngeal cancer may cause pain, as well as alteration in the anatomical and physiological functioning of eating and swallowing. As a result the nutritional status of an individual may be adversely affected.

Effect of surgery on swallowing

This is well documented and can manifest itself in the first few months. The effect of surgery on swallowing depends on site, size of resection, mode of reconstruction, and loss of cranial nerve function. Swallowing problems following surgery are more likely with:

- Pre-treatment swallowing dysfunction.
- Larger resection.
- Posteriorly-placed tumours (e.g. base of tongue, soft palate).
- Existing co-morbidities.
- Reconstruction (may also be due to size, sensate flap may help).
- Combined treatment (e.g. adjuvant radiotherapy).

For glossectomies, ensuring residual tongue mobility is important to maximize function. Patients who have undergone surgery have ↑ oral preparation times (impaired chewing), slower oral transit times, residual food bolus, and risk of aspiration.

Effect of radiotherapy on swallowing

Although there is no removal of tissue the effects of radiotherapy on swallowing occur on a more gradual basis. The effects are dependent on:

- Total radiation dose.
- Fraction size.
- Radiated volume.
- Site and size of tumour.
- Treatment technique.
- Whether patient continues to smoke.
- Combined modalities.

Swallowing is affected acutely (after 10–14 days onwards) because of pain, mucositis, loss of taste, and lethargy. Late complications such as xerostomia, fibrosis, and neuromuscular dysfunction are delayed contributory factors to dysphagia.

Effect of chemoradiotherapy on swallowing

The addition of chemotherapy to radiation is associated with greater acute toxicity side effects in addition to nausea and vomiting. The resultant dysphagia (acutely and possibly more severe long term) are similar to radiotherapy alone, i.e. ↑ oropharyngeal transit times, ↓ tongue base contact with posterior pharyngeal wall, reduced laryngeal elevation, ↑ bolus residue, abnormal oesophageal sphincter function, and aspiration (attributed to xerostomia, fibrosis, and neuromuscular dysfunction).

Dysphagia and aspiration

The main problems following treatment are dysphagia (difficulty in swallowing) and aspiration (penetration of food/fluid through laryngeal inlet into lungs). Both are symptoms of abnormal oral and pharyngeal phases of swallowing. Bolus residue is contributory to aspiration, and a consequence of swallowing dysfunction and altered sensation. In the acute stage the presence of an indwelling tracheostomy tube may exacerbate dysphagia.

Assessment of swallowing

Bedside assessment

A trained SALT:
- Takes a history.
- Assesses the gag reflex, voluntary and reflex cough, vocal quality and volume, reflex and voluntary swallow, posture, respiration, oral motor strength, and range of motions.
- Observes swallowing using a standardized dysphagia evaluation protocol with different food consistencies—the swallow performance can be classified.

Aspiration may be clinically apparent or inferred. However, silent aspiration can still take place leaving the dilemma of whether to restrict oral intake or not.

Methods of further investigation
- **Videofluoroscopy**: this modified barium swallow is the cited gold standard in swallow assessment and allows for a descriptive dynamic study, as well as objective measurements of swallowing functions, such as transit times, detection of bolus residue, and aspiration.
- **Fibreoptic endoscopic evaluation**: this can be used to enhance a bedside assessment, offering a view different from videofluoroscopy. It cannot demonstrate the oral phase, but does not involve radiation. The goal of this assessment is to determine the presence and cause of any aspiration, and determine whether behavioural therapy is available to eliminate aspiration.

Manoeuvres to help improve swallowing
- Chilled food to help re-educate lost sensation.
- Encourage chewing or manipulation of bolus in mouth to facilitate initiation of swallow reflex.
- Altering the temperature, taste, and texture of food in a meal to keep awareness of swallowing process high.
- Place food in parts of mouth where sensation is intact.
- Viscous boluses (e.g. thickened liquid and purees) will enable poorly co-ordinated muscles to produce a more effective swallow than with thin liquids.
- Head or body tilting in the appropriate direction can utilize gravity in the swallowing process.

Hints or risks of aspiration
- Wet or gurgling noises with breathing—fluid in the airways.
- Altered voice during eating—food on vocal cords.
- Cough associated with swallowing.
- Fatigue during a meal.
- Lower cranial nerve palsies.
- Extensive resections.
- Aspiration pneumonia.

It is important to seek urgent advice of SALT if appropriate. Ideally, patients should be continually assessed and followed up throughout their care.

Strategies for reducing risk of aspiration

- Patient should not eat unattended.
- Patient should eat sitting upright—body or head tilt may be useful.
- Avoid distractions at meal times.
- Other techniques (depends on that particular situation):
  - turning head towards paralysed side of face, tongue, or treated neck (encourage passage down competent side);
  - flexing neck while swallowing;
  - double swallow;
  - supra-glottic or super supra-glottic swallow (SALT).

There is variable tolerance of aspiration between individuals and diagnostic groups. The incompetent swallow will need careful evaluation and NBM if considered a serious risk and therapeutic support/interventions.

Strategies to reduce dysphagia

Treatment of established dysphagia is difficult and rarely effective. Methods to prevent or reduce dysphagia include:

- Swallowing exercise regimen (compliance reduces incidence of tube dependency).
- Treatment modifications such as IMRT (sparing salivary glands and other critical swallowing structures, i.e. oral cavity, supraglottic and larynx, and pharyngeal constrictors).
- Radioprotectors—mixed evidence in reducing xerostomia.
- Technical advancements such as volumetric intensity modulated arc therapy and image guide radiotherapy may be beneficial.

Prognosis

There are few qualitative long-term studies in this area. Nevertheless, patients at high risk of swallowing dysfunction should be counselled pre-treatment. Patients are supported for some months following treatment when the healing is completed, residual swelling reduced, and main radiotherapy effects seen. It is concluded when both patient and SALT feel a maximum swallowing potential had been reached.

Alternative feeding routes

If the risk of aspiration is real and significant then the patient cannot take food orally. The enteral feeding routes will need to be used instead, e.g. nasogastric or gastrostomy tubes (see ➔ Nutritional support, p. 126).

The issue of optimal feeding method (nasogastric vs gastrostomy tube feeding) remains unclear in a recent systematic review. There is a variable approach with prophylactic and reactive gastrostomy tube placement instead of nasogastric tube feed. Prophylactic gastrostomy tube placement is associated with earlier better nutrition, earlier weight gains, and less hospital admissions. There are associated risks with procedure. Concerns with prolonged tube dependence and long-term dysphagia are additional reasons for a reactive gastrostomy tube practice.

Psychosocial aspects

Today's society puts increasing emphasis on physical attractiveness and, thus, the face and mouth are central to social interaction. Oral cancer treatment can result in facial disfigurement and alteration of function, e.g. impaired speech, eating, or swallowing, and loss of non-verbal cues due to paralysis. These can have profound effects on the patient through altered body image, loss of self-esteem, negative feelings (e.g. depression, loneliness, anxiety), and loss of sexuality or sexual functioning. People's reaction to facial disfigurement or abnormal communication cues can sometimes be obvious, and in so doing appear rude. This can result in the patient feeling stigmatized. Chronic pain will exacerbate any element of depression. Patients may become more sensitive to adverse reactions, react with aggression, and seek refuge by avoiding social interactions or use alcohol and drugs excessively.

Improving psychosocial outcomes

Depression

Depression is not always easy to detect as it shares some similar symptoms to fatigue and other consequences of cancer treatment. Input from the clinical nurse specialist is invaluable. The use of simple tools, like the Hospital Anxiety and Depression Scale (HADS), concern checklists, and quality of life measurements may help identify patients at risk. These patients should be given appropriate support and coping strategies. If necessary, they can be referred for psychological counselling.

Coping strategies

Psychosocial outcomes can be improved by:
- Developing confidence in performing new self-caring skills, e.g. gastrostomy tube or prostheses care.
- Confronting and acceptance of changed body image.
- Teaching interventions to maximize recovery, e.g. physiotherapy and speech exercises.
- Teaching adaptations (occupational therapy).
- Providing nutritional and communication support (dietician and SALT).
- Rehearsal of public encounters/questions and responses.
- Educating family to improve support.
- Encouraging active participation in support groups.

It has been shown that the majority of head and neck cancer patients have psychological problems and a perceived poorer quality of life compared with other cancer patients. Psychosocial support and interventions are as important as a patient's physical care since improving outcome in these often neglected areas can maximize their level of functioning, social interaction, and therefore quality of life.

Health-related quality of life

Oral cancer and its treatment have a profound effect on patients. They may have physical, functional, psychosocial, and cosmetically disfiguring problems. Traditional outcomes have centred on control of disease and survival. Clinician-centred feedback and questionnaires tended to under-report patient problems and may even have been irrelevant from patients' point of view.

Although ultimate survival remains relevant, an increasingly important measurement of outcome is quality of life (QOL). This commonly used term is recognized by lay people, often implies a sense of well-being, and is associated with patient satisfaction. It is a difficult term to define and is best considered as a multidimensional concept. Even when applied to health its definition remains controversial. In addition to areas such as physical, functional, psychological, and social functioning, other aspects to consider include economic/financial, occupational, and domestic/family (including sexuality) domains.

Many QOL tools have been proposed. There is no ideal QOL questionnaire. In order to measure outcome, the chosen QOL questionnaire should be acceptable, valid, reliable, and respond to the questions being asked, i.e. fit for purpose, as well as practical to use.

Health-related quality of life (HRQOL)

HRQOL is considered to be a specific subset of QOL, assessing symptoms, psychological aspects, and function in a structured way. It is used in many aspects of healthcare including cancer. There are many HRQOL tools available. They are now often questionnaire based and self-completed by patients. They can be used in a cross-sectional or longitudinal manner.

Other methods include semi-structured interviews and qualitative approaches. These are more time-consuming and can be influenced by the interviewer.

HRQOL tools used in head and neck cancer

In addition to global domains, HRQOL questionnaires commonly include head and neck specific domains. Even within the head and neck cancer questions there is recognition that oral cancer (and its subsequent treatment) will have influences on other sub-sites.

There are three commonly used HRQOL questionnaires.

University of Washington Quality of Life (UW-QOL)

- An extensively used (and validated) patient-based, self-administered questionnaire consisting of 15 questions.
- 12 disease-specific items (pain, appearance, activity, recreation, swallowing, chewing, speech, shoulder problems, taste, saliva, mood, and anxiety).
- 3 general items measuring global HRQOL.
- An importance rating section is included, where patients rate which domain changes were most significant to them.

- There is also a free-text section allowing patients to address any issues not otherwise covered, as well as the clinician's insight into patient's concerns.
- Disease-specific questions are scored 0 (worst) to 100 (best) with the 3 global questions being scored separately.
- Considered a broad-based assessment of disease-specific functional status, suitable for routine low-cost use, and remains the most common questionnaire used by head and neck cancer surgeons.

EORTC QLQ Head and Neck-35 (QLQ-H&N 35)

- Another extensively used (and validated) patient-based, self-administered questionnaire to assess head and neck cancer patients.
- 7 domains (pain, swallowing, senses, speech, social eating, social contact, and sexuality) as well as 11 single items inquiring about dental problems, restricted mouth opening, sticky saliva, cough, feeling ill, analgesic use, nutritional supplement use, feeding tube, and weight loss/gain.
- Used in conjunction with EORTC QLQ-C30, making it relatively long and more time-consuming for patients.

Functional Assessment of Cancer Therapy Scale (FACT-HNS)

- This reliable and responsive questionnaire has been used in numerous head and neck cancer studies.
- Contains 11 specific items covering topics, such as eating, swallowing, appearance, smoking, and alcohol habits.
- Scored on a 0–4 Likert scale.

Factors affecting HRQOL in oral cancer

When followed over time the HRQOL of oral cancer patients decreases at 3 months after treatment before recovering to approach or attain pre-operative levels around 1 year after surgery (pattern for most site-specific issues except senses, mouth opening, saliva consistency, and coughing, all of which remain poor in the long term). The 1-year score is indicative and usually stays at that level over the longer term.

Factors associated with poorer HRQOL in treated oral cancer patients include:
- Posterior tumours.
- Advanced overall stage or T stage.
- Pre-treatment depression.
- Presence of co-morbidities.
- RND.
- More complex reconstruction.
- Need for gastrostomy tube feeding.
- Combine treatment (surgery + radiotherapy or chemoradiotherapy).

HRQOL measurements can be used to help:
- In the process of treatment planning (patients and clinicians).
- Provide patients with an overview of their proposed treatment, side effects, and recovery trajectory.

- Evaluate therapeutic (curative and palliative) interventions.
- Identify individual patient's needs for additional supportive interventions, i.e. as a screening tool (e.g. Patients Concerns Inventory).
- Identify areas for audit and research.

HRQOL provides a structured insight into the patient's perspective. It has been demonstrated to be an effective and useful measurement of outcome. However, its use as a routine and universal clinical measurement tool is hampered by time constraints, manpower restrictions, traditional emphasis on survival and complication rates, and difficulty in deciding which validated HRQOL tool to use. This aside, its use in research continues to progress significantly. The ready availability of electronic data capture and immediate analysis with the aid of touch-screen technology along with clinic tools such as the Patients Concerns Inventory will increase the usefulness and acceptability of HRQOL assessment within day-to-day practice. HRQOL measurement will be essential to help evaluate efficacy of newer treatment options, symptom management, and long-term cancer survivor issues.

Palliative care

Palliative care is the active total care of patients whose disease is not responsive to curative treatment. Its aim is to achieve the best QOL for the patients and their relatives. The key principles of palliative care are:
- Management of pain and other symptoms.
- Disease management.
- Provision of psychological, social, and spiritual support.

Oral cancer

The prognosis for oral cancer depends on many factors. Early stage disease if treated effectively has a 5-year survival of 80–90%. Stage 4 disease has a much poorer prognosis, with survivals of <30%. Although loco-regional control has improved with time, the overall survival rates (~55%) have remained static due to distant metastases and second primaries. Recurrence often heralds a poor prognosis.

Problems faced by terminal oral cancer patients

Oral cancer patients with incurable disease often have highly symptomatic problems, poor social or family support, addictive alcohol problems, and their palliative care can be challenging.

General problems
- Fatigue.
- Anorexia.
- Disturbed sleep.
- Weight loss and feeding problems.
- Anxiety and depression.
- Psychosocial problems.
- Existing addictive problems with alcohol and smoking.

Head and neck specific problems
- Pain.
- Shoulder dysfunction.
- Disfigurement and stigmatization (may lead to social isolation).
- Speech, hearing, and communication problems.
- Dysphagia.
- Oral problems:
  - loss of teeth (impact on chewing and eating);
  - dry mouth/sticky saliva;
  - diminished taste;
  - infections, caries, and osteoradionecrosis.
- Fistulae (cutaneous or mucosal).
- Fungating and malodorous tumours.
- Bleeding.

Communication

In order to achieve good palliative care there must be effective communication conducted in appropriate setting. The patient should be given time and space to voice his or her problems and fears. The clinician needs to listen with empathy, clarify the patient's physical, emotional, and psychological needs, allay any fears, and correct any misconceptions. This approach will enable the patient to feel understood and cared for. His or her needs can be met where possible and informed choices made for the future, e.g. resuscitation, etc.

Prognostication of end of life

This is notoriously difficult to predict accurately. There are many good reasons for both patients and clinicians wanting to know when life is likely to end, e.g. for patient and family to plan ahead, provide insight for patient, help clinicians in treatment plan/care, establish patient's eligibility for care programmes, and financial support packages. However, there are many hazards of getting it wrong. There has been a shift in attitudes with increasing patient expectation and, in response, clinicians being more open/candid in their disclosures. It is importance to put emphasis on QOL, rather than merely lengthening it chronologically.

Management of symptoms

Pain

Two-thirds of patients with advanced disease often have pain. Pain in oral cancer can be due to local tumour infiltration causing ulceration or infection, vascular and lymphatic occlusion, nerve involvement, referred pain, or treatment-related (e.g. mucositis). It is important to try and evaluate the type(s) of pain. Pains are often mixed, but mainly:

- **Nociceptive:**
  - arising from stimulation of peripheral nerves transmitted from an undamaged nervous system;
  - often described as aching in skin or deeper tissues (account for three-quarters of pain type in studies).
- **Neuropathic:**
  - arising from damage to the peripheral or central nervous system;
  - may present with hyperalgesia and allodynia;
  - often described as burning or stabbing.

Assessment

Take a detailed history, examine for masses, joint problems, dental and oral causes, cranial nerve involvement, etc. Investigations where appropriate, e.g. radiological.

Management

- **Nociceptive pain:** usually respond to analgesics.
- **Neuropathic pain:** may only partially respond to opioids.

Pain control is aimed at removing cause if possible and pain relief provided in line with the WHO analgesic ladder:

- **Step 1**: non-opioids ± adjuvants:
  - paracetamol 1g every 4–6h regularly, maximum 4g over 24h;
  - if this does not work after 24h move up ladder.
- **Step 2**: weak opioids + non-opioids ± adjuvants. Paracetamol 1g and codeine (30mg not 8mg) or dihydrocodeine regularly every 4–6h.
- **Step 3**: strong opioids + non opioids ± adjuvants:
  - morphine 5–10mg every 4h (NB 60mg codeine equi-analgesic with 5mg morphine every 4h);
  - if pain controlled and no significant side effects (e.g. drowsiness, hallucinations, confusion, vomiting, myoclonus, pin point pupils) titrate dosage upwards (no more than 30–50%) every 24h until pain controlled;
  - give up to 50% more than usual late evening dose if woken up with pain;
  - give prophylactic laxative;
  - if nausea or vomiting give anti-emetics or consider alternative opioid;
  - if acute overdose, e.g. significant respiratory depression, consider naloxone (NB shorter half-life than opioids).

Adjuvants

These co-analgesics if combined with analgesics can enhance pain control:
- **Steroids**: oedema pain.
- **Antidepressant or anticonvulsant**: neuropathic pain.
- **Non-steroidal anti-inflammatory drug**: inflammation.
- **Night sedative**: if lack of sleep/reduced pain threshold.
- **Muscle relaxant**: cramps.
- **Anxiolytic**: anxiety.
- **Antibiotics**: infection.

Breakthrough pain

- If occurs before next dose due consider increasing background dose.
- If associated with predicted activity give analgesia prior to it.
- Consider slow release preparation.
- If poor absorption or unable to take orally consider transdermal or transmucosal preparations, e.g. fentanyl.

Other methods of pain relief

- Tumour mass reduction with surgery, radiotherapy, or chemotherapy.
- Radiotherapy for bone metastases.
- Nerve blocks.
- Transcutaneous electrical nerve stimulation (TENS).
- Acupuncture.
- Psychological interventions.

Oral problems

- Restricted mouth opening and paraesthesia.
- Dry mouth/sticky saliva (xerostomia).
- Mucositis with resultant poor oral hygiene.
- Infections.
- Fungating tumour.

Management

- Oral hygiene care and adequate hydration.
- Relief with sugar-free drops, pineapple chunks/juice.
- Prescription of artificial saliva, sialogogues, pilocarpine.
- Treatment of infection.
- Treatment of mucositis: topical LA preparations, coating agents, steroids, or anti-inflammatory agents plus analgesia.

Communication problems

Problems with speech and hearing are common. Pharyngeal surgery or maxillectomy can cause Eustachian tube dysfunction. Empathy, time, and space are essential to lessen the impact. Regular input from SALT and communication aids are vital.

Dysphagia

Tumour mass or the effect of previous treatments may necessitate consideration of a gastrostomy tube placement. This can be a difficult decision with ethical dilemmas to consider, in particular if the end point is not clear-cut. A systematic evaluation is necessary to ensure treatable causes are not missed.

Respiratory obstruction

Obstruction of a tracheostomy tube may be due to secretions, crusting, displacement, or granulation tissue.

- Prevent with humidification and good tracheostomy tube care.
- Warning signs include:
  - increasing secretions;
  - difficulty with expectoration;
  - bleeding;
  - stridor.

Management of airway obstruction

- Summon help.
- Sit patient up and ask to cough.
- Use suction.
- Manipulate head to reduce any kinking of tube.
- Give oxygen.
- Remove inner tube and apply suction.
- If terminal care advised and obstruction persists sedation should be considered to lessen the impact of the inevitable.

Fungating and malodorous tumours

A visibly fungating tumour will affect the patient, and his or her contacts, both physically and emotionally. There may be fistula formation and salivary leakage. Eating and drinking may become impossible.

Management

- Reduce secretions with medication (but side effects).
- Consider palliative radiotherapy, chemotherapy, or surgery.
- Good wound care is mainstay treatment.
- Debridement and desloughing.

- Saline irrigation and frequent dressing.
- Ensure good room ventilation and external deodorizers.
- Frequent bedsheet or clothes changes.
- Topical antibiotics (e.g. metronidazole gel) or other agents (e.g. flamazine, activated charcoal preparation, live yoghurt, honey).
- Systemic antibiotics if signs of infection.

Major bleeding

Main source of major bleed is usually the carotid artery or its branches. The vessel wall may be breached by direct tumour invasion, post-operative infection, erosion by tracheostomy tube, or may be a late effect of radiotherapy. A sentinel bleed may herald a forthcoming carotid rupture.

Management
- Resuscitation, stenting, or open surgical interventions, but may merely postpone the inevitable.
- Forewarning patients and their carers: a difficult issue (where they can cope, being prepared may lessen the impact).
- Avoid inappropriate resuscitation. This can happen if unfamiliar healthcare personnel are involved.
- Adopt a reassuring confident approach (even if you don't feel it!).
- Prepare enough dressings/towels to contain the spillage (if anticipate).
- Intravenous sedative (5–10mg midazolam) with strong opioid analgesia (diamorphine) to lessen the impact for patient.

Terminal phase

This is defined as the period when day-to-day deterioration, particularly strength, appetite, and awareness, is occurring.

Key aims of terminal care
- Ensure the patient's comfort physically, emotionally, and spiritually.
- Make the end of life peaceful and dignified.
- Provide support to the close ones.

Hospices

The proportion of patients dying at home is declining in the UK, while the proportion dying in hospital is conversely increasing. This shift may be due to increasing reliance on technology, social changes within the family, or the lesser availability of community or pastoral support.

The majority of terminally ill head and neck cancer patients deteriorate gradually with their demise being precipitated by bronchopneumonia or co-morbidity-related issues. Hospices and associated palliative care teams input are important in helping ease suffering for terminally ill patients. Other reasons for admission to hospices include pain and symptom control, respite, or intermediate care, e.g. for convalescence following radical radiotherapy.

Further reading

Bleier, B.S., Levine, M.S., Mick, R., Rubesin, S.E., Sack, S.Z., McKinney, K., et al. (2007). Dysphagia after chemoradiation: analysis by modified barium swallow. Ann Otol Rhinol Laryngol 116(11): 837–41.

Dwivedi, R.C., Kazi, R.A., Agrawal, N., Nutting, C.M., Clarke, P.M., Kerawala, C.J., et al. (2009). Evaluation of speech outcomes following treatment of oral cancer and oropharyngeal cancers. Cancer Treat Rev 35: 417–24.

D'Souza, G., Kreimer, A.R., Viscidi, R., Pawlita, M., Fakhry, C., Koch, W.M., et al. (2007). Case-control study of human papillomavirus and oropharyngeal cancer. N Engl J Med 356: 1944–56.

Feber, T. (2000). Head and neck oncology nursing. Whurr Publisher Ltd, London.

Forbes, K. (1997). Palliative care in patients with cancer of the head and neck. Clin Otolaryngol 22: 117–22.

Grobbelaar, E.J., Owen, S., Torrance, A.D., and Wilson, J.A. (2004). Nutritional challenges in head and neck cancer. Clin Otolaryngol 29: 307–13.

Hansson, B.G., Rosenquist, K., Antonsson, A., Wennerberg, J., Schildt, E.B., Bladstrom, A., et al. (2005). Strong association between infection with human papillomavirus and oral and oropharyngeal squamous cell carcinoma: a population-based case-control study in southern Sweden. Acta Otolaryngol 125: 1337–44.

Harvey, M. (2000). Eating and swallowing problems. In: Feber, T. (ed.) Head and neck oncology nursing, pp. 147–69. Whurr Publishers Ltd, London.

Harvey, M. (2000). Altered communication. In: Feber, T. (ed.) Head and neck oncology nursing, pp. 147–69. Whurr Publishers Ltd, London.

Herrero, R., Castellsague, X., Pawlita, M., Lissowska, J., Kee, F., Balaram, P., et al. (2003). Human papillomavirus and oral cancer: the International Agency for Research on Cancer multicenter study. J Natl Cancer Inst 95(23): 1772–83.

Information and Statistics Division NS. ISD Online. (2007) Edinburgh.

Kumar, B., Cordell, K.G., Lee, J.S., Prince, M.E., Tran, H.H., Wolf, G.T., et al. (2007). Response to therapy and outcomes in oropharyngeal cancer are associated with biomarkers including human papillomavirus, epidermal growth factor receptor, gender and smoking. Int J Radiat Oncol Biol Phys 69(2 Suppl): S109–11.

Mittal, B.B., Pauloski, B.R., Haraf, D.J., Pelzer, N.J., Argiris, A., Vokes, E.E., et al. (2003). Swallowing dysfunction—preventive and rehabilitation strategies in patients with head and neck cancers treated with surgery, radiotherapy and chemotherapy: a critical review. Int J Radiation Oncol Biol Phys 57: 1219–30.

Northern Ireland Cancer Registry. (2007). Cancer incidence and mortality. Northern Ireland Cancer Registry. Belfast.

Office for National Statistics. (2007). Cancer statistics registrations: registrations of cancer diagnosed in 2004, England. Office for National Statistics, London.

Rogers, S.N. (2010). Quality of life perspectives in patients with oral cancer. Oral Oncol 46: 445–7.

Schwartz, S.M., Daling, J.R., Doody, D.R., Wipf, G.C., Carter, J.J., Madeleine, M.M., et al. (1998). Oral cancer risk in relation to sexual history and evidence of human papillomavirus infection. J Natl Cancer Inst 90(21): 1626–36.

Soo, K.C., Tan, E.H., Wee, J., Lim, D., Tai, B.C., Khoo, M.L., et al. (2005). Surgery and adjuvant radiotherapy vs concurrent chemoradiotherapy in stage III/IV nonmetastatic squamous cell head and neck cancer: a randomised comparison. Br J Cancer 93: 279–86.

Urken, M.L., Cheney, M.L., Sullivan, M.J., and Biller, H.F. (1995). Atlas of regional and free flaps for head and neck reconstruction. Raven Press, New York.

Wadsley, J.C. and Bentzen, S.M. (2004). Investigation of relationship between change in locoregional control and change in overall survival in randomized controlled trials of modified radiotherapy in head-and-neck cancer. Int J Radiat Oncol Biol Phys 60: 1405–9.

Watkinson, J.C., Gaze, M.N., and Wilson, J.A. (2000). Reconstruction. In: Stell P.M., and Maran A.G.D. (eds.) Head and neck surgery, 4th edn, pp. 101–57. Butterworth-Heinmann, Oxford.

Watson, M., Lucas, C., Noy, A., and Wells, J. (2005). Oxford handbook of palliative care. Oxford University Press, Oxford.

Webster-Gardy, J., Madden, A., and Holdsworth, M. (2006). Oxford handbook of nutrition and dietetics. Oxford University Press, Oxford.

Support resources

Cancer BACUP. Available at: ℜ http://www.cancerbacup.org.uk
Changing Faces. Available at: ℜ http://www.changingfaces.org.uk
Macmillan Cancer Relief. Available at: ℜ http://www.macmillan.org.uk
Marie Curie Cancer Care. Available at: ℜ http://www.mariecurie.org.uk

Surgical dermatology

Common skin terms

- **Bulla:** a circumscribed elevation of skin of 0.5cm or more in diameter containing liquid. The distinction between vesicle and bulla is arbitrary and depends only on size (vesicles are <0.5cm).
- **Comedone:** a plug of keratin and sebum in a dilated pilosebaceous pore.
- **Crust:** outer layer from the drying of exudate, secretion, or haemorrhage.
- **Cutaneous horn:** exophytic compacted keratin, 20% are squamous cell carcinoma (SCC).
- **Ephelide/freckle:** area of ↑ melanin production from a normal number of melanocytes secondary to solar exposure in genetically susceptible individuals.
- **Erysipelas:** bacterial cellulitis caused by streptococci. Bullae may develop in the area of cellulitis.
- **Impetigo:** an infection of the skin classically caused by *Staphylococcus aureus*.
- **In-transit metastasis:** metastasis found in lymphatic channels >2cm from primary, but not reaching regional lymph nodes.
- **Koebner phenomenon:** the occurrence of a skin condition at the site of trauma. Typically seen in psoriasis and lichen planus.
- **Lentiginous lesion:** linear hyperplasia of melanocytes along the basement membrane of epidermis—solar lentigo, simple lentigo. Remain stable in colour with varied exposure to sunlight.
- **Lichenification:** a chronic thickening of the epidermis with exaggeration of its normal markings, often as a result of (chronic) scratching or rubbing.
- **Macule:** flat lesion defined by an area of changed colour.
- **Melanocytic lesion:** multilevel proliferation or 'nests' of melanocytes—melanocytic naevus. Most are pigmented (unless intradermal).
- **MIN (melanocytic intra-epidermal neoplasia):** melanoma *in situ*.
- **Morphea:** localized sclerosis of the skin.
- **Naevus:** a 'mole'. May be congenital and may contain melanocytes (melanocytic naevus):
  - intradermal naevus—melanocytes in the dermis;
  - junctional naevus—melanocytes at the dermal epidermal junction;
  - compound naevus—melanocytes in both the dermis and at the junction;
  - spitz naevus—pink nodule seen on face of children, grows rapidly and histologically difficult to distinguish from malignant melanoma.
- **Nodule:** raised round lesion >5mm in diameter.
- **Papule:** raised, solid lesion.
- **Plaque:** lesion >5mm in diameter with a flat, plateau-like surface.
- **Pustule:** raised lesion containing purulent exudates.
- **Rosacea:** common facial skin condition with erythema, telangiectasia, pustules with development of rhinophyma in advanced cases.
- **Satellite metastasis:** grossly evident metastatic skin lesion within immediate vicinity of primary tumour (<2cm). A metastasis, not a second primary.
- **Wheal (urticaria, hive):** papule or plaque that is pale pink, pruritic, and may appear annular (ring-like). Wheals are transient, lasting only 24–48h in any defined area.

Skin types

Racial variation in skin pigmentation relates to the amount of melanin produced, not the number of melanocytes in a person's skin.

Fitzpatrick classification

- Type I:
  - very light;
  - also 'nordic';
  - often burns, rarely tans;
  - tends to have freckles, red or blond hair, blue or green eyes.
- Type II:
  - light, or light-skinned European;
  - usually burns, sometimes tans;
  - tends to have light hair, blue/green or brown eyes.
- Type III:
  - light intermediate or dark-skinned European or 'average Caucasian';
  - sometimes burns, usually tans;
  - tends to have brown eyes and hair.
- Type IV:
  - dark intermediate, also 'Mediterranean' or 'olive';
  - sometimes burns, often tans;
  - tends to have dark brown eyes and hair.
- Type V:
  - dark or 'brown' type;
  - naturally black-brown skin;
  - usually has black-brown eyes and hair.
- Type VI:
  - very dark or 'black' type;
  - naturally black-brown skin;
  - usually has black-brown eyes and hair.

Premalignant skin lesions

Actinic (solar) keratosis

- Scaly, hyperkeratotic, often multiple skin lesions.
- Common on head and neck due to chronic sun exposure.
- Histologically show varying degrees of dysplasia.
- When top to bottom change or *in situ* SCC = Bowen's disease or Bowenoid solar keratoses (higher risk of transformation).
- If multiple, ↑ risk of cutaneous SCC and other skin cancers.

Diagnosis: Clinical ± punch biopsy if tumour suspected.

Treatment
- None.
- Sunscreen and avoidance of UV.
- Cryotherapy.
- Topical: diclofenac gel/5F-U cream/imiquimod (see ➋ Basal cell carcinoma, p. 154).
- Photodynamic therapy (PDT).

Lentigo maligna (Hutchinson's melanotic freckle)

- Common, pigmented, often large macule on head and neck (see Fig. 3.1).
- Histologically a proliferation of atypical melanocytes—a melanoma *in situ*.
- Risk of progression unknown.
- Biopsy may be indicated (of darker or changing areas).
- Treatment: none in very elderly?
- Surgical excision is treatment of choice.
- RT/cryotherapy/imiquimod—in larger lesions.
- No need to follow-up surgically excised cases. Others should be reviewed for 3–5 years.

Melanocytic intra-epidermal neoplasia (MIN)

- UK-based histopathological term, not adopted worldwide.
- Melanocytic proliferation confined to epidermis.
- Essentially melanoma *in situ*.

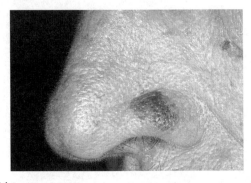

Fig. 3.1 Lentigo maligna.

Skin cancer

Common types

- Basal cell carcinoma (rodent ulcer) (BCC).
- Cutaneous squamous cell carcinoma (cSCC).
- Cutaneous malignant melanoma (cMM).

All types are increasing and related to sunlight exposure.

There are 135,000 cases in England and Wales per annum, but registration of BCC and cSCC (non-melanoma skin cancer (NMSC)) varies widely and thus is under-reported.

Rarer skin tumours include:

- Merkel cell carcinoma.
- Cutaneous T-cell lymphoma.
- Secondary deposits, e.g. lung, breast.

In the UK, NICE published guidance in 2006, 'Improving outcomes for people with skin tumours including melanoma', which outlined how healthcare services for skin cancer patients should be organized, with emphasis on MDTs caring for patients with high-risk tumours. NICE is currently preparing new guidelines specific to melanoma, due to be published in 2015.

Basal cell carcinoma

Background
- Commonest human cancer.
- >80% of skin tumours, and >80% on the head and neck.
- Slowly growing, locally invasive, and destructive, often pearly with telangiectasia.

Risk factors
- Chronic UV radiation.
- Genetic predisposition/fair skin type.
- Male sex.
- Immunosuppression—post transplant, haematological malignancy, anti-tumour necrosis factor (TNF) drugs (e.g. infliximab).
- Exposure to arsenic (rare).
- Gorlin–Goltz syndrome (see ➲ Gorlin–Golz syndrome, p. 401).
- Xeroderma pigmentosum.

Diagnosis
- Usually clinical.
- Incisional/punch biopsy may be of value in cases of doubt.
- Extensive lesions: CT or MRI to determine bone or major structure involvement.

Morphological types
- Cystic.
- Nodular.
- Morphoeic (sclerosing).
- Superficial.
- Combinations of the types, e.g. nodulocystic (Fig. 3.2).

These can all have keratotic, ulcerated, and pigmented variants.

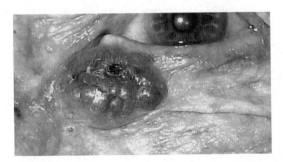

Fig. 3.2 Nodulocystic BCC.

Histological subtypes: less aggressive

- Nodular.
- Superficial (multicentric).

Histological subtypes: more aggressive

- Morphoeic.
- Infiltrative.
- Micronodular.
- Basosquamous.

These types may show the most aggressive features of perineural and perivascular invasion.

High-risk factors for BCCs

- **Site:** midface.
- **Size:** >2cm.
- **Histology:** aggressive features.
- **Recurrent tumour.**

Treatment options

- None: e.g. in the elderly or the medically compromised.
- Surgical: excision or destruction.
- Non-surgical.

Surgical treatment of BCC

Excision with predetermined margins

Recommended treatment by British Association of Dermatologists (BAD):

- In nodular BCC:
  - 3mm margin will give tumour clearance in 85% of cases;
  - 4–5mm margin gives clearance in 95% of cases.
- In primary morphoeic BCC:
  - 3mm margin gives clearance in 66%;
  - 5mm—82%;
  - 13mm—95%.
- Incomplete excision rates of BCC reported as 4–7%, and as high as 40% at medial canthus.

Re-excision

Recommended in:

- Midface/critical site.
- Aggressive histology.
- Deep margin involvement.
- Recurrent tumour.

Mohs micrographic surgery

- Aims to identify and remove all tumour by histologically guided re-excision before reconstruction (Fig. 3.3).
- Labour intensive.
- High rates of cure reported.

- Consider in:
  - recurrent disease;
  - other high-risk tumours;
  - where minimal tissue loss desired, e.g. anatomically sensitive areas such as peri-orbital tissues.
- Also has role to play in the management of some other malignant skin tumours, e.g. cSCC.
- Variations include:
  - excision and intra-operative frozen section;
  - excise, wait for haematoxylin and eosin (H&E) result, and delayed reconstruction (slow Mohs).

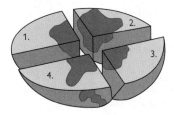

Fig. 3.3 Mohs surgery.

Destructive surgical techniques

Not recommended in high-risk tumours:
- Curettage and cautery: common Tx by dermatologists.
- Cryosurgery.
- Laser.
- Higher recurrence rates than with surgical excision.

Non-surgical treatment of basal cell carcinoma

Not recommended in forms of BCC other than superficial:

Imiquimod
- An immune modulator that stimulates T cells (used in treatment of genital warts).
- 80% cure rate in primary small superficial BCC, used 5 times per week for 6 weeks.

PDT
- Topical methyl aminolevulinate (MAL) greater clearance than aminolevulinic acid (ALA).
- Similar cure rate to imiquimod in superficial BCC.

Radiotherapy
- Treatment of choice where the patient is unwilling or unable to tolerate surgery and treatment is desirable.
- Usually superficial electrons.

- Can be:
  - *single fraction* (higher complications);
  - *fractionated* (commonly 5 doses)—higher cure rate with lower complications.
- Complications:
  - soft tissue radionecrosis; including underlying cartilage;
  - cataracts;
  - up to 5% telangiectasia;
  - secondary RT-induced cancers.
- Higher recurrence than with surgical excision (up to 10% vs 2%).

Advanced/metastatic BCC

- Metastatic BCC vanishingly rare.
- No standard therapy for this group; clinical trials appropriate if available.
- BCCs often exhibit activation of the Hedgehog/PTCH1-signalling pathway.
- Use of oral/topical hedgehog pathway inhibitors currently under investigation in patients with advanced, multiple or metastatic BCC, e.g. vismodegib.

Follow-up of BCC

- Risk of a second BCC is 33–77%.
- Those with completely excised first BCC can be discharged with information.
- Those with more than two BCCs have 70% chance of a further BCC. Consider surveillance by GP or dermatologist.

Cutaneous squamous cell carcinoma

Background

- >10% of skin cancers (second commonest).
- 80% involve the head and neck.
- Locally invasive.
- 5% of all cSCC metastasize.
- Up to 30% high risk, head and neck cSCCs metastasize.

Risk factors

- Chronic UV radiation.
- Genetic predisposition/fair skin type.
- Male sex.
- Immunosuppression (as per BCC).
- Xeroderma pigmentosum, albinism.
- Exposure to arsenic (rare).
- May arise in chronic wounds, scars, burns, sinus tracts.
- Can follow Bowen's disease, actinic keratosis.

Presentation

- Ulcer, nodule, or keratin horn; often rapidly growing.
- Diagnosis: clinical/histological.

High-risk SCC

For recurrence or metastasis:

- **Site:** lip, ear, non-sun exposed sites, those arising in chronic wounds, after RT, and from Bowen's disease.
- **Size** >2cm.
- **Depth** >4mm.
- **Histology:** poorly differentiated, perineural infiltration.
- **Immunosuppression.**

Staging of cSCC

- Continues to evolve.
- American Joint Committee on Cancer (AJCC) 2010 guidance: 'Cutaneous squamous cell carcinoma and other cutaneous carcinomas' (see ➲ Further reading, p. 174).
- Aiming to achieve parity with mucosal SCC TNM staging system.
- Incorporates primary tumour risk factors into T stage.
- Two or more high-risk factors increases primary tumour from T1 to T2.
- Nodal staging now takes into account number and size of nodal disease.
- Nodal burden has been shown to decrease overall survival.
- Main continuing omission is officially recognizing the parotid status.

The role of sentinel node biopsy (SNB)

- Sentinel lymph node biopsy offers another means for identifying lymph node metastases in clinically negative nodal basins.
- Its utility in cSCC is yet unknown, due to a lack of controlled trials.
- It provides a minimally invasive staging procedure that may have a role in high-risk cSCC patients.

Primary tumour treatment

- **Surgical excision:** treatment of choice:
    - **low-risk, well-defined tumours:** margin of 4mm gives clearance in 95%;
    - **high-risk:** margin of 6mm or more (including SCC of the lip);
    - high-risk lesions may recur as in-transit metastases in surrounding skin;
    - consider Mohs surgery in high-risk tumours and recurrence.
- **Curettage and cautery or cryosurgery:** may be appropriate for low-risk, well-defined tumours, by experienced practitioners.
- **Radiotherapy:** treatment of choice where the patient is unwilling or unable to tolerate surgery, and in unresectable disease.
- **Anti-EGFR, cetuximab:** targeted treatment for SCC, can be added to RT for unresectable cSCC.
- **Re-excision:** recommended in incomplete excisions especially in high-risk tumours. Adjuvant RT where re-excision not desirable.

The neck/parotid

- No role for imaging in the clinically N0 patient.
- No evidence for elective lymph node dissection (ELND) in N0.
- Enlarged nodes should have FNA.
- Regional lymph node dissection in node-positive disease.
- Extra caution should be paid to the extrajugular node, facial, occipital, and retro-auricular nodes.
- A more selective approach may be suitable depending on the position of the primary.
- Post-operative regional adjuvant RT—recommended for >N1 disease or extracapsular spread.

The parotid

- The parotid lymph nodes are the most common site for drainage in cSCCs which metastasize, as the scalp is a common site for cSCC and the first echelon nodes are commonly found in the parotid.
- Superficial parotid nodes most commonly involved, therefore superficial parotidectomy is indicated in P+ disease.
- If P+, occult neck disease may be present in 10–35%, therefore ELND recommended.

Follow-up

- 75% of recurrence/metastasis occurs within 2 years in high-risk tumours.
- BAD recommends follow-up of those with high-risk tumours for at least 2 and up to 5 years.

Keratoacanthoma

(See Fig. 3.4.)
- Common, rapidly growing skin tumour.
- Resembles cSCC clinically.
- Central keratin plug.
- Spontaneously involutes.
- Differentiation from cSCC can be difficult clinically (Fig. 3.5).
- Treat as cSCC.

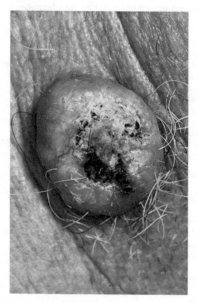

Fig. 3.4 Keratoacanthoma.

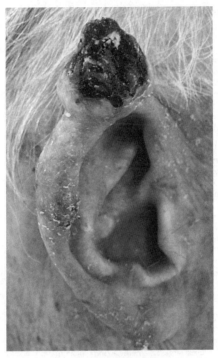

Fig. 3.5 cSCC on superior aspect of pinna on background of actinic keratosis.

Cutaneous malignant melanoma

Background

- A malignant tumour of neural crest-derived cutaneous melanocytes.
- <10% of skin cancers (3rd most common).
- Can arise *de novo*, 30–50% arise from pre-existing naevi.
- Most malignant.
- Commonest sites are lower legs in women and the back in men.
- 75% of skin cancer deaths due to cMM.
- Increasing incidence, but death due to cMM rising more slowly, due to detection at an earlier stage.

Risk factors

- Sunburn in childhood.
- Skin types—red hair, freckles.
- Immunosuppression including anti-TNF drugs (2× incidence).
- >100 moles.
- Lentigo maligna.
- Previous primary melanoma (5% develop second primary).
- Non-melanoma skin cancer.
- Family history (melanoma or pancreatic cancer).
- FAMMM syndrome—familial atypical multiple mole melanoma syndrome.
- Giant congenital pigmented hairy naevus.
- Genetic mutations: *CDKN2A* gene mutations (10–20%).
- Xeroderma pigmentosum.

Diagnosis/clinical features

Glasgow criteria

- **Major features:** change in size, colour, irregular shape, irregular colour.
- **Minor features:** largest diameter >7mm, inflammation, oozing, change in sensation.
- Lesions with any one major feature or three minor features are suspicious of melanoma.
- *ABCDE* checklist is a good aide-memoire:
  - Asymmetry;
  - Border irregularity;
  - Colour variation;
  - Diameter >6mm;
  - Evolving/Elevated.
- Only 30–50% of malignant melanoma arise in pre-existing naevi.
- Dermatoscopy can be useful in diagnosis.

Types

- Superficial spreading: most common (Fig. 3.6).
- Nodular: early vertical growth phase.
- Lentigo maligna melanoma: invasion within a lentigo maligna, most common on face (Fig. 3.7).
- Acral lentiginous: arise on the soles/palms and subungual (under the nails).

- Choroidal and mucosal melanomas.
- Desmoplastic/neurotropic: rare, deeply infiltrating, fibrous, non-pigmented, sun-exposed sites, elderly patients, tends to recur locally.

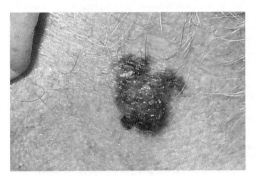

Fig. 3.6 Superficial spreading melanoma.

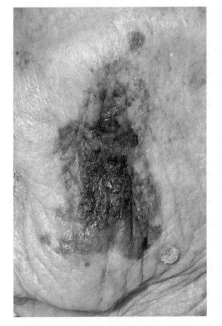

Fig. 3.7 Lentigo maligna melanoma.

Management of cMM

- Suspicious lesions should initially be completely excised and directly closed with a margin of 2–5mm and a cuff of underlying fat.
- If unable to excise, a *full-thickness* 2–4mm punch incisional biopsy should be performed from within lesion (most elevated area) to differentiate lentigo simplex, lentigo maligna, and malignant melanoma.
- Excision of the lesion:
  - gives the diagnosis;
  - determines depth of the lesion and thus the margin for subsequent wide local excision (WLE);
  - aids staging.
- All melanoma patients should be discussed at a skin cancer MDT.
- Two skin cancer networks exist as per NICE guidance:
  - local skin MDT provides core services;
  - specialist skin MDT provides specialist care.

Breslow thickness

Depth of a melanoma in millimetres measured from the top of the granular layer of epidermis to the deepest point of invasion. Correlates strongly with the risk of in-transit micro-metastases, as well as nodal and metastatic disease, and thus survival.

Clark's level: I–V

The skin has five anatomical levels from the outermost epidermis (level I) to the underlying fat (level V). Clark's level refers to deepest portion of the skin invaded by tumour. Since overall skin thickness varies considerably throughout the body (e.g. eyelid skin vs heel skin), the Clark's level of invasion has some prognostic use in certain areas in addition to Breslow thickness but is no longer considered in staging to define T1 melanomas unless mitotic rate cannot be determined.

Wide local excision

This is the secondary excision of a post-excision scar to reduce the risk of local recurrence and metastasis due to the presence of in-transit micro-metastases in the skin surrounding a melanoma. It is carried out after histological confirmation of a melanoma and is determined by the reported Breslow thickness. The histological margin of clearance of the cMM in the primary excision can be taken into account when carrying out WLE.

Present BAD guidelines for WLE

- **Breslow thickness <1mm:** excise scar with margin of 1cm; cMM <0.75mm depth, a narrower excision may be sufficient (5-year survival 95–100%).
- **Breslow thickness 1–2mm:** excise with margin of 1–2cm (5-year survival 95–100%).
- **Breslow thickness 2.1–4mm:** excise with margin of 2–3cm (5-year survival 80–96%).
- **Breslow thickness >4mm:** excise with margin of 2–3cm (5-year survival 50%).

Staging

The most recent 2010 (7th edition) AJCC staging system for melanoma is complex, but TNM based. It continues to evolve under the guidance of the melanoma staging committee, and is based mainly on data from North America, Australia, and Europe. Changes in the recent edition include: mitotic rate, immunohistochemical staining, and no lower threshold for nodal status.

- T = Breslow thickness, ulceration (stage I, II disease).
- N = nodal micrometastasis or palpable disease (stage III disease).
- M = distant metastases (stage IV disease).

Metastatic disease

- No role for imaging in the asymptomatic clinically N0 M0 cMM patient. BAD suggest consider in high-risk primary cMM, i.e. >2mm with ulceration or >4mm.
- No role for ELND.
- SNB:
  - does not protect patient from melanoma-related death but does improve recurrence-free survival;
  - aids staging;
  - can be considered in stage 1B melanoma and upwards in specialist centres after discussion in skin specialist MDT; (<0.75–1mm with ulceration or mitoses ≥1mm^2 or >1mm thickness);
  - positive SNB requires further staging and regional completion lymphadenectomy to be performed.
- Patients at intermediate or high risk of recurrent disease, i.e. stage IIIB (or stage IIIA with a macroscopic sentinel node) and above should have the following staging investigations:
  - CT scan (with contrast) of brain, chest, abdomen, and pelvis;
  - lactate dehydrogenase (a marker of disease burden);
  - FNA of suspicious nodes ± open biopsy if FNA negative.
- Established nodal disease should be treated with regional lymph node dissection (this may include the parotid).

Adjunctive therapy

- The use of adjunctive radiotherapy after lymphadenectomy remains controversial in melanoma.
- Prognosis remains dismal in patients presenting with stage IV disease, but is better for those with delayed metastasis.
- Prognosis improves in direct proportion to time taken for late metastases to develop.
- Resection of late appearing metastases to non-liver intra-abdominal organs or gastrointestinal mucosa can improve disease-free survival.
- Stereotactic radiosurgery for brain metastases may extend survival.
- For palliative chemotherapy, single agent dacarbazine remains the treatment of choice.
- Recent advances have led to the development of cancer immunotherapy.

- ~50% of melanomas harbour activating (V600) mutations in the serine-threonine protein kinase B-Raf.
- The B-Raf kinase inhibitor vemurafenib is licensed in patients with metastatic melanoma.
- Ipilimumab, a CTLA-4 activator, is licensed in stage IV cMM.
- PD-1 kinase inhibitors are in phase 1 trials and show promise of a hope of cure for metastatic cMM.

Follow-up of those with undetectable disease/apparent cure

- All patients with invasive melanoma should be monitored 3-monthly for 3 years.
- Thereafter patients with melanomas <1.0mm in depth may be discharged from routine care.
- Other patients should be followed up for a further 2 years at 6-monthly intervals.
- Those with resected nodal or distant metastases should be further followed annually from 5–10 years.

Rare skin cancers

Merkel cell carcinoma

(See Fig. 3.8.)

- Arises from neuro-endocrine cells in skin.
- Now thought to be caused by Merkel cell polyomavirus (MCV) in ~80%.
- Presents as painless nodule, which ulcerates in later stages.
- Now has specific AJCC staging.
- Mortality >40% at 5 years.
- WLE (after biopsy or excision) with margins up to 2cm, and SNB. Adjuvant RT is indicated to the primary site and nodal basin.
- Primary RT may be used.
- Chemotherapy for systemic disease.

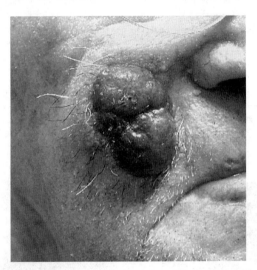

Fig. 3.8 Merkel cell carcinoma.

Cutaneous T-cell lymphoma

- Rare in head and neck.
- Low-grade non-Hodgkin lymphoma includes mycosis fungoides and Sézary syndrome.
- Treatment: psoralen and ultra-violet A (PUVA)/PDT.
- RT/chemotherapy.

Reconstructive options

Following surgical excision of a skin tumour:
- None—healing by secondary intention.
- Direct/primary closure.
- Skin grafting.
- Local flap.
- Other flaps—distant/free.

Healing by secondary intention
- Slow, risk of infection, intensive wound care may be needed.
- Useful in frail/elderly.
- Successful at medial canthus.
- Beware of consequences of contracture, e.g. ectropion.

Direct closure
- Elliptical excision in relaxed skin tension lines (RSTLs).
- Direct closure of a circular defect ± excision of dog ears. Gives a shorter scar than a classical ellipse and works well in younger, thicker skin.
- Closure may be against RSTLs to avoid anatomical distortion, e.g. vertically in peri-orbital area.

Skin graft
- Transfer of a devascularized piece of skin to a recipient wound bed where neovascularization takes place.
- Types:
  - full-thickness (Wolfe/full-thickness skin graft (FTSG));
  - split-skin (Fig. 3.9).

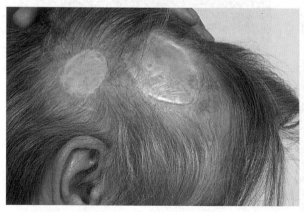

Fig. 3.9 FTSG (smaller area) and SSG.

FTSG donor sites for the head and neck
- Pre-auricular.
- Supraclavicular.
- Upper eyelid.
- Post-auricular.
- Nasolabial.

Split skin
- Upper arm and thigh commonest sites.
- Meshing increases coverage.
- No evidence that meshing or perforations improve 'take rate'.

FTSG vs SSG
- Less donor site morbidity.
- Better aesthetics.
- Less secondary contracture.
- More robust skin.
- Less skin available as donor site needs to be directly closed.
- Lower 'take rate' as skin is thicker.

Graft take relies on:
- Plasmatic imbibition for 24–36h.
- In-growth of capillaries, then lymphatic vessels, later of nerves.

Graft take reduced by:
- Mobility (shearing forces).
- Haematoma under graft.
- Infection (*Streptococcus pyogenes, Pseudomonas* spp.).

Graft take improved by:
- Careful surgical technique: handling, minimal use of diathermy.
- Vacuum dressings.
- Platelet-rich plasma (PRP).

Management of SSG donor site options
- Bupivacaine for analgesia.
- Paraffin gauze.
- Mepitel®.
- Alginate (Kaltostat® dressing).
- Vacuum dressings.
- Moist healing, OpSite® dressings.
- PRP.

Donor site dressings should be left for 10–14 days.

Local flap

A flap is the transfer of vascularized tissue. A local flap includes the margin of the primary defect as one of its edges. Its design imports tissue from an area of local laxity to fill the primary defect and usually allows direct closure of the secondary defect.

Classified by:
- Composition (e.g. cutaneous).
- Blood supply (random pattern vs axial).

- Type of movement:
  - advancement (Fig. 3.10 and Fig. 3.11);
  - rotation (Fig. 3.12 and Fig. 3.13);
  - transposition (one bit of skin crosses over another) (Fig. 3.14).
- Geometric shape of flap, e.g. rhombic, rhomboid (like a rhombus), bilobed, hatchet.

Other terminology includes interpolation flap (where a distant pedicled flap bridges normal tissue and is divided after 3 weeks), e.g. some naso-labial flaps, and the forehead flap to reconstruct the nose.

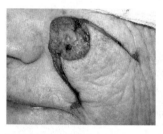

Fig. 3.10 Local advancement flap.

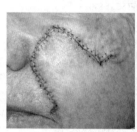

Fig. 3.11 Local advancement flap.

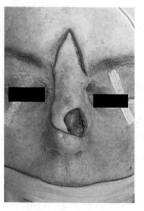

Fig. 3.12 Local rotation flap.

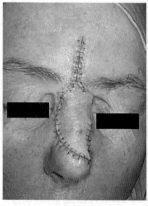

Fig. 3.13 Local rotation flap.

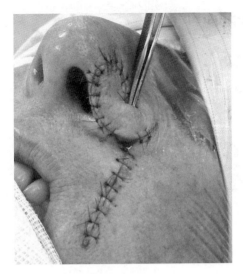

Fig. 3.14 Transposition flap with interpolation.

Skin graft versus local flap

- Grafting is easier if the surgeon is less experienced.
- Aesthetics of grafting are often worse: contour defects, colour match, graft failure, and contracture.
- Flaps can cover bare bone/tendons/ cartilage (non-graftable sites).
- Surveillance for recurrent tumour may be superior if grafted (but there are no studies to show this).

Distant or free flaps may be required for large reconstructions.

Tissue expansion

- Useful in the scalp—insertion is sub-galeal.
- Osmotic expanders remove the need for a port and injection.
- Careful planning is required to avoid complications of infection, dehiscence, and insufficient tissue production to cover the defect.

Dermal template

- Integra® dermal regeneration template has been used for burn reconstruction with great success.
- It has two layers—an outer silicone layer to protect wounds from infection and control heat/moisture and a porous inner layer functioning as a scaffold for regenerating functioning dermis. Once dermis has regenerated, the silicone layer is removed and an epidermal split skin graft is placed.
- Its use in general reconstruction continues to be reported.
- May be useful as an adjunct to other techniques when large defects exist.

Complications

Early
- Infection.
- Bleeding.
- Bruising.
- Graft failure/flap failure (manuka honey dressings are useful).
- Flap failure relates to design. Tension is more important than length to width ratio.

Late
- Scar: hypertrophic scarring remains within the limits of the scar, keloid scarring extends beyond (Fig. 3.15).
- Tissue contraction distorting facial features, e.g. lip snarl, ectropion (Fig. 3.16).
- Recurrence of tumour.

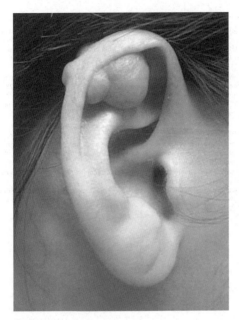

Fig. 3.15 Keloid scarring on pinna.

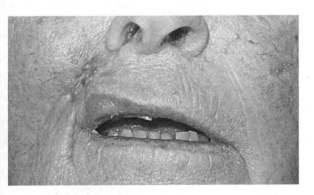

Fig. 3.16 Contracture following flap necrosis.

Further reading

American Joint Committee on Cancer. (2010). Cutaneous squamous cell carcinoma and other cutaneous carcinomas. In: AJCC Cancer Staging Manual, 7th ed., pp. 301–314. Springer, New York.

Marsden, J.R., Newton-Bishop, J.A., Burrows, L., Cook, M., Corrie, P.G., Cox, N.H., et al. (2010). Revised U.K. guidelines for the management of cutaneous melanoma 2010. *Br J Dermatol* **163**(2): 238–56.

Motley, R., Kersey, P., and Lawrence, C. (2002). Multiprofessional guidelines for the management of the patient with primary cutaneous squamous cell carcinoma. *Br J Dermatol* **146**: 18–25. [Updated 2009—see http://www.bad.org.uk/healthcare/guidelines.]

Telfer, N.R., Colver, G.B., and Morton, C.A. (2008) Guidelines for the management of basal cell carcinoma. *Br J Dermatol* **159**: 35–48.

Online resources

American Joint Committee on Cancer website. Available at: http://www.cancerstaging.org

British Association of Dermatologists' Management Guidelines. Available at: http://www.bad.org.uk/healthcare/guidelines

NICE. Skin tumours including melanoma: improving outcomes for people with skin tumours including melanoma. Available at: http://www.nice.org.uk/guidance

SIGN. Clinical guidelines. Available at: http://www.sign.ac.uk/guidelines/published/index.html

Salivary glands

Introduction

There are three main pairs of major salivary glands in the head and neck, namely the parotid, submandibular, and sublingual salivary glands. In addition to these major glands there are numerous minor salivary glands distributed throughout the oral cavity. These minor salivary glands are situated in the adnexal layer of the oral mucosa.

Relevant anatomy

Parotid gland

- Lies in a tight fascial envelope formed by the deep investing layer of cervical fascia that splits to enclose the gland.
- Composed of a superficial and deep lobe. The latter contributes only one-fifth of the total volume of the gland and is separated from the superficial lobe by the plane of the facial nerve as it traverses the gland.
- The facial nerve is the most notable anatomical structure within the parotid gland. The nerve enters the gland soon after leaving the stylomastoid foramen at the skull base. Within the gland the nerve has a short course as a single trunk before dividing into upper and lower divisions. These upper and lower divisions then further divide into the classic five terminal branches:
  - temporal;
  - zygomatic;
  - buccal;
  - marginal mandibular;
  - cervical.
- There is considerable overlap and cross-innervation of the buccal branch.
- The parotid gland also contains lymph nodes which are the first echelon nodes for part of the scalp and ear.
- The parotid duct exits the anterior part of the gland and is closely associated with the buccal branch of the facial nerve:
  - anatomical surface landmark—middle third of a line drawn from the inter-tragal notch of the ear to the midpoint between the upper lip and alar base;
  - lies ~1.5cm below the zygomatic arch;
  - is 4–6cm in length;
  - perforates the buccinator muscle to enter the mouth at the papilla, which lies opposite the second molar tooth;
  - is of smaller calibre than the submandibular duct.
- Gland receives:
  - parasympathetic secretomotor fibres from the inferior salivatory nucleus via the otic ganglion and auriculotemporal nerve;
  - sympathetic supply from the terminal branches of the external carotid artery.

Submandibular gland

- Lies in the submandibular triangle of the neck surrounded by a capsule derived from the deep cervical fascia.
- The triangle is formed by the anterior and posterior bellies of digastric muscle, and lower border of the mandible.
- The submandibular triangle also contains a number of extra-capsular lymph nodes, but in contrast to the parotid gland there are no lymph nodes within the gland itself.
- There are no major nerves within the submandibular gland although:
  - the lingual nerve is closely associated with the submandibular duct;
  - the hypoglossal nerve lies medial to the gland;
  - the marginal mandibular branch of the facial nerve is superficial to the gland separated from it by the thick layer of deep investing cervical fascia.
- The submandibular duct exits from the superior surface of the gland deep to the mandible. As it exits the gland it curves around the mylohyoid muscle to enter the floor of the mouth it travels anteriorly, crossing over the lingual nerve and the sublingual gland to open in the anterior floor of the mouth behind the lower incisor teeth.
- Gland receives:
  - parasympathetic secretomotor fibres from superior salivatory nucleus via the chorda tympani and lingual nerve;
  - sympathetic supply from branches of the external carotid artery.

Sublingual gland

- Lies in the floor of the mouth either side of the tongue.
- Located in the sublingual space, bounded by:
  - mandible laterally;
  - genioglossus muscle medially;
  - mylohyoid muscle inferiorly;
  - mucosa of the floor of the mouth superiorly.
- No surrounding capsule.
- Drains directly into the floor of the mouth through ducts that are multiple (2–5) and small in calibre.

Physiology

- 1–1.5L of saliva secreted per day.
- Resting salivary flow rate ~0.25mL/min.
- Stimulated salivary flow rate ~1mL/min.
- Resting salivary flow is secreted from the glands in following proportions:
  - *parotid*—20%;
  - *submandibular*—75%;
  - *sublingual*—5%.
- The glands vary in their proportion of mucinous/serous secretion:
  - *parotid*—serous;
  - *submandibular*—mixed (10% mucinous);
  - *sublingual*—mixed (10% serous).

History

History of a lump

- How long has the lump been present? The majority of salivary tumours are benign and slow growing.
- Does the lump ever get smaller? The majority of salivary tumours slowly enlarge.

'Meal-time' syndrome

Patients with obstructive salivary gland pathology usually exhibit so-called 'meal-time' syndrome. They have little or no problems when not eating. On eating, salivary gland flow increases causing the gland to enlarge as a result of distal obstruction. Pain results from capsular distension. These symptoms occur as soon as the salivary flow rate is stimulated—to the patient this means immediate pain and swelling on the first sight or taste of food.

Clinical examination

Parotid

Inspection

- Is there parotid swelling?
  - unilateral?
  - bilateral?
- Are there any skin changes over the parotid gland? If seen unilaterally this may indicate infection or malignancy.
- Are there any potentially malignant cutaneous lesions on the ear or scalp?
- Is there any facial nerve weakness?—sign of malignant tumour.
- Is there a swelling in the oropharynx?—sign of a deep lobe tumour.

Palpation

Always ask the patient first and check whether it is a painful lump:

- Is there diffuse swelling of the parotid gland or is there a discrete lump?
- Is the lump mobile?
- What size is the lump?
- Is it possible to express saliva from duct?
- Is there any associated cervical lymphadenopathy?

Submandibular/sublingual

Inspection

- Is there any obvious swelling below the lower border of the mandible?
- Is there abnormal tongue movement or sensation?
- Is there any weakness of the marginal mandibular branch of the facial nerve?
- Is there any swelling in the floor of the mouth?
- Is there any other pathology that could be causing lymphadenopathy in the submandibular triangle?

Palpation

Bi-manually palpate the submandibular gland, with one gloved finger in the mouth and a finger over the submandibular triangle. Compare one side to the other.

- Is there a stone palpable in the submandibular duct?
- If there is a swelling palpable in the submandibular triangle:
  - is it bimanually palpable?—suggestive of a submandibular gland swelling;
  - is it only palpable in the neck?—more suggestive of enlarged lymph submandibular node.
- Is there submandibular vs sublingual swelling? Since the majority of the submandibular gland lies in the submandibular triangle most of the swelling will be in the neck (Fig. 4.1). In contrast, swelling from a sublingual gland will appear exclusively in the mouth.

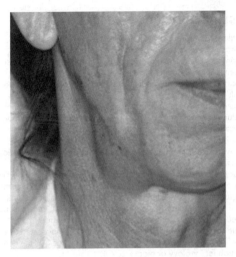

Fig. 4.1 Submandibular salivary gland swelling.

Investigations

- **Plain films:** may demonstrate calcified salivary stones.
- **Sialography:** reveals duct obstruction, sialectasis, filling defects. Pre-contrast, filling, and emptying phase films are taken. Contrast medium is lipiodol (iodine-based).
- **USS:** can demonstrate tumours, lymph nodes, stones. Deep lobe difficult to visualize.
- **MRI:** can demonstrate tumours, nodes, stones. Can be combined with ductal contrast to show obstructive disease. High-resolution visualization of facial nerve is debatable.
- **CT:** as MRI.
- **FNA:** with 23G (blue) needle gives as much diagnostic information as a 21G (green).
  - *arguments against FNA*—no change in management as 'superficial parotidectomy is treatment of choice', risk of seeding (theoretical);
  - *arguments for FNA*—identification of benign vs malignant lump, non-surgical disease (e.g. sarcoidosis/lymphoma), intra-parotid metastatic lymph node disease (e.g. from skin cancer).
- Needle core biopsy with larger needle under USS advocated by some— higher diagnosis rates as architecture preserved (see ➋ Fine needle aspiration for cytology or biopsy, p. 77).
- **Scintigraphy:**
  - radio-isotopic study of salivary gland function undertaken by injecting 40MBq technetium pertechnetate intravenously and collecting a series of images from a gamma camera;
  - during study salivary flow rate is stimulated with lemon juice;
  - results give an idea of total salivary function;
  - can reveal Warthin's tumour (rarely used).
- **Sialadenoscopy:** technique in which an endoscope is passed down the parotid or submandibular duct with a view to diagnosing causes of duct obstruction. It is possible to therapeutically remove calculi or dilate strictures using minimally invasive techniques.

Xerostomia

Definition

Subjective sensation of dry mouth. Not always associated with disease nor clinically apparent reduction in quantity or quality of saliva. More common in ♀ and elderly patients. Has following effects:

- Difficulty in chewing and swallowing (due to limited increase in salivary flow rate from resting levels).
- Erythematous and atrophic mucosa.
- Lobulation and depapillation of the tongue.
- Dental caries (this is most frequently seen around the cervical margins of teeth).
- Oral candidosis and angular cheilitis.

Primary xerostomia: pathology of salivary glands

- Irradiation glands, including radioactive iodine therapy.
- Sjögren's syndrome.
- Sarcoid.
- HIV.
- Cystic fibrosis.

Secondary xerostomia: systemic disease

- Drug therapy.
- Disorders leading to fluid/electrolyte imbalance:
  - dehydration;
  - diarrhoea and vomiting;
  - diabetes;
  - congestive cardiac failure (CCF) and oedema.
- Neurological:
  - organic brain disease;
  - drugs (anticholinergics and sympathomimetics);
  - psychological—mouth breathers.
- Anxiety.
- Drug-induced xerostomia.

Epidemiology

- Most prevalent cause for xerostomia.
- Drugs commonly implicated:
  - antihistamines;
  - antidepressants;
  - anticholinergics;
  - antihypertensives;
  - antipsychotics;
  - anti-Parkinson agents;
  - diuretics;
  - sedatives.

Management
Options for management include drug dose reduction or use of alternative medication with reduced anticholinergic activity. Consider modification of dosing schedule to allow maximum salivary flow at night (xerostomia is often worse at night). Avoidance of sublingual preparations of drug.

Sjögren's syndrome

Definition
Chronic multisystem autoimmune exocrinopathy.

Epidemiology
0.5–2% population affected, ~90% ♀, mean age at presentation 50 years.

Cause
Unknown—thought to be triggered by an environmental agent in person with genetic predisposition (associated with HLA-B8 and DR3).

Classification
- **Primary:** affects salivary and lacrimal glands (= Sicca syndrome).
- **Secondary:** 50–60% of patients have another connective tissue or autoimmune disease, e.g.:
  - rheumatoid arthritis (15% also have Sjögren's syndrome (SS));
  - systemic lupus erythematosus (SLE) (30% have SS);
  - scleroderma;
  - polymyositis;
  - thyroiditis;
  - primary biliary cirrhosis.

Clinical
- Persistent xerostomia and xerophthalmia >3 months.
- Salivary and lacrimal gland enlargement—if unilateral consider B-cell MALT lymphoma as ↑ incidence in SS (particularly Sicca).
- Parotitis/ascending infections.
- Dry skin, nasal, and vaginal mucosa.
- Signs of associated connective tissue disorder (CTD).

Investigation
- Stimulated and unstimulated saliva flow.
- Sialography: punctuate sialectasis and delayed emptying.
- Labial gland biopsy.
- Bloods: erythrocyte sedimentation rate (ESR), autoantibodies (rheumatoid factor, anti-Ro, anti-La).
- Schirmer test:
  - blotting paper test for tear production;
  - <5mm/5min.

Diagnosis
Diagnosis made on the basis of positive findings in four out of the following six categories:
- **Ocular symptoms.**
- **Oral symptoms.**
- **Ocular signs:** positive Schirmer test or positive Rose Bengal score (for corneal ulceration).

- **Histopathological features:** lower labial gland biopsy showing focal inflammatory cell infiltrate replacing acini.
- **Salivary function testing:** unstimulated total salivary flow rate <1.5mL in 15min, positive salivary scintigraphy or sialography.
- **Serum testing—autoantibodies:** presence of at least one of the following antibodies: Ro/SS-A or La/SS-B, antinuclear antibodies, rheumatoid factor.

Management

- Saliva substitutes/stimulation.
- Pilocarpine (muscarinic parasympathomimetic) if some residual functioning salivary tissue:
  - start very slowly and increase gently to avoid side effects;
  - side effects include ↑ BP and pulse rate, gastrointestinal symptoms, and sweating.
- Patients should be treated in a multidisciplinary fashion with input from:
  - rheumatology;
  - ophthalmology;
  - OMFS;
  - general dental practitioner.
- Management of associated disease including low threshold for scanning/ biopsy if risk of lymphoma.

Diffuse gland swelling

Swelling is a common symptom. It most frequently affects the parotid gland and can be classified as follows:
- Inflammatory.
- Autoimmune.
- Drug reactions.
- Metabolic.
- Neoplastic.
- Miscellaneous.

Neoplasia usually produces a focal swelling in the gland. The one notable exception to this is MALToma which often produces diffuse salivary gland swelling and can mimic an inflammatory cause.

Inflammatory

Inflammatory swellings are classified into:
- Acute specific: viral.
- Chronic specific.
- Acute suppurative.
- Chronic suppurative.

Acute specific: viral
- The commonest viral infection to cause parotid swelling is mumps (see ➲ Mumps, p. 455).
- Other viruses implicated in parotid swelling include:
  - coxsackie virus;
  - cytomegalovirus;
  - para-influenze viruses.

HIV
- Associated with generalized lymphadenopathy.
- Parotid enlargement common finding in children with HIV.
- Enlargement is firm, non-tender, and solid.
- Pain is unusual and treatment is not usually required.
- Adult patients with HIV may also present with parotid enlargement. They are prone to developing multiple cysts within the parotid gland.

Chronic specific
Chronic specific inflammatory disorders include:
- Tuberculosis:
  - rare in parotid glands;
  - usually associated with immunosuppression.
- Sarcoidosis:
  - chronic multisystem disease of unknown aetiology;
  - can present as a smooth, firm, non-tender salivary gland swelling;
  - hallmark of the disease is involvement of pulmonary lymph nodes;
  - biopsy reveals non-caseating granulomas;
  - investigate with CXR, calcium levels, serum angiotensin-converting enzyme (ACE);
  - usual treatment is corticosteroids;
  - response to treatment monitored with serum ACE levels.

Acute suppurative
- Most frequently affects elderly or infirm patients.
- Common factor is dehydration resulting in reduced salivary flow and ascending infection.
- Investigated with USS to identify evidence of obstruction or abscess formation within gland—sialography contraindicated in acute phase.
- Treated by rehydration, antibiotic therapy, and removal of any obstruction.
- Usually mixed *Staphylococcus* and *Streptococcus* infection—treatment: co-amoxiclav.
- Pus usually drains spontaneously via the duct such that formal surgical drainage is rarely required.

Chronic suppurative
- Large and heterogeneous group of conditions that is poorly understood.
- Patients present with recurrent symptoms of parotid swelling that appear to settle with good hydration and antibiotics—symptoms are recurrent.
- Cause often unknown. A minority of patients will have salivary stones.
- ↓ function of the gland allowing chronic ascending infection.
- Treatment is initially conservative with antibiotics and massage ± salivary stimulants to encourage gland function.
- Some believe sialography can be therapeutic as well as diagnostic.
- Patients with chronic inflammatory disease who do not respond to conservative measures may benefit from surgery.
- Sub-total or near-total parotidectomy is the treatment most widely advocated—superficial lobe excision with piecemeal removal of the deep lobe from between facial nerve branches.
- Temporary facial nerve palsy higher in surgery for chronic sialadenitis than for benign tumour surgery:
  - *superficial parotidectomy*—30%;
  - *sub-total parotidectomy*—30–40%;
  - *total parotidectomy*—50%.
- Permanent palsy rate 1–3% in all groups.

Autoimmune

SS produces chronic swelling of the parotid and submandibular glands. Patients with SS and salivary swelling are prone to reduction in salivary function, and chronic ascending infections as in chronic suppurative parotitis.

Patients with SS can also develop lymphomas from the mucosal associated lymphoid tissue (MALToma) within the parotid gland. These lesions can indistinguishable clinically from recurrent infection and are best diagnosed with open biopsy of the parotid gland.

Drug reactions

Drugs implicated in parotid enlargement include guanethidine and iodine-containing agents. Drug-related parotid enlargement usually produces a bilateral painless swelling (sialosis).

Metabolic

Chronic asymptomatic enlargement of the parotid also occurs in malnourished communities. This has been observed in pellagra for many years. Other metabolic conditions include

- Liver cirrhosis.
- Diabetes.

Miscellaneous

Parotid duct stenosis

Occasionally chronic trauma to the opening of the parotid duct from a denture can result in chronic parotid duct swelling.

Pneumoparotitis

This condition occurs in glass blowers and players of wind instruments. High pressure within the oral cavity results in inflation of the parotid gland with air. The air is usually absorbed into the gland or escapes back down the parotid duct. Ascending bacterial infection is uncommon.

Localized gland swelling

Benign tumours

- Commonest cause of localized swelling of the salivary glands.
- More common in larger glands, the parotid accounting for most lesions (Fig. 4.2).
- Tumour most frequently encountered is the pleomorphic salivary adenoma (PSA). Produces a slowly growing mass that is clinically recognizable as a firm swelling within the territory of the gland.
- Adenomas can be monomorphic or pleomorphic.
- PSA is the commonest salivary gland swelling of the upper lip.
- Rarely undergo malignant transformation.
- Second most common benign tumour is the Warthin's tumour or adenolymphoma (not a true lymphoma):
  - can be multifocal and/or bilateral;
  - most commonly seen in smokers;
  - ♂ preponderance.

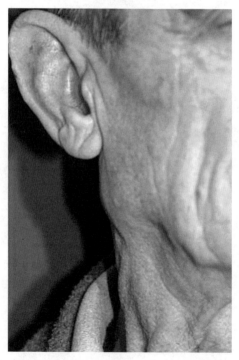

Fig. 4.2 Parotid adenoma.

Management

Main aim in the management of salivary gland tumours is to differentiate benign from malignant disease. The gold standard for this is surgical excision. In elderly or unfit patients diagnosis may have to rely on a combination of imaging and FNA/core biopsy.

Superficial parotidectomy

- Commonest surgical procedure for clinically benign focal parotid disease (Fig. 4.3 and Fig. 4.4).
- Most parotid masses lie in superficial lobe of the gland.
- Conventionally approached via a modified Blair incision starting at the superior border of the ear, continued inferiorly in the pre-auricular crease, under the ear lobe, over the mastoid bone, and into the neck two-finger breadths below the lower border of the mandible.
- Main trunk of the facial nerve can be identified in:
  - anterograde fashion (tragal pointer, posterior belly of digastric, squamotympanic fissure);
  - retrograde manner (buccal branch of facial nerve running with the duct, or marginal mandibular branch).
- Some surgeons advocate facelift incision (minimizes cosmetic impact of scar) (Fig. 4.5).

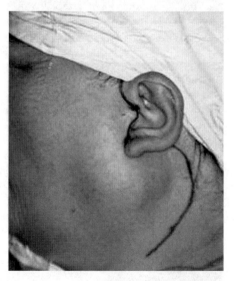

Fig. 4.3 Conventional approach to parotid tumour.

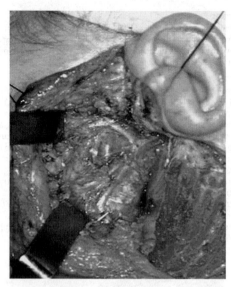

Fig. 4.4 Completed superficial parotidectomy exposing the facial nerve.

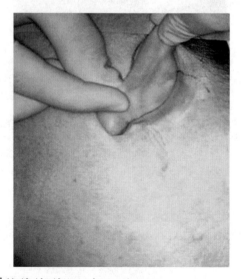

Fig. 4.5 Modified facelift incision for parotid tumour.

Superficial parotidectomy has the advantage of removing the tumour in its entirety with a surrounding cuff of normal parotid tissue. Recurrence after superficial parotidectomy is rare.

Risks of superficial parotidectomy include:
- General risks of surgery in the head and neck, e.g. bleeding, haematoma, infection, scar.
- Facial nerve injury:
  - *temporary nerve injury*—30%;
  - *permanent injury*—1–3%.
- Frey's syndrome:
  - inappropriate re-innervation of the acetylcholine receptors of the facial sweat glands with the preganglionic parasympathetic secretomotor fibres of the auriculotemporal nerve;
  - can be objectively demonstrated with starch iodine test in >90% patients (Fig. 4.6);
  - takes time to develop and may not be present until at least 1 year or more after surgery;
  - subjective symptoms (facial flushing and/or sweating) in around 30% of patients;
  - number of treatment options have been described (tympanic neurectomy, interpositional graft) but is most readily treated with intradermal botulinum toxin.

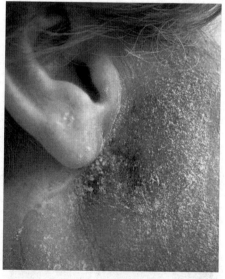

Fig. 4.6 Frey's syndrome revealed by starch iodine test.

- Salivary fistula and sialocoele:
  - occur as a result of continued salivary secretion from the cut surface of the parotid gland;
  - rarely results in pooling of saliva within the wound (sialocoele) or a leak of saliva through the surgical wound (fistula);
  - both are best treated conservatively (botulinum toxin into gland if active treatment required).

Extra-capsular dissection

- Advocated as an alternative to superficial parotidectomy minimizing surgical morbidity.
- Same surgical approach as superficial parotidectomy but no attempt made to identify facial nerve.
- Good for medium-sized lesions in the superficial lobe with no clinical concern about malignancy.
- Advantages:
  - lower rate of temporary (<5%) but not permanent facial nerve palsy (<2%), less Frey's syndrome, minimizes post-surgical defect without compromising recurrence rates (2% for PSA) (Fig. 4.7).
- Disadvantages:
  - if tumour turns out to be histologically malignant salvage surgery with a superficial parotidectomy may be required.

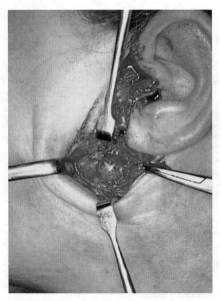

Fig. 4.7 Extracapsular dissection of parotid tumour.

Management of deep lobe tumour
- Deep lobe tumour is defined as the tumour mass arising in the deep lobe of the parotid, deep to the branches of the facial nerve. These are rare as most of the parotid tissue is in the superficial lobe.
- The most commonly used approach is to access the deep lobe parotid via a superficial parotidectomy. The superficial parotid can be left *in situ*, pedicled anteriorly. The facial nerve branches are dissected free and mobilized to allow access to the deep lobe. The deep lobe is then dissected free from the pharyngeal space.
- A variety of different approaches are described for large tumours including the use of mandibular osteotomies to gain access to the parapharyngeal space.

Malignant tumours

- Commonest malignant parotid lump is a secondary metastatic deposit arising from a cutaneous SCC of the ear/scalp.
- Primary malignant neoplasms of the salivary glands are comparatively rare—around 800 cases per annum in the UK (Fig. 4.8).
- Many types, but those most frequently encountered include:
  - adenoid cystic carcinoma (most common overall);
  - mucoepidermoid carcinoma (most common in parotid);
  - acinic cell carcinoma.

Malignant tumours of major glands become more common with decreasing gland size:
- 15% of parotid tumours are malignant.
- 35% of submandibular gland tumours are malignant.
- 85% of sublingual gland tumours are malignant.
- 50% of minor salivary glands tumours are malignant.

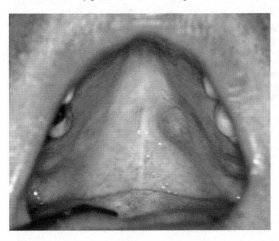

Fig. 4.8 Malignant minor salivary gland tumour.

Management

Patients with salivary gland tumours should be assessed clinically, radiographically, and cytologically with the aim of staging the disease.

Clinical features of malignant neoplasm in the parotid include:

- Facial nerve involvement (only in 20–30%).
- Cervical lymphadenopathy.
- Rapid growth.
- Pain.
- Deep fixation.
- Overlying skin changes.

All patients with malignant tumours should be discussed and treatment planned in an appropriate multidisciplinary manner. The options for treatment are surgery, radiotherapy, or combined modality treatment. Chemotherapy has little role in the treatment of salivary gland malignancy.

Tumours of major salivary glands should be treated by surgical resection:

- Radical resection involving the sacrifice of major structures, such as the facial nerve, is rarely warranted as there is little evidence that survival is improved.
- Combining neck dissection with parotidectomy gains additional staging information and can improve survival. This is particularly the case in larger malignant parotid tumours (>3cm).
- Adjuvant radiotherapy is sometimes indicated but generally only improves local control and does not improve overall survival.
- In many cases the diagnosis of a major salivary gland malignant tumour is retrospective following histological assessment of what was believed at operation to be a benign tumour.
- Further surgery is sometimes required to provide an adequate margin of clearance.

Role of radiotherapy in benign salivary gland tumours

- Some advocate role of RT in PSA spillage. Reduces the chance of recurrence but needs to be balanced with side effects and ↑ risk of inducing further malignant head and neck tumours (1% per decade).
- Proven benefit in recurrent PSA >1 nodule.
- Reduction in subsequent PSA recurrence following RT greatest if subclinical disease at time of delivery, i.e. if possible remove any persistent disease before RT given.

Sialolithiasis

- 90% of salivary calculi occur in the submandibular gland.
- Majority of the rest occur in parotid gland.
- <1% of calculi arise in sublingual gland.
- Bilateral calculi rare.
- Calculi composed mainly of phosphate and oxalate salts.
- Prevalence—1% of population.
- ~50% of cases asymptomatic.
- Slight ♂ predominance.
- No known association with renal calculi.

Management

The options for symptomatic calculi lie between removing the calculi hence relieving gland obstruction or removing the obstructed gland. There is an increasing trend to gland preservation and minimal-access surgical techniques.

Submandibular calculi

- 90% are radiopaque.
- Calculi in the submandibular impact at three points which reflect constrictions in the course of the submandibular duct system:
  - intraglandular;
  - at the hilum of the gland in the region of the mylohyoid muscle;
  - at the submandibular duct papillae (Fig. 4.9).

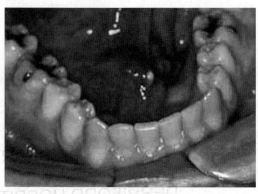

Fig. 4.9 Submandibular calculus impacted at the papilla.

Gland-preserving treatments include:

- Transoral removal near duct papilla:
  - simple procedure performed under LA;
  - duct stenosis can occur following removal of stone but is rare.
- Transoral removal of hilar stone:
  - more demanding procedure which is usually carried out under a GA or LA with sedation;
  - main limitation of the procedure is 'palpability' of the stone—if the stone is palpable transorally on bimanual examination then it can usually be successfully retrieved (bimanual palpation advised to avoid confusion with the hyoid bone).
- Endoscopic/radiologically guided stone retrieval:
  - sialadenoscopy has an emerging role in the management of obstructive salivary gland disease and can be useful from a diagnostic point of view in terms of visualizing the site of obstruction;
  - in similar fashion to renal stones it is also possible to apply intracorporeal lithotripsy to calculi via an endoscope;
  - calculi can be retrieved with a basket although care must be taken to ensure that the distal duct diameter is wide enough to retrieve the stone.

Submandibular gland removal

In cases of intraglandular calculi or where gland preservation techniques are not possible then the recommended treatment is submandibular sialoadenectomy. This is a surgical procedure performed via a transcutaneous cervical incision.

Three cranial nerves can be injured during submandibular gland excision:

- Marginal mandibular branch of facial nerve:
  - supplies depressor anguli oris resulting in elevation of the angle of the mouth;
  - temporary palsy occurs in ~30% of patients, permanent damage is rare.
- Lingual nerve (rare).
- Hypoglossal nerve (rare).

Parotid calculi

- Rare.
- Most obstructive parotid salivary gland pathology is not secondary to calculi but results from mucous plugs or casts of epithelial cell debris in the ductal system.
- Parotid duct is of a narrower calibre than the submandibular duct and as such is more readily obstructed.
- Parotid calculi are often small and may be difficult to see on ultrasound and plain radiography (90% are radiolucent).
- Same general principals apply to management of parotid calculi as those in the submandibular gland:
  - removal of calculi carries far less morbidity than parotidectomy;
  - endoscopic and interventional radiological techniques have an increasingly important role to play.

Ranula

- Mucous extravasation cyst of the floor of the mouth (source of mucous most commonly sublingual gland).
- Often presents in childhood.
- May be a history of minor trauma to the floor of the mouth that is thought to damage the numerous delicate ducts that drain the sublingual gland.
- Only rarely, as in the case of a plunging ranula, is there any swelling in the submandibular triangle.

Management

- Ranulas can be conservatively managed if they are small and not causing any problems.
- Larger ranulas, and those causing symptoms, are best treated surgically.
- Attempts to partially excise or marsupialize a ranula (the so-called 'deroofing' procedure) is rarely successful as it tends to produce scarring of the floor of mouth and further damage to the ducts draining the sublingual gland.
- Definitive treatment of a ranula is surgical excision of the ipsilateral sublingual gland.

Disorders of minor salivary glands

Mucocoele

Mucocoeles of the minor salivary glands are extremely common. They form as a result of trauma to the mucosal surface that damages the delicate minor salivary glands and associated ducts in the submucosa. The result is a recurrent cystic swelling. They have the following characteristics:

- **History:** recurrent swelling and mucous discharge with an intermittent cystic swelling. There is often a preceding history of trauma to the lower lip.
- **Site:** lower lip mucosal surface most common (Fig. 4.10). Be suspicious of an alternative diagnosis at other sites, such as upper lip where minor salivary gland tumours are more common.
- **Examination:** appears translucent or bluish in colour due to its mucous content. On palpation is soft. If large, then diagnosis can be confirmed by transillumination.

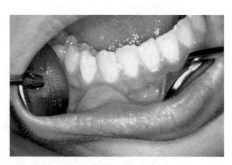

Fig. 4.10 Mucocoele of the lower lip.

Treatment

Mucocoeles are treated by simple surgical excision of cyst and associated minor salivary gland, usually under LA. Complications are unusual, although it is possible to injure some of the terminal branches of the mental nerve resulting in localized reduction in sensation of the lip.

Tumours

- Tumours of the minor salivary glands are important as ~50% are malignant.
- Commonest malignant tumour is adenoid cystic carcinoma; commonest benign is PSA.
- Present as firm masses.
- Sites with high malignancy rates:
  - retromolar;
  - floor of mouth.
- Upper lip tumours are usually benign (Fig. 4.11, Fig. 4.12, Fig. 4.13).

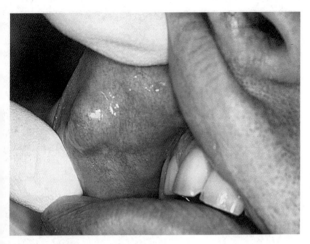

Fig. 4.11 Minor salivary gland tumour of upper lip.

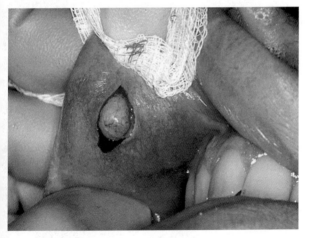

Fig. 4.12 Removal of minor salivary gland tumour of upper lip.

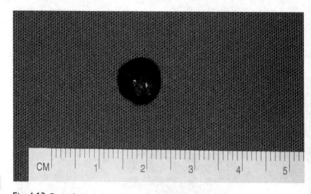

Fig. 4.13 Excised specimen—minor salivary gland tumour of upper lip.

Orthognathic surgery

Introduction

- Orthognathic (from the Greek *orthos* (straight) and *gnathos* (jaw)) surgery is surgery to treat facial disproportion.
- ~20% of the population is affected by a dentofacial deformity.
- Successful management of this group of patients requires a MDT involving orthodontists and maxillofacial surgeons, together with restorative dentists, hygienists, psychologists, and technicians.
- Accurate diagnosis and appropriate treatment planning are both essential to a successful outcome.

Aetiology

The pathogenesis of anomalous facial development is complex, multi-factorial, and, in many cases, simply represents the extremes of variation of normal development. Some cases are associated with recognized syndromes.

Treatment objectives

- **Function:**
  - establish a functional occlusion aiming to achieve normal overbite/overjet and transverse relationships;
  - improve airway and correct sleep apnoea.
- **Aesthetics:** normalize facial balance and proportions in three dimensions.
- Provide stable results in the long term.

Other possible benefits

- ?Temporomandibular joint dysfunction syndrome (TMJDS). (No firm evidence.)
- Mouth opening.
- Traumatic occlusions and dental health.

Diagnosis

Patient concerns

Patient motivation is of key importance and presenting complaints tend to fall into two broad categories:

Functional disturbance

- Actual or potential.
- Commonest complaints relate to difficulty in biting or chewing, e.g. significant reverse overjet or anterior open bite.
- Traumatic overbite in Class II division 2 malocclusions.
- TMJ-related symptoms. Care must be exercised in promising a cure with orthognathic surgery.
- Sleep apnoea and snoring.

Aesthetic concerns

- More difficult to assess.
- Subjective/objective assessment.
- May be immediately obvious to the clinician (a prominent chin or very hypoplastic maxilla).
- Understanding the patient's aesthetic concerns and what they wish to achieve is essential.

Consider the possibility of body dysmorphic disorder, and try and identify this group of patients before embarking on treatment.

Clues to body dysmorphic disorder

- Patient concerns appear out of proportion to extent of deformity.
- Patient unable to clearly express what they see as the deformity, descriptions are often vague or non-specific.
- Patient concerns have led to significant distress, anxiety, or depression.
- Withdrawal from or avoidance of social contact and employment.
- May attribute failed relationships or inability to find employment to facial appearance.
- May have had previous cosmetic type surgery, and may be dissatisfied with results.
- May have sought numerous opinions.

Obstructive sleep apnoea (OSA)

OSA is a common condition affecting ~4% of middle-aged individuals, with a slight predominance in σ. The condition is more common in individuals with a history of snoring, and has an association with obesity. Patients experience a repetitive obstruction of the upper airway during sleep, during which time arterial oxygen saturation usually (but does not always) fall. This may lead to sleep fragmentation and result in daytime sleepiness.

Diagnostic criteria require an apnoea/hypopnoea index of >5 events per hour of sleep. There is mounting evidence that significant OSA is associated with metabolic syndrome. Metabolic syndrome comprises hypertension and type 2 diabetes, with associated disturbances of lipid metabolism, and central obesity that predisposes to cardiovascular disease, including MI and stroke. Survival data demonstrates clear evidence that patients who are not compliant with treatment for OSA survive less long than those who are either compliant or those who do not have the condition. Sleep disruption causes excessive daytime sleepiness and patients may be a danger to themselves or others, especially when driving. Patients may present for ENT or maxillofacial surgery as part of the management of the condition, but the group at greatest risk comprises those who are unrecognized and therefore untreated, who present for surgery for an unrelated condition.

Screening questionnaires have been developed to help identify at-risk patients. The Epworth Sleepiness Scale (ESS) is the most popular and is used for assessing the level of daytime sleepiness that such patients experience and, whilst being rather unsophisticated, it has worldwide acceptance as a rough and ready guide to impaired daytime function. Other tools used to identify patients include the Karolinska, Berlin, and Pittsburgh sleep questionnaires. More recently, the 'STOPBang' questionnaire has been developed to screen patients at risk of OSA, and is proving to be useful in general practice.

Although simple clinical observation of the patient during sleep is often enough to make a diagnosis, investigations usually include overnight respiratory or full polysomnography, encompassing the multichannel monitoring of a number of parameters that assess breathing and physiological arousal from sleep.

Treatment includes submitting the patient either to continuous positive airway pressure, use of a mandibular advancement device, or to surgical osteotomy of the jaws (Fig. 5.1).

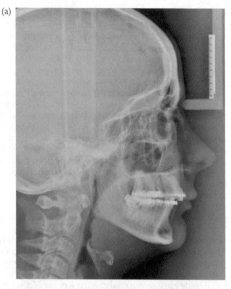

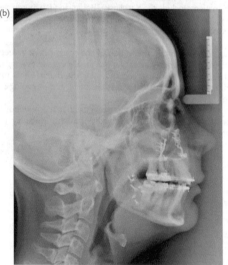

Fig. 5.1 (a) Pre- and (b) post-operative lateral cephalogram showing the change in the dimensions of the airway in a patient who has undergone bimaxillary surgery for sleep apnoea.

History

Medical history of particular relevance in orthognathic surgery

- Co-existing medical conditions may contribute to facial deformity, e.g. chronic juvenile arthritis (severe Class II) or acromegaly (Class III).
- Medical conditions that impact on suitability for treatment and the likelihood for developing complications.
- Oral contraceptive pill—should be discontinued 4 weeks before elective surgery.

Dental history

- Consider caries, periodontal disease, and TMJ disorders.
- Pattern of orthodontic extractions may be influenced by the prognosis of carious or restored teeth.
- Orthodontic and orthognathic surgery contraindicated in the presence of active or advanced periodontal disease.
- Pre-existing TMJ conditions may predispose to condylar resorption and relapse.

Growth and timing of treatment

- Surgical correction is usually deferred until growth has ceased. Most importantly in cases of asymmetry and Class III and open bite cases.
- Assess at what age the deformity first become apparent. Development of a class III malocclusion in adulthood may, for example, point to systemic disease such as acromegaly.
- Childhood TMJ trauma may result in abnormal growth.
- Developing an anterior open bite after the cessation of growth points to condylar resorption or sometimes periodontal disease.
- In asymmetric cases establish whether or not the condition is progressive, e.g. in unilateral condylar hyperplasia interventional surgery may be indicated at an early stage to reduce later secondary changes in the occlusal plane.
- Most asymmetries become apparent during the adolescent growth spurt.
- In general, treatment is deferred until a stable situation is reached, often best assessed with serial records.

Clinical examination

The patient is best assessed sitting upright in good light with the head in the natural head position and the Frankfort horizontal parallel to the floor. Patients, particularly those with asymmetric deformities, may present with an abnormal head position habitually developed for either functional reasons or to mask their deformity. It is important to compensate for such abnormal head posture if a true assessment is to be carried out.

Facial proportions

Profile view
See Fig. 5.2.

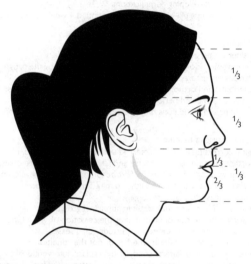

Fig. 5.2 Profile view of the face showing division into upper, middle, and lower thirds.

Maxilla
- Either normal, over-projected, or hypoplastic (suggested by para-nasal hollowing).
- Naso-labial angle 100 ± 10°—influenced by the degree of lip support derived from the upper incisors.
- Obtuse naso-labial angle associated with maxillary hypoplasia or upper incisor retroclination.
- Angulation of upper incisors to maxillary plane.
- Lip competency.

Mandible
- Can be normal, prognathic/progenic, and retrognathic/retrogenic. (Fig.5.3).

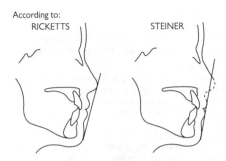

According to:
RICKETTS   STEINER

Fig. 5.3 Ricketts and Steiner's lines. Allows an assessment of the antero-posterior relationships of the lips. Reproduced with permission from Henderson D. (1986). *Colour Atlas and Textbook of Orthognathic Surgery*. Book Medical Publisher Inc. with permission of Elsevier.

Vertical proportions

The normal face is divided into equal thirds (Fig. 5.4):
- **Upper face:** hairline to glabella.
- **Mid-face:** glabella to subnasale.
- **Lower face:** subnasale to soft tissue menton.
- The lower third of the face is further divided:
  - upper third extending from subnasale to the upper lip stomion;
  - lower two-thirds running from the lower lip stomion to the soft tissue menton.
- These vertical proportions are applied in both the frontal and profile views.

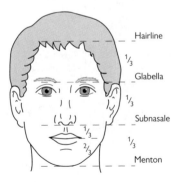

Fig. 5.4 Frontal view of the face showing division into thirds and further sub-division of lower third.

Vertical measurements
- Upper lip length.
- Alar base width = intercanthal distance = intercanine width.
- The inter-pupillary distance equals the width of the mouth.

Intra-oral examination
- Assess the general condition of the dentition and periodontal condition.
- Note the dental relationship, crowding, and spacing.
- Delineate the degree of dental compensation.
- Look for cross bites, and transverse arch discrepancies.
- Measure:
  - overbite and overjet;
  - upper incisor show at rest 2–3mm;
  - upper incisor show when smiling;
  - any occlusal cants;
  - maxillary dental centre line position with relation to the facial midline;
  - mandibular dental centre line position with relation to the facial midline;
  - mandibular dental centre line position with relation to the central chin point.
- Check for displacements on closing, which may either mask or enhance the true degree of skeletal discrepancy.

Records

Photographs
Standard facial views include full face at rest and smiling, right and left lateral views, and three-quarter views. Include intra-oral views to show occlusion, frontal view of teeth in occlusion, right and left lateral views, and mirror shots of the upper and lower dental arches (Fig. 5.5).

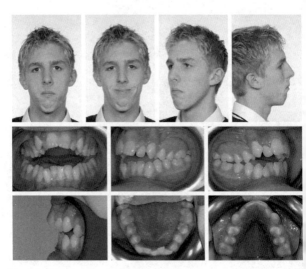

Fig. 5.5 Set of standard photographic views for orthognathic records.

Study models
Surgical planning for most procedures requires mounted models on some form of adjustable anatomical articulator.

Radiographs
- OPT: for pathology, wisdom teeth, etc.
- Lateral cephalogram for cephalometric analysis and treatment planning.
- Occlusal or peri-apical views as required.
- Postero-anterior (PA) cephalogram in cases of asymmetry.
- Special investigations.

Cephalometrics

- Cephalometric analysis (Fig. 5.6) forms the basis of orthognathic assessment and treatment planning, and underpins all current computer planning applications and profile prediction software.
- The lateral cephalogram:
  - *positioning with the Frankfort plane horizontal*—essential that the patient does not posture the teeth into an abnormal position;
  - *avoid patient forward posturing the mandible*—commonly seen in Class II patients.
- A multitude of different analyses are available and orthodontic texts should be consulted for more details.
- Most commonly used for orthognathic planning are those of the Eastman, Downs, and Rickets.

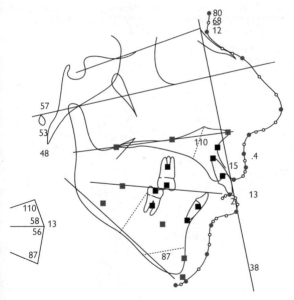

Fig. 5.6 Lateral cephalogram showing one of a number of available analyses.

Useful cephalometric relationships
- SNA is an indication of the relationship of the maxilla to the cranial base in the sagittal plane. Normal range 78–84°, mean 81°.
- SNB is an indication of the relationship of the mandible to the cranial base in the sagittal plane. Normal range 77–82°, mean 79°.
- ANB is an indication of the relationship of the mandible to the maxilla. Normal range 1–3° with A point anterior to B.
- SNPo is an indication of the relationship of the chin to the cranial base, independently of SNA/SNB.
- NPo is the facial plane and is an important reference plane for establishing facial convexity.
- Frankfort horizontal passes through both orbitale and porion. It has traditionally been used to define high- and low-angle cases relating the angle of the mandibular plane to the cranial base—the FM angle (high is >40°).
- SN–MP sella and nasion are reliable points subject to less plotting error than the Frankfurt horizontal hence SN–MP is a good index of the slope of the mandibular plane. Mean angle 32°.

Linear measurements
See Fig. 5.7.

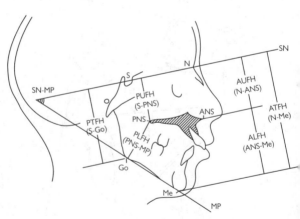

Fig. 5.7 Linear measurements. Traced lateral cephalogram showing anterior and posterior face heights, and the ratio of upper to lower face height. Reproduced with permission from Henderson D. (1986). *Colour Atlas and Textbook of Orthognathic Surgery*. Book Medical Publisher Inc. with permission of Elsevier.

Vertical proportions
ALFH is normally 55% of the total with AUFH being 45%.

Special investigations
In complex deformities, those with a significant asymmetry or a syndromic aetiology, CT scanning can be particularly useful. 3D-re-formatting allows a rapid appreciation of skeletal morphology.

Construction of accurate skeletal models facilitates both diagnosis and surgical planning. Bone scans may have a role to play in some cases (for example, condylar hyperplasia) to establish whether or not active growth is taking place.

Treatment planning

Checklist: essential clinical information for planning

- Class I/II/III occlusion.
- Skeletal base relationship.
- Maxilla AP—hypoplastic/normal.
- ?Vertical maxillary excess.
- Chin position normal/retrogenic/progeny.
- Upper incisor show at rest.
- Upper incisor show smiling.
- Centre lines—upper dental/lower dental/chin point.
- Overjet/overbite.
- Occlusal cant—yes/no?
- Naso-labial angle.
- Upper lip length.
- Alar base width.

Pattern recognition

Pattern recognition is important in orthognathic surgery. With experience one will learn to recognize a number of familiar presentations and these in turn suggest predictable treatment plans.

Common examples

- Class III patient with maxillary hypoplasia and mandibular prognathism with an average face height and no open bite—Tx: following pre-surgical orthodontic preparation, a maxillary advance and a mandibular set-back.
- Class III patient with a long face and high FM plane angle often with an open bite—Tx: following pre-surgical orthodontic preparation, maxillary impaction and advance with greater posterior impaction to correct open bite and mandibular set-back.
- Class II division 2 patient with retrogenia, a deep overbite, and a ↓ lower face—Tx: orthodontic conversion to a Class II division 1 malocclusion maintaining the curve of Spee and a subsequent mandibular advance to a three-point landing, which establishes a Class I occlusion and increases the lower anterior face height.
- Class II patients with a long face (vertical maxillary excess), retrogenia, and an anterior open bite—Tx: maxillary impaction (greater posterior than anterior) to close the open bite along with autorotation and advancement of the mandible.
- Class II patients with retrogenia and good maxillary position—Tx: simple mandibular advance.
- Severe class II patients with significant retrogenia and bird-face type deformity—Tx: depending on severity suggests mandibular advance with advancement genioplasty, inverted 'L' osteotomies or distraction osteogenesis.

Definitive surgical planning

Planning is essentially a clinical exercise and cannot be successfully achieved without the patient. A logical and systematic approach is essential and

outlined is a scheme which can be universally applied to all cases. Whilst by
no means exhaustive this scheme will give reliable results in the vast majority of patients and certainly be more than adequate for any exam situation.

Determine the position in which to place the upper incisor tip, defined in three
dimensions (AP, vertical, and lateral)
- The vertical position of the incisor tip is defined by the degree of
  vertical maxillary excess and the upper incisor show at rest.
- Normal incisor show is 2–3mm.
- Advancement of the maxilla increases upper incisor show, any AP
  change in the maxilla must therefore be considered in relation to the
  desired vertical position of the incisor tip, i.e. a patient with normal
  incisor show of 3mm who requires a maxillary advance of 1cm will in
  addition require a degree of maxillary impaction in order to maintain
  the incisor show at current levels.
- The AP position of the incisor tip is determined by:
  - AP position of the maxilla;
  - naso-labial angle;
  - degree of lip support;
  - lateral relationship is determined by the upper dental centre line in
    relation to the facial mid-line. If correction of the maxillary dental
    centre line is required surgically one must consider whether to
    rotate the maxilla or move it bodily sideways. Introduction of a 'yaw'
    deformity may result in facial asymmetry or difficulties in positioning
    the mandible.

Next determine the position of the posterior maxilla
- AP movement and rotational movement of the posterior maxilla must
  equal the movement of the incisor tip (unless segmental surgery is being
  considered).
- Vertical movement of the maxilla, however, may differ between the
  anterior and posterior.
- In AOB cases a differential impaction with greater impaction of the
  maxilla posteriorly is often required.
- Differential posterior impaction may also be indicated to deliberately
  alter the maxillary occlusal plane.
- Lateral width discrepancies may be treated with:
  - surgically-assisted rapid maxillary expansion (SARPE);
  - maxillary midline widening;
  - mandibular narrowing.

Finally determine mandibular movements
- Mandibular movements are those required to achieve a
  Class I relationship.
- Consider the lower dental centre line in relation to the upper dental
  centre line and facial midline.
- Note whether or not the lower dental centre line is coincident with the
  centre line of the chin. If they are coincident then aligning the dental
  centre lines will deliver the chin point to the facial midline. If they are
  not the chin point must be addressed separately.

Lastly look at the chin
- The chin position can be altered by genioplasty.
- Consider the movement required in three dimensions: AP, vertically, and laterally.
- The antero-posterior position of the chin can be influenced by the maxillary occlusal plane. In patients for whom advancing the mandible would render them prognathic, one treatment strategy is to alter the maxillary occlusal plane. Posterior impaction of the maxilla forces clockwise rotation of the mandible and minimizes chin advancement.

Planning considerations in sleep apnoea

There are a number of decisions to be made specifically in relation to those patients with sleep apnoea. 👁 It is generally considered that to correct sleep apnoea it is necessary to advance the mandible by 1cm, although the literature to support this particular figure is somewhat lacking.

Sleep apnoea patients generally present at an older age than most orthognathic patients. They may or may not have any pre-existing malocclusion (indeed can have perfect class I occlusions) and often have no aesthetic concerns. There may be pressure to offer treatment as quickly as possible. Some of these patients may have limitations placed on their employment as a result of their sleep apnoea. This desire for expeditious treatment is at odds with a prolonged period of pre-surgical orthodontics. It is often wise in these patients to have had a trial of treatment with a mandibular advancement splint. If this is effective in managing their symptoms then it offers reassurance that surgical advance will be equally effective.

These patients must be assessed as would any other orthognathic patient. If per chance they are significantly retrognathic then mandibular advance may offer both resolution of their sleep apnoea as well as aesthetic improvement.

The fundamental decision in treatment planning is whether to go down a conventional orthognathic route with pre-surgical orthodontic preparation or simply to offer bimaxillary advance whilst maintaining their existing occlusion. If orthodontic preparation is undertaken the aim is to achieve an overjet which will allow either a 1cm advance of the mandible or an overjet which if combined with a small maxillary advance would facilitate the same. If patients are willing to combine orthodontics and surgery it is likely they may have a better aesthetic outcome. Accepting the existing occlusion and advancing both jaws may involve more of a compromise on the final facial aesthetics although this is often acceptable to this group of patients, particularly in view of the accelerated treatment.

Patients who have bimaxillary advance with the aim of maintaining their existing occlusion often adapt more slowly, perhaps because even the very smallest change in the occlusion is perceived to be different whereas if the occlusion is expected to change then adaptation appears quicker.

Hard to soft tissue relationships

Orthognathic surgery moves the bones of the facial skeleton, but the aesthetic result is determined by the soft tissue profile. An understanding of how the soft tissues move relative to the underlying bone is therefore of importance in the planning of surgery.

Nasal tip relative to A point

Moves in a ratio of approximately:

- 1:3 for osteotomies at the Le Fort I level.
- 1:2 for Le Fort II.
- 1:1 for Le Fort III.

Upper lip

- At the Le Fort I level the upper lip moves forward ~80% of the amount of maxillary advancement.
- When the maxilla is set-back the lip moves by ~50% of the skeletal move.
- For maxillary impaction the lip moves up between 10–40% of the bony impaction and lengthens by ~50% of any downward movement.
- The morphology of the lip will affect these predictions with a thick fleshy lip moving relatively less than a thin lip.
- A tight scarred lip as may occur in a cleft patient may move in a ratio of 1:1.

Lower lip

The movement of the lower lip is altered by many factors and does not follow the lower incisor teeth in any predictable pattern, although estimates of ~85% of the skeletal move in advancement and 60% with set-back are quoted.

Chin

Soft tissue pogonion moves consistently in a 1:1 fashion with either mandibular advance or set-back.

Adjuncts to planning

The planning process can be refined by:

- cephalometric prediction tracing;
- photo-cephalometric planning;
- computerized programmes.

Ensure that patients do not interpret these images as more than a prediction or imply any guarantee regarding the final outcome.

Certain features are difficult to record accurately from the patient. One such example is a maxillary occlusal cant the true extent of which can be difficult to measure clinically. Planning using 3D reconstructions of CT data can offer significant benefits in these cases and facilitates accurate assessment of the true extent of any cant. Similarly, mid-line discrepancies can be accurately measured off the scan. This computer-assisted planning leads to greater fidelity in the planning of surgical moves, especially in complex cases.

Computer-aided design/manufacturing (CAD/CAM) techniques allow the construction of skeletal models from CT data by procedures such as stereo-lithography or fused surface deposition. Such models greatly assist in the visualization of the true extent and location of abnormality and can be used to facilitate surgical planning.

CAD/CAM technology now allows surgical wafers to be constructed directly from 'virtual' surgical plans. These modern techniques potentially eliminate the need for model-surgery.

Pre-surgical orthodontics

Orthodontic treatment carried out prior to jaw surgery to facilitate a correct jaw position, usually achieved with fixed appliances, which allow precise positioning of teeth in all dimensions. Orthognathic surgery patients should be assessed in multidisciplinary joint clinics.

The joint clinic

- Successful surgical correction of jaw discrepancy involves a close working relationship between surgeon and orthodontist.
- Patients should be assessed in joint clinics where an individualized treatment plan must be agreed with clear aesthetic and functional goals.
- Radiographs, plaster models and photographs must be available, including an appropriate tracing of lateral skull radiograph. Records are increasingly likely to be in digital format simplifying access and storage. The development of 3D imaging and CBCT is further advancing treatment planning.
- Develop a problem list matched to patient concerns and expectations.
- Consider ethnic facial morphology.
- Explain and record the risks vs benefits of treatment, and possible alternatives.

Pre-surgical preparation (12–18 months)

High-quality pre-surgical orthodontics is essential to obtaining good results from combined orthodontic/surgical treatment. Pre-surgical orthodontics should enable the desired skeletal and soft tissue changes to be achieved by the planned surgical procedures.

The aim of pre-surgical orthodontics is to eliminate any existing dental compensation and, hence, reveal the true jaw discrepancy in all three dimensions. Dental movements aim to align and upright teeth with respect to each arch using a period of fixed appliance therapy that permits full 3D control. If possible tooth movements are planned in the opposite direction to surgical movements to allow for post-surgical change, for example, is prudent that any pre-surgical orthodontic preparation increases rather than decreases any open bite present at the beginning of treatment. In this way any orthodontic relapse will be in a beneficial rather than detrimental direction.

Pre-surgical orthodontics goals

- Relieve crowding.
- Level and align arches.
- Decompensate.
- Allow stable arch co-ordination.
- Achieve root divergence at the site of any segmental osteotomy.

Relieve crowding
- Crowding relieved by extractions, expansion, interproximal reduction, or a combination of approaches to achieve the pre-surgical objectives.
- Detailed analysis of space needed and discrepancies between tooth size and arch length carried out by the orthodontist.

Arch alignment
- Relief of crowding.
- Correction of rotations and occlusal interferences.
- Arch expansion or extractions.

Levelling
- Commonly accompanies arch alignment in conventional orthodontics but is not always desirable in surgical cases.
- By not levelling the arch and maintaining the curve of Spee one can achieve an increase in lower anterior face height when the mandible is advanced to a so-called 'three-point landing' with occlusal contact at the incisors and molars (leaving lateral open bites, which are closed down post-operatively by over-eruption).
- This manoeuvre is commonly adopted in Class II division 2 malocclusions and those with a ↓ lower anterior face height.

Decompensation
- In patients with severe Class III discrepancies the lower incisors are often retroclined and upper incisors are typically proclined.
- These incisor positions camouflage the underlying Class III jaw discrepancy.
- The upper jaw may be narrow with inclined upper molars. Correcting tooth positions will influence both AP and transverse relationships.
- The effect of a planned surgical move on the incisor angulation must also be borne in mind when planning the degree of decompensation.
- A differential posterior impaction of the maxilla is commonly carried out in open bite cases to upright the upper incisors. When this move is planned it is desirable to leave the upper incisors proclined and achieve full decompensation surgically.
- When planning the degree of decompensation the amount of labial bone is a key consideration. This may limit the degree of decompensation that can be achieved without moving the roots out of the available bone.
- It must be pointed out to patients that decompensation often exaggerates the pre-existing deformity and, therefore, makes them look worse as the pre-surgical orthodontics progresses. This effect is generally more obvious in Class III patients with an increase in reverse overjet and apparently greater chin prominence.
- In Class II cases lower incisor proclination and upper incisor retroclination can be present providing camouflage to the underlying skeletal pattern.

- Transverse dimension:
  - Transverse decompensation of inclined molars is common. The upper jaw may be narrow with buccal inclined upper molars and the lower arch with lingual inclined molars. Pre-adjusted orthodontic appliances and rectangular wires can upright these molars to express a much larger discrepancy in transverse dimension;
  - Post-surgical change in tooth positions following surgical correction can influence both AP and transverse relationship;
  - Consider if orthodontic appliances alone can achieve stable transverse correction—is surgical expansion (either by SARPE or segmental osteotomy) indicated if dental expansion risks periodontal health and stability?

At the end of pre-surgical preparation study models, radiographs, and photographs are used to agree the final surgical plan. It is important to consider

- What will the incisor inclination be post-surgery?
- Are changes in occlusal plane likely?
- Is maxillary width sufficient to accept the post-operative position of the mandible?
- Is surgical overcorrection planned?

Prior to surgery the orthodontist must ensure that:

- The overjet allows appropriate AP movement of upper and or lower jaw to achieve the desired aesthetic as well as occlusal result.
- Incisors are in the planned position.
- Arches are co-ordinated to create compatible inter-canine widths with coincident centrelines.
- Arches are stabilized with large rectangular archwire (minimum 019 × 025-inch stainless steel) 4–6 weeks prior to surgery.
- Surgical hooks are attached to the archwire to aid surgical inter-maxillary fixation (IMF) and post-surgical elastic traction.

Post-surgical orthodontics

Immediate review with the surgeon following operative intervention is important to plan the post-surgical phase of treatment. Teeth move rapidly in the post-operative phase and intermaxillary elastics can be used to refine jaw position. Initially, light elastics can be used and the patient reviewed at weekly intervals. It is important to consider force and direction.

After 6 weeks post-surgical orthodontic detailing commences. Usually, heavy rectangular archwires are replaced with lighter settling wires and intermaxillary elastics to fine tune the occlusion.

Surgical management

Timing of surgery

- Orthognathic surgical treatment is usually carried out at any time after the cessation of growth (prevents unfavourable post-operative change taking place as a result of further jaw growth).
- Growth usually ceases at the age of 17 in girls and 18 in boys.
- If growth has ceased, or there are extenuating social or psychological circumstances, consideration may be given to earlier surgery.
- In cases of condylar hyperplasia or asymmetrical growth, early intervention may be considered to reduce secondary occlusal changes.

Pre-operative assessment

- Routine haematological investigations should include a full blood count.
- Some units will recommend grouping and saving blood in maxillary surgery.
- Other pre-operative tests are ordered only if specifically indicated on the basis of the patient's medical history.

Peri-operative management

- Antibiotic prophylaxis.
- Steroids: various regimens exist.
- DVT prophylaxis.
- Some advocate anti-fibrinloytics, e.g. tranexamic acid.
- Minimize intra-operative blood loss (also aids operative field):
  - use of LA;
  - cutting diathermy;
  - hypotensive anaesthesia (may help to reduce post-operative oedema).

Post-operative care

- The advent of miniplate fixation means that rigid IMF is not required post-operatively. Benefits patients in terms of airway management, early function, and comfort.
- Most surgeons, however, advocate some form IMF often in the form of light guiding elastics.
- Nursing in the immediate post-operative period should ideally be carried out in a high dependency unit where close monitoring of the patient is possible. Invasive monitoring is not generally required.

Maxillary procedures

Maxillary osteotomies are based on the Le Fort fracture lines. Unlike fractures, however, osteotomies terminate at the posterior maxillary wall and aim to separate the pterygoid plates from the posterior maxilla (fracture lines run across the plates, see Fig. 5.8).

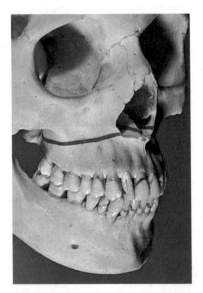

Fig. 5.8 Le Fort I bone cuts *in vitro*.

Le Fort I
- The most popular of all the maxillary orthognathic procedures.
- Total maxillary osteotomy sectioning through the lateral walls of the maxillary sinus and lateral wall of the nose just above the apices of the teeth (Fig. 5.9).
- The nasal septum is divided from the maxillary crest.
- Once mobilized, the maxilla can be repositioned in three dimensions:
  - anteriorly;
  - posteriorly (less common);
  - superiorly;
  - inferiorly;
  - rotated or moved bodily to right or left.
- After down-fracture modifications of the procedure allow for segmentalization of the maxilla to correct discrepancies of width, occlusal plane, or dento-alveolar relations.

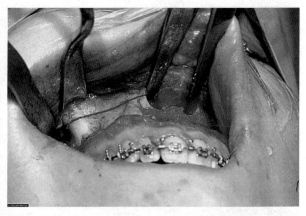

Fig. 5.9 Operative view of the lateral bone cut of a Le Fort I maxillary osteotomy.

Exposure
- Via a sulcus incision, which runs from second premolar/first molar region.
- Incision is curved upwards slightly as it approaches the zygomatic buttress.
- Identification of the zygomatic buttress, infraorbital nerve, and piriform aperture.
- Posteriorly the dissection continues sub-periosteally to enter the pterygopalatine fissure.
- Dissection of the floor of the nose.

Bone cuts
- Some surgeons place a K-wire in the nasal dorsum to act as a reference point for vertical movements.
- Bone cut runs from the posterior aspect of the zygomatic buttress at a point 5mm above the apices of the teeth forwards across the lateral wall of the maxillary sinus to cross the lateral rim just above the base of the piriform aperture (Fig. 5.10).
- Completion of the bony cuts requires:
  - division of the lateral nasal walls;
  - separation of nasal septum from the maxillary crest;
  - pterygomaxillary dysjunction.
- Down-fracture.
- Mobilization.
- Trimming of bony interferences.
- Insertion of wafer and IMF.
- Fixation.

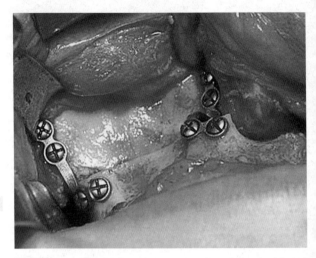

Fig. 5.10 Fixation of Le Fort I maxillary osteotomy with miniplates at the piriform aperture and the zygomatic buttress.

Le Fort I variants

Le Fort I with mid-line expansion

- Orthodontic preparation provides space between the roots of the central incisors.
- The maxilla is divided anteriorly in the mid-line between the incisor teeth.
- Division is continued in midline or preferably in a U-shape:
  - a cut is made in the palate running from the region of the greater palatine foramen on one side round anteriorly to the foramen on the opposite side;
  - palatal mucosa is thinnest and tightly bound down to the underlying bone in the midline, and it is easy to perforate this mucosa with the possibility of subsequent fistula;
  - adherent nature of the midline mucosa also limits the amount of bony separation and hence expansion that can be achieved;
  - 'horseshoe' osteotomy places the bony cut in the region of the lateral palatal mucosa, which is thicker and more fibro-fatty in texture making perforation less likely; as this mucosa is less adherent to the underlying bone a greater degree of expansion can be obtained (Fig. 5.11);
  - fixation is unchanged for these cases, but the expansion should be supported with an auxiliary archwire or an acrylic plate to maintain width.

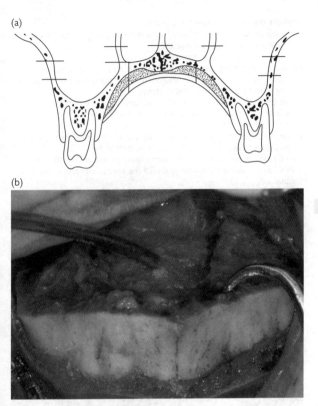

Fig. 5.11 (a) Schematic illustration of the para-sagittal cuts of a horseshoe osteotomy. (b) Operative view from above of a horseshoe osteotomy of the palate.

Surgically assisted rapid palatal expansion
- An adjunctive surgical procedure to widen the maxilla—a Le Fort I osteotomy without down-fracture.
- Form of distraction osteogenesis.
- Indicated in patients in whom the mid-palatal suture has fused (at around 14 years of age) and who are thus not suitable for rapid palatal expansion by orthodontic means alone.
- The bony cuts are made in an identical fashion to a Le Fort I osteotomy—the pterygoid plates may be left attached or separated.
- The maxilla is split in the mid-line.
- Expansion of the maxilla is achieved by a tooth or bone-borne palatal expansion device (TPD = transpalatal distractor; Fig. 5.12).
- Activation of the device begins after a latent period of 3–5 days and the maxilla is widened ~1mm per day until the desired increase in width is obtained.

Stepped Le Fort I
- The lateral wall of the maxilla can be cut in a stepped fashion, rather than a simple horizontal osteotomy as is the norm (Fig. 5.13).
- Modification was described by Wolford and results in advancement of the paranasal area at a higher level than the standard osteotomy.
- The step also provides a reference point to measure horizontal advance, and a further site for potential fixation or bone grafting should this be required.
- The lateral wall cut begins conventionally in the posterior maxilla, but is continued anteriorly only as far forward as the molar region at which point a vertical component is introduced. The horizontal cut then continues anteriorly to the piriform aperture at a higher level.

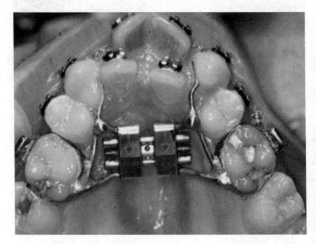

Fig. 5.12 Tooth-borne expansion device for surgically assisted rapid palatal expansion.

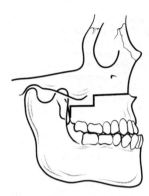

Fig. 5.13 The lateral maxillary cut of a stepped Le Fort 1 osteotomy, showing the anterior maxilla being sectioned at a higher level. Reproduced with permission from Ward-Booth *et al.* (2007). *Maxillofacial Surgery*, Vol. 2, Churchill Livingstone, with permission from Elsevier.

Segmental maxillary procedures

Historically, a wide variety of segmental maxillary procedures have been described mostly with eponymous names, such as Wassmund and Wunderer (anterior segmental osteotomies), or Schuchardt's buccal segment osteotomy. These procedures all have in common surgical approaches through limited incisions. With ↑ experience and understanding of the blood supply these procedures are largely obsolete, with the majority of surgeons performing segmental maxillary osteotomies via a Le Fort I down-fracture technique.

Indications
- Transverse discrepancies.
- Vertical discrepancies.
- Asymmetry.
- Severe open bite deformity.
- Accentuated occlusal curves, which cannot be levelled orthodontically.
- Severe bi-maxillary protrusion.
- Elimination of spacing within an arch.

Technique
- Segmentation of the maxilla requires inter-dental osteotomies to be performed.
- Maxilla may be divided into several segments if required.
- Anterior segmental surgery is the most common form, generally employed in the management of severe open bite deformity.
- Inter-dental osteotomy is most commonly carried out in the canine/first premolar region, or between the canine and lateral incisor.
- If the labial segment is being set-back, a premolar may be extracted and the extraction space closed by retraction of the anterior segment.
- The inter-dental osteotomy is carried out from above following down-fracture of the maxilla using fine burs or micro-saws.

- Orthodontic preparation facilitates these osteotomies by diverging the roots of the adjacent teeth and providing space (Fig. 5.14a).
- When down-fracture technique is employed, the blood supply of the segment is derived primarily from the palatal mucosa and great care must be taken to preserve this.
- Tears may lead to localized periodontal defects, tooth loss, or even avascular necrosis of a segment.
- Segmental surgery requires greater attention to stabilization and an acrylic occlusal wafer is used to tie in the segments at the occlusal level (Fig. 5.14b).
- The orthodontic archwire must be sectioned at the time of surgery to allow for positioning of the segment and should be replaced either with a new archwire pre-bent on the model surgery or with a supplemental archwire.

(a)

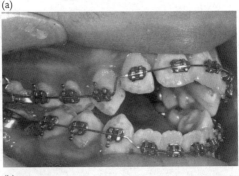

(b)

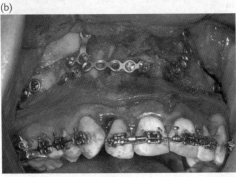

Fig. 5.14 (a) Orthodontic preparation of a patient with a large anterior open bite for an anterior segmental osteotomy. Note the step in the occlusal level between the lateral incisor and canine, and also the reverse curve of Spee in the lower arch. (b) The completed osteotomy showing levelling of the occlusal plane and the fixation of the segments.

Le Fort II

Indications

- Naso-maxillary hypoplasia.
- Mild deficiency of the infraorbital rim.
- Pseudo-proptosis.

The procedure is less versatile than a Le Fort I osteotomy. Anterior movement with a degree of downward rotation of the maxilla is possible, but impaction of the maxilla and rotation to any significant extent cannot be achieved. Unlike the Le Fort III osteotomy, this cannot be combined with a Le Fort I osteotomy.

Exposure

- Intra-oral exposure is as for a Le Fort I osteotomy with a sulcus incision running from first molar to first molar.
- Two para-nasal or 'Lynch' incisions gain access to:
  - nasal bones;
  - upper anterior maxilla;
  - orbital rim;
  - medial orbit.
- The skin is raised sub-periosteally over the glabellar region.
- The lacrimal apparatus must be identified and protected with vessel sloops passed around the lacrimal ducts.

Bone cuts

- Pyramidal osteotomy of the mid-face.
- Posterior aspect identical to a Le Fort I osteotomy from the pterygoid region forward to the zygomatic buttress.
- From this point the bony cut passes upwards to the orbital rim medially to the infraorbital nerve.
- After crossing the orbital rim, the cut runs posteriorly across the orbital floor at right angles to the rim before turning medially to run behind the lacrimal sac as far as the upper part of the lacrimal groove.
- The cut turns forwards to cross the frontal process of the maxilla and the nasal bridge, becoming continuous with the contralateral side.
- The nasal septum is divided at a higher level than in a Le Fort I running from the nasal bones downward and backwards towards the posterior part of the septum at the posterior nasal spine (Fig. 5.15).
- Down-fracture.
- Mobilization of the Le Fort II is more difficult and much less mobility is obtained than with a Le Fort I because of the larger size of the maxillary block.
- Fixation.
- Achieved with miniplates at the zygomatic buttress and across the nasal bridge. The bony defect at the nasal osteotomy can be grafted with a cortico-cancellous block.

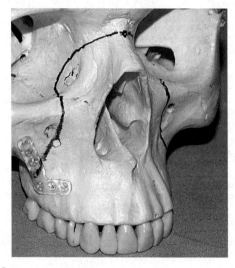

Fig. 5.15 Bony cuts in Le Fort II osteotomy.

Modifications of the Le Fort II

Pyramidal naso-orbital osteotomy
- Limited to the anterior maxilla.
- Combines the upper part of a Le Fort II along with an anterior maxillary osteotomy.
- Anterior mid-face is moved anteriorly *en bloc* maintaining the posterior occlusion and opening space in usually the premolar region.

Kufner osteotomy
- Cuts do not involve the nasal bridge and run anterior to the lacrimal apparatus crossing the upper part of the piriform aperture medially.
- Osteotomy runs laterally across the zygoma and down the postero-lateral aspect of the maxilla to the pterygoid region.
- Indicated in patients with a good nasal bridge projection, but in whom the infraorbital rims and maxilla are retruded.

'Winged' Le Fort I
- Often confused with a Kufner or used synonymously.
- The 'winged' Le Fort I osteotomy divides the maxilla at a higher level than a conventional Le Fort I osteotomy and extends laterally onto the body of the zygomatic bone (Fig. 5.16).

(a)

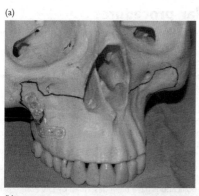

(b)

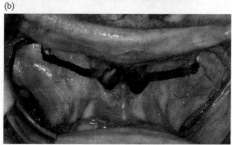

Fig. 5.16 (a, b) Illustration and operative view of a 'winged' Le Fort I osteotomy.

Le Fort III

- Described by Tessier in 1971.
- Le Fort III advances the entire facial mass by separating it from the cranial base.
- Indications for this procedure lie in craniofacial surgery.
- Advances the maxilla and simultaneously increases orbital volume.
- Osteotomy cuts pass across:
  - medial orbital wall;
  - orbital floor;
  - lateral orbital wall;
  - fronto-zygomatic suture.
- The frontal process of the zygomatic bone is split sagittally and continued inferiorly to complete the division of the zygoma.
- The two sides are connected in the midline through the fronto-nasal area as per a Le Fort II.
- Pterygomaxillary and septal separation are also as for a Le Fort II (see ➜ Craniofacial procedures, p. 282).

Mandibular procedures

Osteotomies have been described at almost every part of the mandible in order to achieve forward, backward, or rotational re-positioning.

Bilateral sagittal split osteotomy (BSSO)

The BSSO of the mandible is the workhorse of mandibular orthognathic surgery. It can be used to:
- Advance or set-back the mandible.
- Correct rotations and other asymmetric adjustments.
- Close small open bite deformities by rotation of the mandible in a counter-clockwise direction around a sagittal split, utilizing bi-cortical screws as fixation.
- Introduced in 1957 by Trauner and Obwegeser.
- In the original description the split was confined to the vertical ramus with two parallel horizontal cuts—one buccal and one lingual.
- Subsequent modifications have been described by Dal Pont, Epker, and Hunsuck:
  - Dal Pont brought the buccal cut to a vertical position in the molar region thus increasing the area of bone contact for healing;
  - Hunsuck described the short split whereby the horizontal lingual cut is extended posteriorly to a point just behind the lingula. This latter modification prevents the lingual aspect of the distal fragment impinging in the pterygomasseteric sling in large mandibular set-backs. It also makes it less likely that the condyle will remain on the distal fragment during splitting of the osteotomy (Fig. 5.17).
- A natural cleavage plane between buccal and lingual cortical plates is utilized to develop a sagittal split separating the proximal (condylar-carrying) and distal (dento-alveolar) fragments.
- Following splitting of the cortical plates the distal fragment can be advanced, set-back, or rotated.
- If advanced a gap is produced in the buccal cortical plate and, if set-back, a portion of buccal cortical plate has to be removed. The proximal fragment remains in its pre-operative AP position, but may rotate a small amount around a vertical axis.

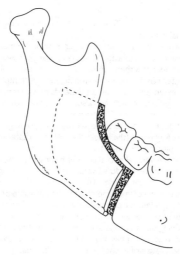

Fig. 5.17 Sagittal split osteotomy as most commonly practised, showing long buccal cut and short lingual split (Hunsuck). Reproduced with permission of Professor K. F. Moos.

Exposure

- Intra-oral incision options:
  - straight incision extending down the external oblique ridge and running forward in the buccal sulcus to a point roughly adjacent to the first molar tooth;
  - conventional third molar incision where the incision runs into the disto-buccal aspect of the terminal molar;
  - in either case a cuff of mucosa is left to facilitate suturing.
- The incision is carried straight down to bone. The vertical extent up the external oblique ridge is limited to avoid the buccal fat pad.
- As the flap is developed postero-superiorly a notched ramus retractor is introduced, and used to strip the soft tissue attachment off the external oblique ridge and anterior edge of the ascending ramus.
- At this point the temporalis insertion is encountered and must be stripped upwards to a point above the level of the lingual.
- A Kocher's forceps may be applied to the anterior edge of the ramus to act as a retractor.
- The lingual soft tissues are now dissected with a thin periosteal retractor being introduced sub-subperiosteally to permit identification of the lingula (Mitchell's trimmer with its sharp end facing downwards and angled slightly forwards is a useful means by which to reliably identify the position of the lingula). The assistant on the opposite side of the patient often gets a better view of the lingula than the operator.

Bone cuts
- Surgical bur (Lindemann or Toller fissure) or reciprocating saw.
- Perform lingual cut first.
- The bur or saw is placed against the lingual side of the mandible just above the level of the lingua and with the tip just posterior to it.
- The lingual cortex cut is then continued down the external oblique ridge—the latter can first be delineated in 'postage stamp' fashion.
- The anterior extent of this latter cut depends on whether the mandible is being advanced or set-back, and also, to a certain extent, upon what type of fixation is envisaged. The greater the advance, then the further forward the buccal cut needs to be in order to achieve good bony overlap of the fragments (the longer the split the greater may be the technical difficulty in achieving it).
- The final cut is the vertical buccal cut which runs from the anterior end of the external oblique cut downwards, parallel to the long axis of the teeth, to cross the lower border. The cut must be deep enough to fully perforate the buccal cortex remembering that, at some point on the buccal surface, the inferior alveolar nerve is at risk of transection.
- Ensure that the full thickness of the cortical bone is divided at the lower border; removing mouth props and using a channel or Awty retractor greatly assists in achieving this. Failure to do divide the lower border is the commonest cause of a 'bad' or unfavourable split.

Splitting
- A fine curved chisel is placed into the lingual cut and tapped backwards until the tip emerges from the lingual cortex just behind the lingula.
- This manoeuvre begins a split propagating down the lingual cortex of the mandible and minimizes the chance of leaving the condyle on the wrong fragment.
- Completion of all the bony cuts is confirmed by tapping a fine osteotome along all the cuts. Tapping out the cuts in such a fashion often begins the process of splitting such that the cortical plates can be seen to separate.
- A Smith's spreader at the upper border in conjunction with a Howarth's periosteal elevator or chisel at the lower border, working strictly from anterior to posterior, separates the two cortices.
- The shorter the distance between the two instruments the less the leverage that needs to be applied to the buccal plate, thus minimizing the chance of fracture.
- The split is thus completed from front to back.
- The two common points of hold-up are anteriorly at the lower border and posteriorly, low down at the angle.
- Once the split has been achieved, the proximal and distal fragments can be easily moved independently of each other. One must be able to obtain shortening of the ramus.
- The position of the nerve must be checked. It should lie on the distal fragment, but often lies entrapped in the buccal aspect of the proximal fragment crossing the osteotomy gap and, at this point, must be dissected free.

Fixation

Plates or bi-cortical screws (Fig. 5.18a):

- Fixation by means of bi-cortical screws is more rigid and thus less forgiving than plates in terms of any post-operative adjustment.
- Plates have a higher removal rate.
- Bi-cortical fixation is by means of position screws and not lag screws (lag screws by only engaging on the lingual cortex provide compression between the fragments and have been associated with a greater incidence of nerve damage).
- Three screws are placed in an 'L' or triangular configuration.
- Some advocate the placement of four bi-cortical screws when operating for sleep apnoea. The rational being that these patients are often of a stockier build generating high bite forces.
- IMF in the desired occlusal position is required prior to fixation.
- Positioning of the proximal fragment requires experience and is largely determined by 'feel'—the condyle must be fully seated in the glenoid fossa.

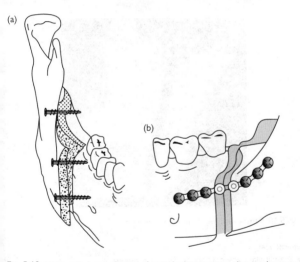

Fig. 5.18 (a) Bi-cortical screw fixation of sagittal split osteotomy, showing the most mechanically advantageous arrangement of three screws in a tripod fashion. (b) Plate fixation of sagittal split osteotomy. Reproduced with permission of Professor K. F. Moos.

Vertical subsigmoid osteotomy

- The vertical subsigmoid osteotomy (VSS) is one of the simplest osteotomies of the mandible.
- It became less widely used with the introduction of semi-rigid fixation when patients were no longer routinely placed in IMF post-operatively (VSS requires IMF during the healing phase).
- With current technology it is now possible to fix these osteotomies intra-orally and obviate the need for IMF.
- In theory eliminates the risk of inferior alveolar nerve damage that accompanies sagittal splitting.
- Has been shown it to be more stable than sagittal splitting for mandibular set-back.
- May be indicated where appropriate in patients with pre-existing TMJ problems.
- Can be carried out either extra- or intra-orally (in both cases bone cuts are the same; Fig. 5.19).

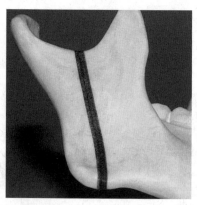

Fig. 5.19 Vertical subsigmoid osteotomy bone cut.

Indications
- Mandibular excess where set-back is required.
- Relieving osteotomy to allow rotations of the mandible (when used in this fashion it may be combined with a sagittal split on the contralateral side).

Informed consent
It is now considered that for consent to be truly informed and valid not only should the procedure and its attendant complications be explained to the patient in detail but such alternative procedures that are available should also be discussed. One can argue a very strong case that a patient requiring a mandibular set-back should have the advantages and disadvantages of

both a BSSO and a VSS explained to them and be offered a choice. Not only is the incidence of nerve damage lower with a VSS but there is evidence that for set-back it is more stable than a BSSO.

Exposure—extra-oral

- Approached via a standard submandibular skin crease incision.
- Entire lateral surface of the ramus is exposed sub-periosteally.
- Muscle attachments at the posterior border are not stripped in order to maintain blood supply.
- Sigmoid notch is identified and a long channel retractor inserted into it.
- Anti-lingula is identified (represents the point behind which the bony cut must be made).

Exposure—intra-oral

- Perhaps more than any other osteotomy procedure, this benefits from specially designed instrumentation to gain adequate access and exposure.
- Incision is the same as that for a sagittal split.
- Periosteum is incised along the external oblique ridge of the ramus and the lateral aspect of the ramus is exposed sub-periosteally.
- Anti-lingula is identified.

Bone cut

- Vertical cut running from the sigmoid notch above downwards to cross the lower border at a point just anterior to the angle.
- If the procedure is being carried out via an extra-oral approach this cut is easily made under direct vision with a reciprocating saw.
- The intra-oral approach:
  - technically challenging;
  - requires the use of an oscillating saw;
  - cut is started at the mid-point of the ramus just behind the anti-lingula, then extended upwards to the sigmoid notch and downwards to the lower border.
- When the bone cut is completed a periosteal elevator is introduced into the cut and the proximal fragment mobilized laterally to overlap the distal fragment.
- Any remaining medial pterygoid muscle attachments are stripped from the medial aspect of this fragment.

Fixation

- Temporary IMF is used to position the fragments.
- Traditionally IMF is used post-operatively.
- A suture is placed through a hole drilled in the lower part of the proximal fragment and sutured to the buccal periosteum to prevent medial displacement.
- IMF is maintained for first 2 weeks, followed by strong elastics.
- It is possible to fix this osteotomy either by means of a bi-cortical screw placed via a transbuccal trocar or to plate the fragments using a right-angled screwdriver.

Inverted-L osteotomy

The inverted-L osteotomy is a variant of the VSS (Fig. 5.20).

Indications

- Mandibular hypoplasia where there is significant deficiency of the ramus, both vertically and horizontally.
- To increase posterior facial height as it allows lengthening of the ramus without significant effects on the masticatory muscles.
- 'Bird-face' deformities are often best treated by this procedure.
- The procedure can be used as an alternative to either VSS or BSSO, where intra-oral access is severely limited.
- In most cases bone grafting is required.

Technique

- Extra-oral or intra-oral approach may be used.
- Extra-oral approach offers greater access and allows for easier positioning of bone grafts and application of fixation.
- Fixation with miniplates (if an intra-oral approach is employed this can still be achieved with a transbuccal technique or using a right-angled screwdriver).

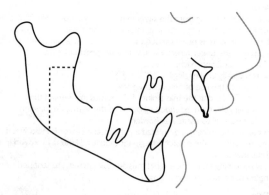

Fig. 5.20 Inverted L osteotomy. Reproduced from Ward-Booth *et al*. (2007). *Maxillofacial Surgery*, Vol. 2, Churchill Livingstone, with permission from Elsevier.

Total subapical osteotomy

Indications

Good facial profile with the chin in the desired AP position relative to the cranial base, but anterior positioning of the entire lower dentition is required (sagittal advancement of the mandible would render the patient prognathic and addition of reduction genioplasty results in flat featureless chin).

Exposure
- Sulcus incision is carried from one external oblique ridge to another maintaining a wide cuff of mucosa at least 1cm from the muco-gingival junction.
- Mental foramen identified bilaterally.

Nerve dissection
- ID nerve must be dissected free in order to safely carry out the osteotomy (Fig. 5.21).
- Dissection of the nerve begins at the mental foramen.
- A series of small perforations are placed around the foramen with a fine bur in postage stamp fashion to form a circumferential osteotomy—this ring of bone is then divided and removed.
- The nerve can then be traced posteriorly by removing a parallel portion of cortical bone overlying the canal.
- The nerve is traced backwards until the ramus at which point it traverses the mandible from a buccal to a lingual position as it approaches the lingula.

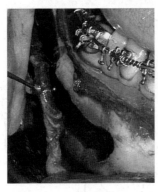

Fig. 5.21 Exteriorization of inferior alveolar nerve from its canal prior to a total subapical osteotomy.

Bone cuts
- Once the nerve is dissected free, the bone cut is completed.
- No lingual dissection is performed, but a finger placed in the lingual sulcus as the cut is made avoids damage to the mucosa.
- The horizontal transverse cut is taken into a vertical cut as the posterior body joins the ramus.
- Mobilization of the entire dento-alveolar segment is relatively simple.

Fixation
- Fixation of the dento-alveolar segment to the basal bone of the mandible is by means of plates and screws.
- Bone graft may be placed in the osteotomy site and increase in lower face height achieved by inter-positional grafting.
- The amount of advancement that may be achieved is limited by the thickness of the bone as direct bone-to-bone contact is required for healing.

Segmental mandibular osteotomies

A wide variety of segmental mandibular procedures have been described the principles of which will be outlined. For detailed description of indications and techniques specialist texts should be consulted.

Body ostectomy

- These osteotomies are carried out in the mandibular body either anterior or posterior to the mental foramen (Fig. 5.22).
- If posterior to the mental foramen the nerve has to be dissected free from its bony canal and exteriorized to avoid damage to the nerve.
- A pre-planned segment of bone is removed, either to close an edentulous space or following extraction (usually a premolar), allowing the anterior segment of the jaw to be set-back.
- 3D skeletal models can be particularly useful in planning these cases, cutting templates may be constructed.
- The proximal segments often rotate internally somewhat to narrow the posterior occlusion.

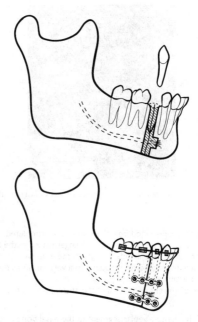

Fig. 5.22 Body ostectomy. A premolar tooth has been removed to allow removal of a section of the body and the anterior mandible is set-back. Reproduced with permission from Ward-Booth et al. (2007). *Maxillofacial Surgery*, Vol. 2, Churchill Livingstone, with permission from Elsevier.

Lower labial segmental osteotomies
- Have in common the separation of a segment of labial bone carrying the lower anterior teeth generally from canine to canine, or first premolar to first premolar.
- Blood supply to the fragment is derived from the lingual soft tissue attachments and it is crucial that these are not compromised during the procedure.
- Lower labial segment may be re-positioned vertically (to close an open bite), inferiorly or posteriorly.
- Inferior and posterior re-positioning require the removal of a portion of bone.
- Posterior re-positioning is often at the expense of the extraction of a premolar tooth.
- Where vertical alveolar osteotomies are carried out between teeth, it is essential that orthodontic preparation opens sufficient space between the roots of the teeth.
- Indications:
  - some cases of anterior open bite;
  - exaggerated curve of Spee;
  - reverse curve of Spee;
  - inferior alveolar protrusion;
  - some cases of bi-maxillary protrusion.

Kohle procedure
- Used in Class III patients with:
  - reverse curve of Spee;
  - downward inclination of the mandibular occlusal plane;
  - increase in lower anterior face height.
- Procedure includes an anterior segmental osteotomy in conjunction with a genioplasty.
- The gap created by the upward movement of the lower labial segment is closed by using the wedge of bone removed from the genioplasty.

Sowray–Haskell Procedure
- Indicated when there is a degree of mandibular protrusion and an associated molar cross bite (Fig. 5.23).
- Procedure combines:
  - *lower labial segmental osteotomy*—often with extraction of premolars to allow setting-back of the labial segment;
  - *narrowing of the mandible*—achieved by removing a midline segment of bone from the subapical osteotomy line to the lower border of the mandible.

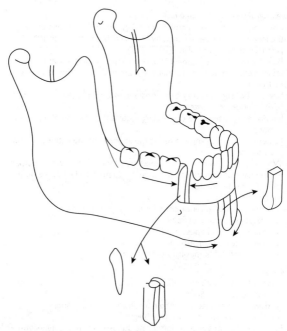

Fig. 5.23 'Sowray–Haskell' procedure. This combines an anterior segmental osteotomy with removal of a section of bone from the mid-line to narrow the mandible. Reproduced with permission of Professor K. F. Moos.

Genioplasty

Genioplasty may be performed either as a solitary procedure or as an adjunct to other orthognathic or craniofacial procedures. The chin may be
- Advanced or set-back in the AP plane.
- Augmented or reduced in its vertical dimension.
- Rotated to the left or right to correct a centre line discrepancy.
- Widened or narrowed in the transverse dimension.
- Altered in all three dimensions in cases of asymmetry combinations.

Beware the set-back genioplasty! This procedure if not very carefully planned may result in poor aesthetic outcomes as a result of flattening of the labio-mental groove producing a flat featureless looking chin.

Surgical technique

Incision
- A wide labial approach avoiding the depth of sulcus running from the region of the canine/first premolar tooth bilaterally.
- Incision is made in a slightly bevelled fashion with either a scalpel or a needle point diathermy.
- Incision is deepened through the mucosa, submucosal tissues, and the mentalis muscle to reach the periosteum.
- The periosteum is incised initially in the midline and subperiosteal dissection is carried out on either side to reach the lower border of the mandible.
- Dissection is continued posteriorly along the lower border beneath the mental nerve foramen allowing identification and protection of the nerves to a point, which corresponds to the posterior extent of the proposed bony osteotomy.
- In the region of the midline, it is not necessary to fully expose the lower border of the chin point and superior aesthetics can be achieved if some mentalis attachment is preserved.

Bone cuts
- For vertical reduction a segment of bone is removed from the chin.
- In asymmetric chins a wedge may be removed from one or other side in order to gain symmetry (in some cases, the wedge removed from one side is reversed and used to augment the contralateral side).
- Vertical augmentation procedures require grafting with bone or a suitable alloplastic material.
- The standard sliding genioplasty employs a horizontal cut, made about 5mm below the level of the mental foramen to avoid inadvertent injury to the nerve, which often loops below the foramen prior to exiting the bony canal. The cut should be carried as far posteriorly on the lower border as possible to ensure a smooth lower border contour.
- Once complete the lower border of the chin should be freely mobile without any bony interferences.
- Care should be taken to ensure adequate haemostasis of any vessels, particularly on the lingual aspect, which could be damaged by the saw.
- Attachments of the geniohyoid and genioglossus muscles should be maintained to preserve the blood supply to the chin segment.

Fixation
(See Fig. 5.24.)
- Fixation with miniplates or screws.
- Plates may be used to fix the segment. Chin plates are now available that are pre-bent to achieve the desired pre-determined advance.
- Lag or bi-cortical screws offer a secure means of fixation with little in the way of palpable fixation, but generally require greater stripping of the lower border anteriorly to permit the required angulation.

Soft tissue closure
- Accurate closure in two layers is essential.
- A genioplasty pressure dressing is applied to support the soft tissues for the first 24–48h.

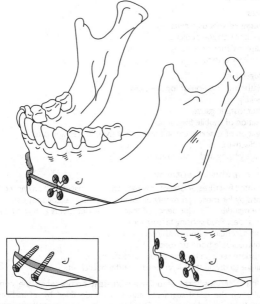

Fig. 5.24 Various methods of fixation in genioplasty. Reproduced with permission of Professor K. F. Moos.

Complications

Haemorrhage

Risk reduced by:
- LA with adrenaline.
- Use of cutting diathermy.
- Hypotensive anaesthesia.
- Efficient operating resulting in shorter surgical time.
- Use of anti-fibrinolytics.
- Care at pterygomaxillary dysjunction—correct positioning, small osteotome.
- Some advocate a posterior transmaxillary osteotomy through the tuberosity.

Sources
- Pterygoid venous plexus.
- Greater palatine pedicle.
- Naso-palatine vessels.
- Maxillary artery.

Management
- Diathermy/ligation of local vessels.
- Packing.
- Haemostatic gauze.
- Fixation of mobile fragments.
- Ligation of external carotid artery (rarely indicated and often ineffective).
- Angiography and embolization.

Unfavourable osteotomy

Unwanted fractures or osteotomy patterns may arise during any procedure, but are by far most commonly encountered in the sagittal split osteotomy of the mandible. The incidence of 'bad' split varies, but is as high as 23% in some series. Predisposing factors include:
- Thin ascending ramus with no cancellous bone.
- Unfavourable bone texture.
- Wisdom teeth in the line of the osteotomy.
- Failure to divide the lower border at the buccal cut.

The most serious form of unfavourable split occurs when the condyle remains on the distal segment—this can be identified by an inability to reduce the height of the ramus. Should this occur, it is essential to complete the split and separate the condyle from the distal fragment. This may require a low subcondylar osteotomy. If at all possible the condyle should be fixed as per a condylar fracture and the osteotomy completed, although in most cases this complication will require the use of post-operative IMF.

Undesirable fractures are not common in maxillary osteotomies, although pterygomaxillary disjunction may result in unfavourable fractures propagating up towards the base of the skull. If pterygoid disjunction is incomplete then difficulty in advancing the maxilla may be encountered.

Nerve damage

Mandible

- Inferior alveolar nerve is at particular risk during sagittal splitting of the mandible.
- Immediately post-operatively paraesthesia is almost universal, although the majority of patients go on to recover sensation.
- The rate of long-term paraesthesia varies in the literature from 3–25%, although sporadic reports of up to 85% are published.
- Age is a risk factor for nerve damage with those patients over 40 being at significantly greater risk of some form of permanently reduced sensation.
- Lag screws increase the incidence of nerve damage.
- Bi-cortical position screws avoid nerve damage, although care is required in their placement.
- Intra-oral VSS has much lower risk of damage to the inferior alveolar nerve than BSS—long-term paraesthesia is rare.
- Simultaneous BSS and genioplasty carries an ↑ risk of sensory disturbance compared with BSS alone.
- Facial nerve damage during mandibular ramus osteotomies is rarely reported (0.5–1%)—most cases resolve spontaneously.

Maxilla

- A number of nerves may be damaged during maxillary osteotomy, although long-term sensory loss is most unusual.
- The exception to this is the sensation of the labial gingival and the anterior palatal mucosa—long-term sensory disturbance at these sites is not infrequently seen.
- Cranial nerves II, III, IV, VI, X, and XII are all reported to have been damaged during maxillary surgery, presumably by unfavourable fracture patterns propagating up to the base of the skull.

Condylar positioning

The position of the condyle within the fossa differs between the awake, upright patient and the supine patient on the operating table. This positional change is exaggerated by muscle relaxation or paralysis induced by anaesthesia.

- In BSSO if the condyles are incorrectly positioned then a malocclusion will result.
- Condylar positioning devices have been described, which preserve the relation between the condyle and fossa, but have never gained widespread acceptance and are rarely used.
- Significant mandibular rotation causes:
  - rotation of the condyle;
  - winging out of the proximal fragment;
  - inability to get the two fragments to lie passively (some degree of this may have to be accepted to prevent excessive torquing of the condyle).

During Le Fort I maxillary osteotomy (especially impaction) if excessive force has to be applied to position the maxilla the maxilla can rotate around any bony interference. This causes the condyles to be distracted out of the glenoid fossae. If the maxilla is fixed in this position an anterior open bite will be present on release of the temporary IMF. To avoid this complication it is essential that the maxilla can be positioned passively, and that any upward pressure is applied at the mandibular angles and not at the chin.

Tooth damage
- Not common in orthognathic surgery.
- Due to direct surgical damage or loss of vitality as a result of ischaemic change.
- Surgical damage to teeth is most likely to occur during segmental surgery.
- Le Fort I cut that is placed too low may damage apices.
- Fixation screws may perforate roots if inappropriately placed.

Genioplasty complications
- Nerve damage resulting in loss of sensation in the distribution of the mental.
- Damage to the roots of the anterior teeth either by the bone cut or by fixation screws.
- Post-operative infection may necessitate the removal of plates and screws.
- Mal- or non-union.
- Excessive stripping of the segment may result in avascular necrosis.
- Scarring can result in tethering of the lower lip and reduction in the depth of the labial sulcus.
- Inadequate repair of the mentalis muscle will result in ptosis of the lower lip with ↑ lower incisor show and deepening of the labio-mental groove.

Soft tissue changes

Nasal changes

After Le Fort I osteotomy:
- The alar base widens.
- The nasal tip is upturned.
- The naso-labial angle decreases with maxillary advance.
- A combination of maxillary impaction and advancement has the greatest effect on nasal aesthetics.

Reduction of nasal septum

In maxillary impaction it is essential to reduce the nasal septum by an amount equivalent to the impaction, in order to prevent buckling of the septum with consequent nasal deviation and airway obstruction.

Cinch sutures/hollowing of nasal rim

Various techniques are described to try to prevent or minimize adverse effects (Fig. 5.25). The cinch suture engages fibro-cartilaginous tissue at the alar base on either side and is tied in the midline to achieve the desired width (Fig. 5.26). This suture:
- Controls the transverse dimension of the alar base.
- Improves tip projection.
- Decreases shortening of the upper lip.
- Maintains the thickness of the upper lip.
- ?Is effective only in the short term.

An alternative approach is to remove bone from around the piriform aperture.

V–Y closure

V–Y closure of the anterior sulcus incision may help minimize lip shortening and maintain lip thickness. A set amount of vertical closure is carried out prior to closing the remainder of the horizontal incision (Fig. 5.27).

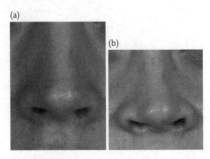

Fig. 5.25 (a, b) Adverse aesthetic result in the nose following maxillary advance and impaction at the Le Fort I level. Note the flaring of the nostrils, widening of the alar base, and upturned nasal tip.

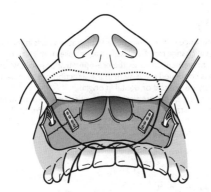

Fig. 5.26 Alar 'cinch' suture. A non-resorbable suture is used and picks up the fibro-fatty tissue at the alar base on either side of the nose. It is tied to adjust the width of the alar base.

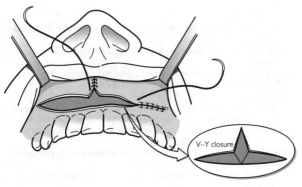

Fig. 5.27 V–Y closure of the anterior sulcus incision.

Stability

- The maintenance of the achieved post-operative result in the long term.
- Post-surgical change may be classified as relapse or migration.
- Relapse is movement towards the pre-operative position, whereas migration is continued movement in the direction of the initial move.
- Relapse may be skeletal or dental in origin.
- Careful planning of pre-surgical orthodontics aims to build in relapse.
- A hierarchy of stability has been described by W.R. Proffit, T.A. Turvey, and C. Phillips from longitudinal data collected over many years at the University of North Carolina.

Most stable to least stable

- Maxillary impaction.
- Mandibular advance.
- Maxillary advancement.
- Maxillary impaction with mandibular advancement.
- Maxillary advancement with mandibular set-back.
- Mandibular set-back.
- Increase in maxillary width.
- Inferior positioning of the maxilla.

Maxillary surgery

- Impaction is the most stable of all the maxillary movements, but stability is decreasing if combined with advancement.
- Rigid fixation with plates offers improved stability over wire osteosynthesis.
- Larger moves exhibit greater post-operative change and moves of >8mm should be considered potentially unstable.
- A period of IMF may aid stability.
- Grafting of an advancement with blocks placed between the pterygoid plates and the posterior maxilla does not appear to increase stability.
- Inferior positioning is the least stable movement and relapse rates of around 30–50% are reported.
- Inferior repositioning of the maxilla can be accompanied by grafting to enhance stability and a good bony union.
- Mal- or non-union of the maxilla is most commonly seen after inferior repositioning.

Transverse dimension

- In younger patients with a small transverse discrepancy orthodontic means via rapid palatal expansion (RPE) can achieve stable results (before the age of 14).
- Older patients or those requiring a greater degree of expansion. The most stable results are achieved with SARPE.
- Surgical widening of the maxilla is generally considered to be an unstable move, but a number of techniques can be utilized to minimize relapse:
  - horseshoe osteotomy of the palate, rather than a simple mid-line split;

- expansion should be supported for at least 6 weeks post-operatively, either by a colleted acrylic plate worn in the palate or by an accessory archwire on the bucco-labial side;
- consider bone grafting of the expansion gap in the palate to aid stability.

Cleft patients

- Present particular challenges.
- Maxilla may be grossly hypoplastic both horizontally and in a vertical dimension requiring therefore advancement and down-grafting.
- Move may be significant and optimum aesthetics often require that ideally this move is achieved in the maxilla and not by combining a mandibular set-back.
- Scarring may make advancement of the maxilla very difficult and it may not be possible to achieve the desired position.
- Scarring may cause early relapse in the first few weeks post-operatively.
- Incidence of mal-union is higher in this group of patients than non-cleft patients.
- IMF may improve stability and the use of a 'Delaire' mask in early post-operative period may help to reduce relapse.
- Distraction osteogenesis has been used widely in cleft patients to achieve maxillary advancements that could not be achieved by conventional orthognathic surgery.
- It was hoped that the results obtained by distraction osteogenesis would be stable but relapse still occurs.

Mandibular surgery

BSSO advancement

- Stability depends on the degree of advancement and method of fixation.
- Wire osteosynthesis is inferior to semi-rigid fixation with either bi-cortical screws or mono-cortical screws and miniplates in terms of stability.
- Little evidence whether screws or plates offer greater stability.
- Compression or lag screws confer no increase in stability.
- Three screws placed in a triangular or inverted-L pattern offer greater stability than three screws placed in a linear fashion along the upper border.
- To correct an anterior open bite the use of four screws has been recommended.
- Larger advancements show greater degrees of relapse irrespective of the method of fixation—for advances in excess of 10mm, the addition of supplemental skeletal fixation with suspension wires for 1 week post-operatively has been shown to improve stability.

Mandibular set-back
- Different degrees of stability between a BSSO and intra-oral VSS. Sagittal split tends to relapse forwards, whereas the VSS tends to migrate further posteriorly.
- Large movements are more unstable and are attributed to impingement of the posterior border against the pterygomasseteric sling.
- The Hunsuck modification of the sagittal split mitigates against this problem by having a much shorter lingual segment.

Condylar resorption
- Presentation is generally between 6 and 18 months post-surgery.
- Incidence reported between 2% and 8%.
- Horizontal relapse often occurs, with development of an anterior open bite due to clockwise rotation of the mandible.
- Radiography reveals:
  - flattening of the condylar head;
  - posterior angulation and shortening of the condylar neck.

Risk factors
- ♀ patients.
- Class II malocclusions.
- High Frankfort mandibular plane angle.
- Pre-existing TMJ symptoms.
- Large mandibular advances (>10mm).
- Counter clockwise rotation of the mandible to close an anterior open bite.

Aetiology: theories
- ↑ pressure on the posterior surface of the condylar head (especially in large advances) increases the load on the joint and stimulates a process of resorption possible by adverse effects on blood flow.
- Alteration of the position of the condylar head in the glenoid fossa may induce remodelling changes.

Management
- Most cases 'burn out' after a time and then remain stable.
- Some postulate a splint that postures the mandible forward and unloads the joint may be of benefit.
- Secondary corrective surgery is controversial. Patients certainly have to be made aware that condylar resorption is unpredictable and may occur again after further surgery.
- ?Corrective surgery should be confined to the maxilla in order to avoid further insult to the condyles if at all possible.
- Others argue that further mandibular surgery can be stable.

Distraction osteogenesis

Introduction

- A biological process of new bone formation between two bone surfaces, which are gradually separated by incremental traction.
- Traditionally, a corticotomy is used to provide the two bony surfaces, although in maxillofacial practice a full osteotomy is often employed.
- A latent period ensues, which allows the formation of early callus between the bone ends before entering the distraction phase.
- During this phase the bones ends are separated by the application of a distraction force.
- Forces are generated away from the bone ends.
- Once the desired lengthening has been achieved, there follows a period of consolidation during which time ossification of the callus is completed.
- One of the advantages of distraction osteogenesis is the simultaneous lengthening of the soft tissues that occurs.

Biology of distraction

- Osteogenesis associated with distraction occurs primarily by the recruitment of primitive mesenchymal cells (membranous ossification).
- Haematoma forms in the gap between the bone ends along with a marked inflammatory reaction.
- Vascular response occurs along with the appearance of mesenchymal cells and the synthesis of type 1 collagen.
- A fibrovascular bridge is formed between the bone ends with the collagen fibres being aligned along the axis of distraction.
- Bone first appears around day 10–14.
- Growth factors and cytokines are involved in the regulation of bone formation—these include bone morphogenic proteins, insulin-like growth factors, and members of the transforming growth factor family.

Terminology of distraction

- **Corticotomy**: division of cortex.
- **Latency period**: period of time between the osteotomy and placement of the distractor before active separation of the bone ends begins. It is recommended that this phase lasts from 3–7 days according to the clinical situation.
- **Distraction phase** (Fig. 5.28):
  - phase of active distraction when the bone ends are being separated;
  - rate of distraction should be 1mm per day with an ↑ rate of 1.5mm per day in children under the age of 6 to prevent premature consolidation;
  - not only is the rate of distraction important, but also the rhythm with 0.5mm twice a day being more effective than 1mm per day;
  - research suggests that gradual continuous distraction is likely to be most effective and miniaturized motorized distracters are under development.
- **Consolidation phase**: period during which maturation and ossification of the callus takes place (distraction device remains in situ often 'locked-off' to prevent any change in position).

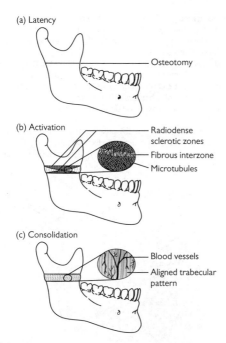

Fig. 5.28 Schematic illustrating the phases of distraction osteogenesis. Latent period, activation or distraction, and finally consolidation.

Indications

Distraction is generally indicated in cases of syndromic deformity:
- Hemifacial microsomia.
- Treacher Collins syndrome.
- Pierre–Robin sequence.
- Mid-face hypoplasia.
- Apert's syndrome.
- Crouzon's syndrome.
- Cleft palate.
- Extremes of conventional orthognathic surgery.

Mandibular distraction
- Achieved with either intra-oral or extra-oral devices.
- Intra-oral devices are fixed directly to the bone with screws just like miniplates:
  - may be completely intra-oral in which case the activation rod usually lies in the buccal sulcus;
  - may be a transcutaneous external port (generally just beneath the angle of the mandible) (Fig. 5.29);

- have the advantage of producing no external scarring, but are limited in as much as they require a minimum volume of bone to allow adequate fixation and are hence unsuitable for very small mandibles;
- removal of these devices may be very difficult.
- Extra-oral devices are easier to place, especially on the diminutive mandible, and also much easier to remove at the end of treatment.
  - osteotomy may be carried out through either an intra-oral or a skin incision, with the pins being placed via a trocar;
  - distraction vector is easier to control than with intra-oral devices (Fig. 5.30);
  - main disadvantages are the obvious appearance and most significantly the scarring, which results from the fixation pins being dragged through the tissues (can be reduced by pushing the soft tissues towards osteotomy site prior to pin insertion).

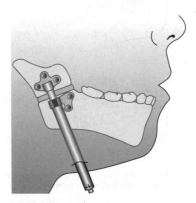

Fig. 5.29 Internal single vector mandibular distractor with external activation.

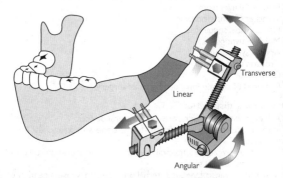

Fig. 5.30 Extra-oral multi-vector distractor. © 2008 Synthes, Inc.

Maxillary distraction
- Used for mid-face advancement in craniofacial cases or for cleft patients with significant maxillary hypoplasia.
- Considered to be less detrimental to speech in patients with potential velo-pharyngeal incompetence than conventional maxillary osteotomy.
- Like mandibular distraction, can be carried out with an extra-oral tooth-borne device such as the rigid external distractor (RED) or with buried intra-oral devices (Fig. 5.31).

(a)

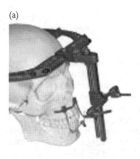

(b)

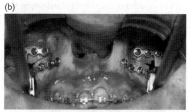

Fig. 5.31 (a) External 'RED' maxillary distractor. (b) Internal buried maxillary distractors *in situ* at the Le Fort I level.

Complications
- Damage to unerupted tooth germs or the inferior alveolar nerve by fixation pins.
- Inadequate bone volume may limit the options for device placement and, hence, lead to an undesirable distraction vector.
- Device failure can occur resulting in an inability to achieve the desired distraction or necessitating replacement of the device.
- Loosening of pins may also lead to failure.
- Condylar pain may be felt during active distraction as the reciprocal effect of the lengthening of the mandible is to push the mandibular condyle up into the glenoid fossa. This may also cause re-modelling of the condylar head.

Stability

Initial hopes for distraction osteogenesis were that it would be free of relapse due to the gradual increase in the length of the tissues over time. Although relapse rates may often be better than obtained with conventional surgery, there is no doubt that relapse may in some cases still be considerable.

Adjunctive procedures

Following successful orthognathic treatment some patients may be left with residual deformity. This is most commonly seen in patients who have presented with significant asymmetry. Bowing of the lower border of the mandible in patients with hemi-mandibular hypertrophy may result in noticeable residual asymmetry following orthognathic surgery even when all the mid-line structures have been correctly positioned in the facial mid-line (Fig. 5.32).

The treatment options in this scenario are either to reduce the lower border on one side or augment the other in order to achieve symmetry. Reduction of the mandible is generally complicated by the inferior alveolar nerve which has to be dissected free and re-positioned in order to allow the required bony reduction. An alternative approach is to utilize CAD/CAM technology, mirror imaging the other side to custom fabricate an onlay with which to augment the deficient side. PEEK (polyethyl-ether ketone) is a high-density plastic which can be custom fabricated and has good bio-compatibility (Fig. 5.33 and Fig. 5.34).

This technique can be used in a variety of situations to help achieve symmetry between two sides or to restore bony deficiencies as a result of congenital or post-traumatic deformity or post-resection defects.

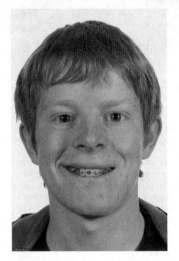

Fig. 5.32 Shows asymmetry of the lower borders of the mandible in a patient with hemi-mandibular hyperplasia.

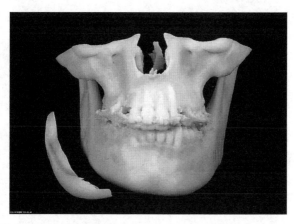

Fig. 5.33 3D skeletal model showing the mandibular asymmetry with the proposed custom-made onlay fabricated by mirror imaging the left side.

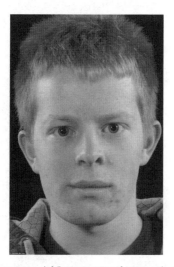

Fig. 5.34 Post-operative result following insertion of custom onlay to lower border of right side of mandible of patient in Fig. 5.32.

Further reading

Cheney, M.L. (1997). *Facial surgery (plastic and reconstructive)*. Williams & Wilkins. Baltimore, MD.
Henderson, D. (1986). *Colour atlas & textbook of orthognathic surgery*. Wolfe Medical, London.

Craniofacial

Introduction

Craniofacial surgery is the sub-specialist area of surgery that diagnoses and manages a large heterogeneous group of both congenital and acquired conditions. The common factor is the involvement of the cranium (and its contents) and the face. Craniofacial surgeons are usually either oral and maxillofacial or plastic surgeons working with neurosurgeons. Because of the complexity and range of conditions managed the overall care is provided by an extensive MDT (see ➲ The craniofacial team, p. 295). Craniofacial units usually provide care to both paediatric and adult patients.

Classification

Numerous classifications exist with little agreement as to which offers the best approach. Each has advantages and disadvantages (see ➲ Further reading, p. 296 for more information).

For the purposes of simplicity the following classification will be utilized:

- **Craniosynostosis:** group of conditions characterized by the premature closure of the skull vault sutures.
- **Craniofacial clefting disorders:** characterized by a failure of the developing branchial arches (or other structures) to fuse or possibly the breakdown of previously-fused structures.
- **Craniofacial tumours:** only specific to craniofacial surgery because of their location and the necessity to utilize craniofacial techniques for their surgical management.
- Head and neck vascular anomalies.

Craniosynostosis

Craniosynostosis is the premature fusion of one or more of the skull vault sutures. Termed 'simple' synostosis if single suture involved and 'complex' if multiple sutures are involved. Most complex cases are syndromic whereas most single suture synostoses are not. However, there are rare single-suture synostoses associated with syndromes, e.g. unilateral coronal synostosis associated with *FGFR3* gene mutations (Muenke syndrome).

- Premature fusion of a suture can result in:
  - restricted growth at right angles to the affected suture;
  - degree of compensatory overgrowth (or bossing) in other areas of the skull vault;
  - raised intracranial pressure.
- In multiple suture or syndromic craniosynostoses head shape is determined by the number and site of the involved sutures. Can result in severe restriction of skull vault growth along with:
  - raised intracranial pressure;
  - exophthalmos;
  - optic dislocation (globes herniate anterior to eyelids);
  - restricted mid-face growth (upper airway and feeding difficulties).

The severity of functional problems varies from case to case, as does age of onset. Thus babies born with such conditions need early referral and close monitoring so that intervention is timely to minimize long-term effects. With the syndromic craniosynostoses other related abnormalities (e.g. cardiac, skeletal, renal) will vary from syndrome to syndrome.

Craniosynostosis can also be the by-product of a variety of other conditions, so-called 'secondary' synostosis. There is a higher incidence of raised intracranial pressure in this group which therefore require close monitoring.

Single-suture synostosis

Presentation
- Appears soon after birth or in early infancy, after the effects of birth canal moulding should have resolved.
- Most obvious feature is an abnormally shaped head, which is determined by affected suture (Table 6.1).

Table 6.1 Suture and resulting head shape

Suture	Approximate frequency	Descriptive term	Resultant head shape
Sagittal	1 in 5000	Scaphocephaly	Long and narrow
Metopic	1 in 15,000	Trigonacephaly	Pointed forehead
Unicoronal	1 in 2300	Plagiocephaly	Asymmetrically flattened forehead
Bicoronal	Rare	Brachycephaly	Bilaterally flattened forehead
Lambdoid	Very rare	Posterior plagiocephaly	Posterior asymmetric flattening

Signs
- Examine for raised intracranial pressure:
  - palpate fontanelles;
  - fundoscopy.
- Affected suture often ridged.

Investigations

Plain radiology
- Not particularly helpful since images are commonly poor quality and difficult to interpret.
- In the case of a unilateral coronal synostosis the shape of the orbit ('harlequin eye') may be helpful.

CT, MRI, or USS
- Of more use.
- In some units CT reserved for complex cases and those who decline surgery.

Management
- Refer all patients to a craniofacial team for comprehensive care (allows full diagnostic assessment and formulation of management plan).
- Indications for treatment:
  - to improve appearance;
  - small percentage of patients have associated raised ICP.
- Some evidence that surgical treatment results in better intellectual outcomes (but not universally accepted).
- Intervention involves:
  - removal of affected suture ('suturectomy');
  - remodelling of skull shape.
- Exact procedure and degree of remodelling will vary from case to case and craniofacial unit to unit.
- Cases involving the forehead: the key procedure is a fronto-orbital advancement:
  - recontoured skull components are plated into position with resorbable fixation;
  - in selected cases distraction osteogenesis is used.
- In general, surgery at about the age of 1 year in uncomplicated cases is the norm.
- For sagittal synostosis surgery can be performed at 6 months (some centres advocate earlier surgery).
- For straightforward single-suture cases follow-up after surgery is usually when the child starts school with the anticipation of no further intervention being necessary.
- In unilateral coronal synostosis there may be residual facial asymmetry that should be managed conventionally as for other facial asymmetries. Longer-term follow-up may be indicated.

Syndromic synostosis

There are numerous syndromes associated with synostosis. The most common are discussed, although management principles are the same for all.

Crouzon's syndrome

- Autosomal dominant condition associated with the *FGFR2* gene mutation.
- Commonly presents with a bicoronal synostosis but other sutures may also be involved.
- Extent of mid-face hypoplasia and degree of exorbitism variable.
- Incidence of raised ICP much higher than non-syndromic bicoronal synostosis.
- Presenting problems vary as does the time of presentation but commonly the diagnosis is suspected at birth or soon after.
- There are often subtle skeletal abnormalities affecting the limbs but these are rarely obvious or symptomatic.

Apert's syndrome

- Also an autosomal dominant condition caused by a mutation of the *FGFR2* gene.
- Craniosynostosis often affects the bicoronal as well as other sutures, resulting in a tall skull flattened anteriorly and occipitally.
- Variable hypertelorism with downward slanting of palpebral fissures.
- Variable exorbitisim.
- Shallow orbits and shortened skull base.
- Most obvious extra-cranial feature is a variable degree of hand and foot abnormalities with complex syndactyly. It is this feature that usually makes clinical diagnosis straightforward.
- As the child develops, the face takes on the shape of an inverted triangle:
  - hyperteloric eyes form the wide base;
  - hypoplastic maxilla often with crossed central incisors form the apex.
- Cleft palate is a common (17–43%) association and in those without a cleft the palate is narrow and high-arched.
- Intellectual impairment is more common than in Crouzon's syndrome.

Saethre–Chotzen syndrome

Presentation much more variable.
- Autosomal dominant.
- Late presentation (adulthood) common.
- Asymmetric complex bicoronal synostosis that may be mild (accounting for late presentations).
- Ptosis.
- Tear duct abnormalities.
- Low hairline.
- Parrot-beaked nasal shape.

Pfeiffer syndrome

- Autosomal dominant.
- Variable presentation of complex synostosis, the most severe being the clover-leaf skull (Kleeblattschädel) deformity.
- The digits (particularly thumbs and big toes) are broad and short.

Principles of management

Diagnosis

- Prenatal diagnosis becoming more commonplace.
- Diagnosis in early postnatal period still the norm.
- Clinical assessment confirmed with genetic testing.

Initial management

- Aimed at assessing and minimizing effects of the condition on vital functions:
  - breathing;
  - eating;
  - scleral cover;
  - presence of raised ICP.
- In some cases urgent tracheostomy and eyelid surgery is necessary.
- Consider feeding via a NGT.
- Systematic approach to investigate for additional abnormalities.
- Significant amount of time needs to be devoted to counselling parents and other family members about the condition and its implications.

Early management

- In general, approach to the cranial abnormalities similar to single-suture cases.
- Surgery aimed at increasing cranial vault volume and improving the overall shape, thus dealing with the potential raised ICP and aesthetic concerns.
- Number of different designs of procedure for each type of abnormality and different units utilize different approaches.
- Surgical principle—re-assembled skull bones held in position with resorbable fixation.
- In some units there is a move away from initial fronto-orbital advancement. Instead a posterior skull vault expansion is carried out delaying any further aesthetic procedures to the anterior of the skull until the craniofacial complex is further developed.
- For some cases, particularly those with significant symptomatic exorbitism, a monoblock procedure can be carried out:
  - fronto-orbital bar left attached to the mid-face;
  - whole unit is advanced, bringing the maxilla, orbital rims, and forehead forward.
- Distraction osteogenesis has been used as an alternative to conventional osteotomies and plate fixation.

- In terms of timing the initial cranial vault expansion, a balance between a number of factors needs to be reached:
  - if the infant is developing signs of raised ICP then surgery should not be delayed;
  - in elective cases the general state of development, co-morbidity, and size should be taken into account;
  - in most craniofacial units surgery is proposed from 6–15 months of age with the tendency for earlier surgery for sagittal synostosis.

Infancy to adolescence
Monitoring for re-synostosis.

Treatment of associated problems
- Proactive management of vision and hearing.
- Genetic assessment and counselling of parents should they be considering having more children.
- Consideration of further mid-face surgery and/or hypertelorism correction.
- Orthodontic input.
- Management of obstructive sleep apnoea. This can occur as a result of mid-face retrusion and, therefore, mid-face advancement may be helpful. Investigation with formal sleep studies and appropriate imaging will help identify and quantify the problem, as well as aid in localizing the level of airway obstruction.

Adolescence to the completion of growth
- Emphasis should be on final aspects of surgery to mid-face and skull.
- Regular monitoring for the functional manifestations of raised ICP (clinical features as well as papilloedema and formal optic field assessment).
- Developmental and psychological issues.
- Patients should be assessed and managed as for other facial abnormalities:
  - conventional orthognathic surgery;
  - distraction osteogenesis;
  - other aesthetic surgery techniques, e.g. rhinoplasty, forehead recontouring.

Torticollis and positional skull deformity

Both of these conditions deserve mention because they are often mistaken for craniosynostosis, particularly a unilateral coronal synostosis. In addition the management of deformational skull deformity is controversial with a variety of experts utilizing helmet moulding to improve the head shape.

Torticollis

- Damage to the sternocleidomastoid muscle (either inter-uterine or as a result of birth trauma) results in shortening.
- Occasionally a mass forms in the muscle—'sternomastoid tumour'.
- Diagnosis is clinical:
  - baby's head tilted to the affected side;
  - restriction of head rotation to the contralateral side.
- USS can be helpful.
- The asymmetric pull can cause a skull base torsion and plagiocephaly.
- Treatment initially with active physiotherapy, although a small number (up to 10%) benefit from a surgical release of the tight sternomastoid muscle.

Positional skull deformity

- Thought to be the result of inter-uterine and birth canal moulding compounded by the adoption of a preferred head side whilst the baby is lying supine.
- The 'back to sleep' campaign encouraging parents to let babies sleep supine to reduce the incidence of sudden infant death syndrome (SIDS) has resulted in an ↑ incidence of positional/deformational plagiocephaly.
- Typically results in posterior (occipital) skull flattening with one side being more affected than the other and ipsilateral frontal bossing giving a parallelogram shaped head.
- No evidence that the condition predisposes to facial or temporomandibular joint disorders.
- 💣 *Management is controversial:*
  - most craniofacial surgeons believe that the condition is largely self-correcting and tends to improve as the child gains head control, with any resultant deformity being posterior and not likely to be obvious. Therefore management is expectant with head positioning away from the favoured side and 'tummy time';
  - other experts treat more actively with helmet moulding therapy. These devices are worn for a significant proportion of the day over several months and are most effective if treatment is started between the ages of 6 and 12 months;
  - to date, no RCTs assessing the efficacy of latter treatment (only case series reporting good outcomes).

Craniofacial procedures

Le Fort III osteotomy
- Used for significant facial retrusion.
- Allows advancement of the whole face.
- Can be a conventional procedure with bone grafting, plate and screw fixation, or the advancement can be attained with distraction osteogenesis.
- Distraction can utilize buried internal devices (with the activation rods exiting transcutaneously) which push the maxilla into its new position or external devices (halo frame) that pull the maxilla.

Surgical access
- Bicoronal scalp incision.
- Orbital floor approach (not always necessary) via lower eyelid or transconjunctival.
- Intra-oral approach for pterygoid dysjunction (may be approached from bicoronal incision).
- See Chapter 5 for operative details; ➜ Maxillary procedures, p. 232.

Hazards
- Encroachment of cranial cavity with low anterior fossa and high cut through bridge of nose.
- Excessive bleeding particularly from pterygoid venous plexus.

Modifications
Can be combined with a simultaneous Le Fort I osteotomy to optimize aesthetic and occlusal result.

Fronto-orbital advancement and cranial remodelling
- Standard procedure for the management of craniosynostosis.
- Numerous modifications and adaptations using both conventional fixation techniques (resorbable) and distraction osteogenesis.
- In addition there are procedures that involve remodelling without fronto-orbital advancement that are used for sagittal synostosis or posterior skull procedures (Fig. 6.1).

Surgical access
- Bi-coronal scalp incision.
- Craniotomy to access the areas being recontoured.

Bone cuts
- Determined by the particular procedure in use.
- Multiple modifications described.

Hazards
- As the procedure is often performed on infants blood loss can be significant even with the use of techniques such as cell savers.
- Dural tears can occur particularly in those cases with raised ICP.

Monoblock advancement

- Modification of the fronto-orbital advancement that incorporates the maxilla with the forehead (Fig. 6.2).
- Carried out conventionally or as a distraction osteogenesis procedure.
- Can be performed as part of an initial skull vault expansion procedure or as a second later procedure.

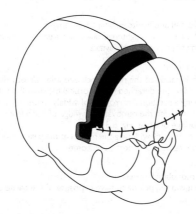

Fig. 6.1 Fronto-orbital advancement.

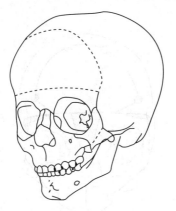

Fig. 6.2 Monoblock advancement.

Surgical access
- Bicoronal scalp incision.
- Orbital floor approach (not always necessary) via lower eyelid or conjunctiva.
- Intra-oral approach for pterygoid dysjunction (may be approached from bi-coronal incision).
- Frontal craniotomy.

Hazards
- As for Le Fort III and fronto-orbital advancement.
- The risk of infection is heightened due to inherent communication between the nasal and cranial cavities.

Facial bipartition
- Further modification of the monoblock operation already described.
- Involves dividing the detached fronto-orbital bar/maxilla in the sagittal plane allowing a rotational narrowing of widely spaced orbital cavities (hypertelorism) with the removal of a wedge of bone from the forehead/bridge of nose (Fig. 6.3).
- Also has the effect of widening the maxilla at the palatal level.
- Used in management of Apert's syndrome.

Surgical access
- As for the monoblock procedure.
- In addition it is often helpful to have exposure of the palate to facilitate the palatal cut.

Hazards
- As for the monoblock procedure.
- Risk of oronasal fistula if palatal access obtained.

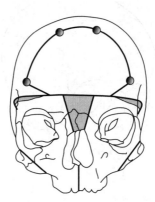

Fig. 6.3 Facial bipartition.

Box osteotomy for hypertelorism

Used for symmetrical or asymmetrical hypertelorism, as well as vertical orbital discrepancies that involves the whole orbit.

Surgical access

- Bicoronal scalp incision.
- Frontal craniotomy.
- Orbital floor approach (transconjunctival or lower eyelid).
- Intra-oral access is often helpful via an upper buccal sulcus incision.

Bone cuts

- A cut through the orbital roof, medial wall, floor, and lateral orbital wall is made.
- Zygomatic arch is sectioned and the nasal bones cut.

Hazards

- As for the monoblock procedure.
- Infraorbital nerve injury.

Craniofacial clefting disorders

The most commonly used classification of the various complex craniofacial disorders is that proposed by Paul Tessier who is rightly regarded as the father of craniofacial surgery. He proposed a simple numerical system ascribing a number to the soft tissue component and bony component of the cleft (Fig. 6.4).

Remarkably, in an era before cross-sectional imaging, Tessier predicted clefts before he had seen clinical examples of them. There is always an association between a soft tissue cleft and the bony clefts, but the severity of each is variable.

Principles of management

- Overall management planned to deal with the particular functional and anatomical abnormalities that each patient exhibits.
- In general, functional issues are dealt with in the first instance, e.g. if there are problems with scleral coverage which may result in corneal scarring and blindness. These must be addressed to prevent further complications.
- If the cleft involves a communication between the cranial cavity and the aerodigestive tract then surgery to separate the two should be considered.
- In terms of surgery to correct the cleft and/or hypertelorism delay tends to produce better outcomes and limits the number of surgical interventions.
- Surgery always remains a balance between optimal outcome and the particular functional, developmental and psychological issues that the patient and his or her family are facing.

Encephalocoeles

- Neural tube defects where neural tissue herniates through or causes a skull defect.
- If herniating tissue only contains meninges the defect is termed a meningocoele.
- Usually mid-line lesions with posterior encephalocoeles causing more in the way of functional problems.
- Craniofacial encephalocoeles may be frontal, ethmoidal, orbital, or sphenoidal.
- Herniated tissue usually comprises non-functioning glial tissue and can be removed without significant impairment.
- Resultant defects can be closed with a variety of techniques depending on size and location.
- In the frontal and ethmoidal group hypertelorism is a common feature. Facial bipartition is a useful technique to normalize the orbital position and close the cleft.

Craniofrontonasal dysplasia

- Clefting condition characterized by a mid-line facial cleft.
- Usually has an X-linked inheritance pattern.
- ♀ are usually more severely affected.
- Hypertelorism and cleft nose can be treated following the principles of management described in ➔ Craniofacial procedures, p. 282.

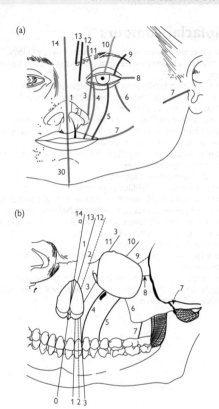

Fig. 6.4 (a) Tessier classification of facial clefts. (b) Bony clefts of the face.

Craniofacial tumours

- Tumours that are defined by anatomy rather than pathology.
- By their nature a heterogeneous group of malignant and benign tumours.
- May be facial (or orbital) tumours that originate outside the cranial cavity and then grow to involve it, or they may originate from within the cranial cavity to involve the face.
- Each tumour must be managed on an individual basis taking into account its anatomy and pathology. In addition the therapeutic objective (curative or palliative) must be decided.
- Access may be with wide exposure and craniofacial bone disassembly, or using endoscopic techniques.
- Surgical approach can be classified as:
  - transoral (including mid-face degloving);
  - transnasal (endonasal, lateral rhinotomy or total rhinotomy);
  - transfacial (allows access to maxillary/sphenoid/ethmoid sinuses and pterygomaxillary space, via incision from medial canthus along nasojugal groove and through upper lip);
  - transcranial (anterior craniotomy);
  - lateral (posterior lateral/pterygoid fissure/petrosectomy approaches).
- Key reconstructive consideration is sealing the cranial cavity from the aerodigestive tract. This can be achieved with local pericranial/muscle/galeal flaps or free tissue transfer.

Vascular malformations of the head and neck

The classification of vascular malformations is often complex with multiple terms for the same pathology and similar terms for differing pathology.

Vascular malformations

The endothelial turnover is normal and, therefore, usually only gradually increase in size. However, may be prone to more rapid growth with hormonal changes such as pregnancy. High-flow lesions can increase in size due to recruitment of adjacent vessels probably as a result of the ↑ blood flow.

Low-flow malformations

Venous malformations

- Can occur at any site and present with symptoms related to the site of origin.
- Usually head and neck lesions are obvious with skin or mucosal discolourations that blanch on pressure. Often they become more prominent on straining, lying down, or in a head-down position as the venous pressure increases ('turkey wattle' sign).
- Present at birth but may only become evident in infancy.
- Diagnosis is both clinical and radiological.
- Variety of imaging modalities are used:
  - duplex Doppler—simple, non-invasive method of differentiating high-flow from low-flow lesions;
  - MRI/MRA;
  - CT/CTA;
  - conventional angiography.
- Management primarily with interventional vascular radiological techniques utilizing sclerosant agents, such as absolute alcohol, sodium tetradecyl sulphate (STD), and bleomycin.
- Surgery has a minor role in the complete excision of suitable lesions and debulking of larger lesions.

Capillary malformations

- Seen as superficial port wine stains.
- Often confined to the distribution of a single branch of the trigeminal nerve.
- May form a component of Sturge–Weber syndrome.
- Treatment can improve the appearance of the lesions. Usually carried out with a pulsed dye laser.
- Surgery has minimal role.

Lymphatic malformations

- Often termed cystic hygromas.
- Can be divided histologically into micro- and macro-cystic lesions.
- Aggressive surgical debulking may be necessary in the very large lesions but their site often precludes surgical intervention.

- Infections, such as upper respiratory tract infection (URTIs) often cause dramatic and painful swelling of the lesion. Such infections should be treated aggressively with antibiotics and surgical drainage when a collection is identified.
- Injection of the lesion with sclerosant agents or OK423 (lyophilized Group A haemolytic *Streptococcus*) are newer treatment modalities that may be useful.

Mixed lesions

- Not uncommon.
- Presentation will depend on the proportions of the mix.
- Management as previously described.

For many of the lesions complete cure is unattainable and offering support to help deal with the consequences of the resultant facial disfigurement is very important. Camouflage make-up techniques may also be helpful.

High-flow malformations

Arterio-venous malformations

- Present as pulsatile mass.
- Spontaneous haemorrhage and skin ulceration indicate a more aggressive lesion.
- The pathology is usually an abnormal connection between the arterial component and venous drainage missing out the damping effect of the capillary bed. This forms the nidus of the lesion.
- As flow increases the veins dilate and often become tortuous with additional small vessels being recruited to aid the venous drainage.
- In very large lesions a steal effect or high-output failure may occur.
- Curative management is pre-operative embolization (utilizing beads, coils, glue or Onyx®) followed by surgical resection of the lesion.
- In some cases surgical resection is not possible and embolization alone can be carried out. However, this carries the risk of recurrence and the development of collateral vessels that may make subsequent endovascular intervention more difficult.

Vascular tumours

- Haemangioma is the commonest childhood tumour.
- Not present at birth but develop rapidly (proliferative phase) and present as a red, vascular lesion (strawberry naevus).
- Can occur at any site through head and neck.
- Skin lesions common (60%).
- Proliferative phase usually reduces at 7–10 months.
- Lesion gradually regresses until age of 7–10 years.
- Treatment is expectant unless the lesion interferes with development, e.g. obstructing vision, on the developing vocal cords or is causing significant symptoms (recurrent bleeding).
- Initial active treatment is with beta-blockers (propranolol).
- Intra-lesional and/or systemic steroids, interferon as well as surgery can be used for lesions that do not respond.
- If lesion does not fully involute laser treatment and/or surgery may also be useful.

Hemifacial microsomia

- Commonest facial abnormality after cleft lip and palate.
- Also known as:
  - craniofacial microsomia;
  - first and second arch syndrome;
  - Goldenhar syndrome;
  - oculo-auricular-vertebral syndrome.
- Some experts reserve the term Goldenhar syndrome for those cases where there are significant cervical spine and visceral organ abnormalities.
- Characterized by a 3D failure of growth affecting the orbit, mandible, ear (auricle), facial nerve, and overlying soft tissues.
- Severity of abnormality for each component is variable so that it is possible, for example, to have a severely affected mandible with normal facial nerve function.
- Can occur bilaterally.
- May be associated with cleft palate and macrostomia.
- Pathogenesis unclear. It has been suggested that an intra-uterine vascular event affecting the stapedial artery is responsible.
- Majority of cases are thought to be sporadic and multifactorial.
- Small proportion may have an autosomal dominant or recessive inheritance pattern.
- Number of classification systems used to score the severity and, hence, aid treatment:
  - OMENS;
  - OMENS+;
  - Pruzanski as modified by Kaban (this only scores the mandibular abnormality).

Management

- Aimed at dealing with functional problems first (associated cleft palate is treated as usual).
- In early life, and in severe cases, breathing and feeding may be compromised. If these are problems and result from a very small mandible, intubation, feeding tube placement, and/or tracheostomy may be necessary. In such cases early mandibular distraction may have a role.
- The affected child should be monitored for developmental progress. Hearing assessments are mandatory. Increasingly the use of bone-anchored hearing aids is being advocated, even if contralateral hearing is normal.
- As child develops (particularly towards the end of the mixed dentition) consideration to:
  - mandibular reconstruction (utilizing costochondral grafting);
  - mandibular lengthening (utilizing distraction osteogenesis);
  - simultaneous Le Fort I osteotomy or active orthodontics to level developing maxillary cant.

- As the child enters early teens consider ear reconstruction:
  - dependent of the degree of pinna abnormality and patient wishes;
  - autologous reconstruction vs implant-supported prosthesis.
- As growth reaches completion, final stages of management should be considered:
  - conventional orthognathic surgery with pre- and post-surgical orthodontics;
  - malar augmentation techniques;
  - finally soft tissue augmentation (fat transfer techniques, free tissue transfer, and fillers).

Treacher Collins syndrome

- Autosomal dominant disorder with variable penetrance.
- 1/50,000 live births.
- Characteristic features include:
  - zygomatic bone abnormalities with bony clefting;
  - mandibular hypoplasia;
  - abnormally formed pinnae, external auditory canals, and middle ears;
  - high-arched maxilla with clefts (30% of cases);
  - anti-mongoloid slanting of the palpebral fissures;
  - inferior placement of the lateral canthal ligaments;
  - true colobomas (25% of cases)—a coloboma is a gap in part of the structures of an eye;
  - pseudocolobomas (50% of cases).

Management

- Similar to that of hemifacial microsomia.
- Early priorities are to deal with functional problems, particularly airway compromise secondary to mandibular hypoplasia.
- Distraction osteogenesis has a significant role.
- In severe cases early tracheostomy may be necessary.
- A MDT addressing all the different aspects of care best provides the management.
- Malar reconstruction is best delayed until the age of ~9 years of age.
- Definitive orthognathic surgery should be performed at the completion of growth.

The craniofacial team

Key to the provision of modern craniofacial care is the multi-disciplinary craniofacial team that provides not only surgical skills but also a wide range of equally important talents to provide comprehensive care to this group of patients. The model of organization will vary from unit to unit, but the patient will need regular input from the following specialties:
- Neurosurgery.
- Craniofacial surgery (maxillofacial or plastic surgery).
- Ear, nose, and throat surgery.
- Genetics.
- Ophthalmology.
- Psychology.
- Speech and language therapy.
- Orthodontics.

In addition, most patients may require intermittent input from one or more of the following specialties:
- Paediatrics (general).
- Respiratory medicine.
- Audiological medicine.
- Endocrinology.
- Paediatric dentistry.

There is significant overlap between the craniofacial team and the cleft lip/palate team in some units, particularly in the USA. On occasion the teams are merged to operate as a cleft craniofacial team.

Key to the functioning of all craniofacial teams are clinical nurse specialists and psychologists, who provide much of the support and help that families need.

Organization of craniofacial services in the UK

Craniofacial services in England and Wales are provided by four supra-regional craniofacial centres. They are funded to provide services for the congenital paediatric cases requiring transcranial surgery, although extend their services to adults and a wider case mix. In Scotland the centre in Glasgow provides both adult and paediatric services. In Northern Ireland single-suture synostoses are treated locally, while complex disorders are referred to the Department of Craniofacial Surgery in Birmingham.

Further reading

Hayward, R., Jones, B., Dunaway, D., and Evans, R. (eds) (2004). *The clinical management of craniosynostosis.* Cambridge University Press, Cambridge.

Posnick, J. (2000). *Craniofacial and maxillofacial surgery in children and young adults.* WB Saunders Company, Philadelphia, PA.

Useful contacts

Department of Craniofacial Surgery, Birmingham Childrens' Hospital, Steelhouse Lane, Birmingham B4 6NH, UK. Tel: +44 121 333 8073. E-mail: elizabeth.mcalister@bch.nhs.uk

Great Ormond Street Hospital NHS Trust, 24 Great Ormond Street, London WC1N 3JH, UK. Tel: +44 207 813 8445; Fax: +44 207 813 8446.

Oxford Craniofacial Unit, Level LG1, West Wing, Childrens' Hospital, John Radcliffe Hospital, Headington, Oxford OX3 9DU, UK. Tel: +44 1865 231085; Fax: +44 1865 231091. E-mail: craniofacial@orh.nhs.uk

Regional Maxillofacial Unit Glasgow, Southern General Hospital, 1345 Govan Road, Glasgow G51 4TF, UK. Tel: +44 141 232 7510; Fax: +44141 232 7508. E-mail: Louise.Morgan@ggc.scot.nhs.uk

Royal Liverpool Children's NHS Trust, Alder Hey, Eaton Road, Liverpool L12 2AP, UK. Tel: +44151 228 4811.

Online resources

Headlines (patients' support group): Gil Ruff, 128 Beesmoor Road, Frampton Cotterell, Bristol BS36 2JP, UK. Tel: +44 1454 850557. E-mail GilRuff@headlines.org.uk; ℘ http://www.headlines.org.uk/index.htm

Changing Faces (support group for patients with disfigurement): The Squire Centre, 33–37 University Street, London WC1E 6JN. E-mail: info@changingfaces.org.uk. ℘ www.changingfaces.org.uk. For young people: ℘ http://www.iface.org.uk. *Scotland* Tel: 0845 4500 640. *Northern Ireland* Tel: 0845 4500 732. ℘ http://www.changingfaces.org.uk/Home

Cleft lip and palate

Incidence

- Commonest facial anomaly in UK. ~1:1000 live births per year.
- Cleft lip (CL), with or without cleft palate (CP), and isolated clefts of the palate are two distinct conditions.

Cleft lip

- May or may not be associated with CP.
- Wide range of potential problems ranging from incomplete unilateral cleft lip through complete unilateral cleft to bilateral cleft involving lip, alveolus, and palate.
- Accounts for 60% of cleft lip and palate (CLP) cases:
  - 25% cleft lip alone (unilateral or bilateral);
  - 25% unilateral cleft lip and palate (UCLP);
  - 10% bilateral cleft lip and palate (BCLP).
- Racial variation in incidence:
  - common in Chinese people (~1:500);
  - less common in Afro-Caribbean people (~1:2000).
- Concordance rate in monozygotic twins ~60%.
- 15–30% have cleft as part of a syndrome:
  - Van der Woude;
  - hemifacial microsomia;
  - 22q11 micro-deletion known as velocardiofacial syndrome (VCF) or DiGeorge syndrome;
  - *EEC*—ectrodactyly ectodermal dysplasia and clefting syndrome.

Cleft palate

- Accounts for other 40% of CLP.
- Range from complete clefts of hard and soft palate to partial incomplete clefts of the soft palate.
- No racial variation, but ↑ association with syndromes:
  - Stickler syndrome;
  - 22q11 microdeletion (VCF);
  - trisomy 13;
  - trisomy 18.

Aetiology

Multifactorial

Genetic and environmental factors implicated.

In utero/maternal environmental factors

- Anti-convulsants, such as phenobarbital and phenytoin (10-fold increase).
- Alcohol use.
- Cigarette smoking (2-fold increase).
- Folic acid deficiency.
- Corticosteroids (3-fold increase).
- Hypoxia.
- Retinoids (vitamin A).

Chromosome abnormalities

- Methylenetetrahydrofolate reductase (*MTHFR*) gene on chromosome 1.
- *IRF6* on chromosome 1.
- *TGFA* on chromosome 2.
- *MSX1* on chromosome 4.
- *BCL3* and TGF-B on chromosome 10.
- *TGFB3* on chromosome 14.
- *RARA* on chromosome 17.
- Point mutations in genes *FOXE1*, *GL12*, *MSX2*, *SK1*, *SATB2*, and *SPRY2* may contribute to 6% of isolated CLP cases.

Genetic and environment interaction may increase risk

- 6-fold ↑ risk if mother smokes cigarettes and has *TGFA* genotype on chromosome 2.
- A *MSX1* defect on chromosome 4 increases the risk for mothers who drink alcohol or smoke cigarettes.
- Mothers are more susceptible to folate deficiency if they have MTHFR deficiency.

Diagnosis

Ultrasound

- Possible to diagnose clefting as early as 12 weeks of gestation by transvaginal ultrasound.
- Diagnosis is made by obtaining coronal and frontal planes of fetal face.
- Full anatomical survey is indicated if an oral cleft is diagnosed to rule out other associated syndromes.
- Detection rate dependent on a number of factors:
  • experience of operator;
  • gestational age at the time of the study;
  • indication for the study;
  • technology used.
- Cleft Lip and Palate Association (CLAPA) survey (2006) reported that 45% of respondents had an antenatal diagnosis compared with only 15% in 1996.
- 3D USS has been shown to increase diagnostic accuracy especially using the reverse face or 'flip face' view.
- Ultrasound is more accurate in diagnosing isolated CL and CLP (67–93%), but is limited in making the diagnosis of isolated CP (7–22%).
- Detection rates improve markedly after 20 weeks of gestation; therefore, patients with ↑ risk of clefting and a normal early ultrasound should have a repeat scan after 20 weeks.
- Clefts may be classified on ultrasound into five types:
  • *type 1*—isolated cleft lip;
  • *type 2*—unilateral cleft of the lip and palate;
  • *type 3*—bilateral cleft of the lip and palate;
  • *type 4*—median cleft lip;
  • *type 5*—clefts associated with amniotic banding of limb-body-wall complex.
- The type of the cleft has been correlated with chromosomal abnormalities, structural anomalies, and fetal death.
- The more severe the cleft the greater the risk is of associated chromosomal abnormalities, structural anomalies, and fetal death.
- Once diagnosis has been made antenatally parents should immediately be referred to the local cleft team for appropriate counselling and support.
- False positive diagnoses do occur and patients should be informed accordingly.

At birth

- In those cases where an antenatal diagnosis has not been made, the aim is to diagnose all clefts at birth and for parents to be contacted by a member of the local cleft team within 24h.
- A recent CLAPA survey reported that 45.3% of clefts were diagnosed antenatally, 41% at birth, 4.4% within 24h, and a further 9.3% after 24h with one patient only diagnosed after 12 months.

- Designated cleft nurse specialist should be available to give further counselling and support to the family, where necessary including advice by telephone and home visits.
- Appropriate psychological support should be provided (see ➔ Psychology, p. 328).
- Specialist feeding and nursing advice should be implemented at the time of birth.
- The child and parent should be seen in a multidisciplinary outpatient clinic soon after birth by team members who will be involved in their long-term care.
- Details of surgery should be discussed at this outpatient visit and dates for surgery provided where appropriate.
- The parents should be taken to see the ward to familiarize them with the hospital facilities.

Genetic advice
- All parents given the option of genetic counselling at birth (particularly important if syndromic diagnosis is suspected).
- Traditionally risk has been given as a percentage:
  - risk of having a second child with cleft lip and/or palate—4%;
  - risk of having a third child—10%;
  - risk if a member of the family has CLP to a first-degree relative—2%;
  - risk if a member of the family has CLP to a second-degree relative—0.7%;
  - risk if a member of the family has CLP third-degree relative—0.3%.
- Norwegian study has shown:
  - relative risk of cleft recurrence in first-degree relatives is 32 for any cleft lip and 56 for cleft palate alone;
  - risk of clefts in children of affected mothers is similar to the risk of clefts in children of affected fathers;
  - the parent–offspring risk is similar to the sibling–sibling risk;
  - association between cleft severity and patient's sex;
  - does not affect the risk of having a cleft.
- Genetic counselling recommended to young adults with cleft lip and/or palate.

Management of lip

Principles

- Clefts of the lip cause cosmetic and functional problems.
- Functional problems include impairment:
  - in the production of bilabial sounds (pa, pi);
  - of maxillary growth because of scar constriction.
- Babies with isolated cleft lip can usually feed normally, although they may have difficulty creating an adequate lip seal.

Anatomical defects in UCLP include:

- Discontinuity of skin, muscle, and oral mucosa of the upper lip on cleft side.
- Vertical soft tissue deficiency on medial aspect of the cleft.
- Abnormal muscle insertions into nasal spine and alar base.
- Alveolar cleft in region of the canine tooth.
- Defect in primary palate anterior to the incisive foramen.
- Rotation of septum, columella, and nasal spine away from the cleft.
- Separation of domes of the alar cartilages at the nasal tip and kinking of the lateral crus on the cleft side.
- Dislocation of lower and upper lateral cartilages on the cleft side.
- Displacement of alar base in all three planes of space.
- Displacement and flattening of the nasal bone on the cleft side.

Anatomical defects in BCLP include:

- Discontinuity of skin, muscle, and oral mucosa of the upper lip bilaterally.
- Bilateral defect of alveolus and anterior palate.
- Central segment consisting of prolabium and pre-maxilla with short columella.
- Lack of orbicularis oris continuity.
- Collapse of lateral palatal segments behind pre-maxilla.
- Alar domes and middle crura are splayed, caudally rotated (bucket handle), and subluxed from their normal anatomic position overlying upper lateral cartilages.

Surgical options

- Lip repair is usually carried out at 3–5 months in UK.
- Neonatal lip repair, while still practised in some units abroad, has fallen into disrepute in the UK.
- Many different protocols for lip and palate repair worldwide.
- The following protocols and timings reflect practice in most UK cleft centres.

Unilateral cleft lip and palate

- The lip, nose, and anterior palate are repaired at the first surgery at 3–5 months of age in healthy children.
- Anterior palate is repaired with an unlined turnover flap from the vomer (popularized by surgeons in Oslo, Norway) (Fig. 7.1).

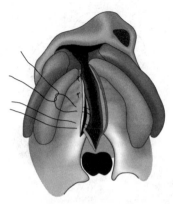

Fig. 7.1 Vomer flap for hard palate repair in a right unilateral cleft of the lip and palate.

Important steps in lip repair include:
• Skin incision design.
• Subperiosteal mobilization.
• Muscle repair.
• Nasal floor restoration.
• Alar base positioning and primary nasal dissection.

Design of skin incisions important to accomplish:
• Symmetry.
• Equal lip length.
• Natural appearance of the cupid's bow.
• Inconspicuous scarring and restoration of the nostril floor.

Many different techniques have been described for lip repair:
• Straight-line techniques (Rose–Thompson).
• Rotation advancement techniques (Millard, Delaire).
• Lower lip Z-plasties (Tennison–Randall).
• Combinations of these.

Individual techniques have advantages and disadvantages:
• Millard (Fig. 7.2):
  • scar mimics philtral column on cleft side;
  • reconstructs nasal sill;
  • allows some leniency in surgical technique (cut as you go);
  • may result in short lip on cleft side;
  • scar crosses philtral column at nasal base.
• Tennison (Fig. 7.3):
  • useful for repairing a wide cleft;
  • may result in a long lip;
  • scar crosses philtral column inferiorly.

Many now use a combination of these two techniques to take advantage of the strengths of each technique and discard the weaknesses (Fig. 7.4).

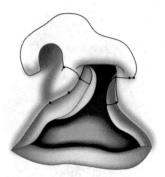

Fig. 7.2 Millard lip repair.

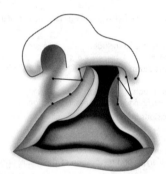

Fig. 7.3 Tennison lip repair.

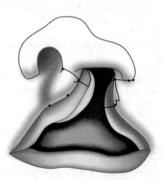

Fig. 7.4 Combination of Millard and Tennison repair.

- Radical subperiosteal mobilization of tissues of the cleft side (which includes incision through inelastic periosteal layer) to orbital rim, zygomatic process, and pyriform rim. It is important to ensure that muscle and skin is closed without undue tension; this also aids in accurate repositioning of the alar base.
- Dissection and repair of orbicularis oris muscle.
- Skin of the lip is dissected off the muscle medially and laterally.
- Muscle repaired with resorbable or non-resorbable sutures.
- Primary bone grafting or gingivoperiosteoplasty (GPP; at the time of lip repair) is not widely practised in UK.
- Primary bone grafting is thought to impair growth.
- GPP requires pre-surgical orthopaedics to bring the alveolar segments into close apposition.
- Pre-surgical orthopaedics for unilateral cleft lip and palate patients is not routinely carried out in UK.
- Repair of the nose (not done by all in UK) is carried out by:
  - separating skin from the alar cartilage on the cleft side (as described by McComb and Andel);
  - approached both from lateral and medial aspects of the alar cartilage through the skin incisions already made for the lip repair;
  - repositioned structures of the nose are maintained using either buried slow-resorbing sutures (e.g. PDS) or external tie-over splints.

Bilateral cleft lip and palate
- Very little conformity (2008 surgical interest group meeting) in UK about:
  - use of pre-surgical orthopaedics;
  - technique for repair;
  - timing of repair.
- Formal surgical repair is often preceded by pre-surgical orthopaedics to reposition the premaxilla posteriorly and align the lateral alveolar segments.

Principles of repair
- Symmetry should be maintained meaning that repair of both sides should occur simultaneously (asynchronous lip repair is practised by three units in UK and Ireland).
- Establish primary muscle continuity (if undue muscle tension exists at time of primary repair then final muscle repair is deferred for about 9 months to a year).
- Median tubercle may be reconstructed from either the prolabium (if patient has a well-developed white roll on the prolabium) or from the lateral lip elements (if there is a poorly developed white roll on the prolabium).
- Reconstruction of the labial sulcus from the prolabial mucosa and lateral lip elements (some rely on muscle action to create a labial sulcus and do not formally reconstruct the sulcus).
- Hard palate repair varies widely and includes:
  - complete closure with a vomer flap on both sides;

- complete closure on one side with a full vomer flap and partial repair of the opposite side with a vomer flap raised up to the pre-vomerine suture;
- complete closure on one side only leaving the contralateral side open.
- Variation in hard palate repair exists because raising a full bilateral vomerine flap may compromise blood supply to the pre-maxilla, but raising the flap to the pre-vomerine suture and no further is thought to maintain the blood supply to the pre-maxilla. If only one side is repaired at the first surgery then the child is brought back after approximately 6 weeks to close the contralateral side with a vomer flap.
- The nose is repaired as previously described for unilateral patients except both sides of the nose are dissected and primary positioning of the alar cartilages is carried out to construct the nasal tip and columella.

Incomplete lip

- Principles are the same as for complete cases and a functional repair should always be carried out.
- It is also important to address the nose in incomplete cases as there is usually a lip/nose deformity.

Management of palate

Principles

- Functional palatal repair is important for speech and may be important for Eustachian tube function.
- Timing of palatal repair is controversial:
  - early closure prior to 1 year has been shown to benefit speech;
  - delayed hard palate closure has only shown consistently improved growth when delayed into adolescence, but this results in unacceptably poor speech.
- Common practice in UK is to close the soft palate in cleft lip and palate patients and the entire palate in isolated cleft palates between 6–9 months.
- Underlying deformity includes (Fig. 7.5):
  - narrow and vertically displaced palatal shelves;
  - abnormal insertion of palatal muscles;
  - abnormal muscle in syndromic patients.

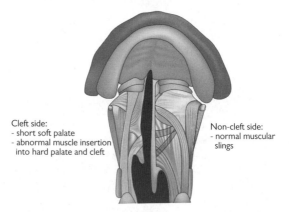

Cleft side:
- short soft palate
- abnormal muscle insertion into hard palate and cleft

Non-cleft side:
- normal muscular slings

Fig. 7.5 Palatal muscles—normal vs cleft side.

Surgical options

- Hard palate in complete cleft lip and palate patients is repaired in the UK using a vomer flap (see ➲ Management of lip, p. 302 and Fig. 7.1).
- Many different techniques have been used to close the palate including:
  - Von Langenbeck;
  - Widmaier;
  - Veau–Wardill–Kilner;
  - Bardach two-flap technique with intravelar veloplasty;
  - Furlow double opposing Z-plasty;
  - Sommerlad radical micro-dissection.

- Von Langenbeck releasing incisions are still used in wide clefts.
- Veau–Wardill–Kilner push-back techniques still widely used in some countries, but abandoned in UK because of:
  - unfavourable mid-facial growth;
  - compromised dental arch form;
  - difficult to manage fistulae;
  - excessive palatal scarring;
  - poor speech outcome.
- Sommerlad repair of the palate with microscopic magnification recreation of the levator veli palatini sling is widely practised in UK. Procedure involves:
  - incision along cleft margin at junction of oral and nasal mucosa;
  - mobilization of mucoperiosteum of hard palate in subperiosteal plane;
  - separation of oral mucosa with minor salivary glands from muscles and nasal mucosa;
  - division of oral insertion of tensor veli palatini tendon;
  - suturing nasal layer with soft palate muscles still attached;
  - separation of tensor veli palatini and palatopharyngeus from the back of the hard palate;
  - dissection of levator veli palatini from the nasal mucosa keeping the nasal mucosa intact;
  - alignment of the levators transversely and suture of the levators together in the midline to reconstitute the levator sling;
  - closure of oral layer using resorbable sutures;
  - lateral releasing incisions in the oral layer (Von Langenbeck) are used to reduce tension on the oral repair in <15% of cases (usually only) in extremely wide clefts;
  - 5% of patients repaired using the Sommerlad technique have required secondary speech surgery.
- The Bardach double flap:
  - widely practised in USA;
  - hard palate is raised as two flaps subperiosteally giving access to soft palate musculature, which is repaired with an intravelar veloplasty;
  - secondary speech surgery needed in >20% of patients.
- Furlow double-opposing Z-plasty:
  - widely practised in USA;
  - lengthens the palate and re-aligns levator veli palatini muscles;
  - difficult in wide clefts;
  - asymmetrical repair;
  - normal or near normal speech reported in >85% of patients.

Management of alveolus

Aims of alveolar bone graft
- Stabilize alveolar arch.
- Restore arch integrity.
- Allow teeth to erupt into optimal position.
- Permit orthodontic alignment of arch.
- Simultaneous oronasal fistula repair.
- Creation of a platform for prosthetic replacement, e.g. implants.
- Optimize maxillary surgery.
- Create support for the nose (alar base) and lip.

Assessment
- OPT and occlusal radiograph.
- Periapical radiograph if necessary.
- CBCT scanning (becoming more popular).
- Important to decide whether tooth extractions need to be done. At the time or at least 3 months before to allow attached gingiva to heal.
- Pre-surgical orthodontic treatment to align alveolar segments and optimize position of teeth adjacent to the cleft.

Principles of surgery
- Pioneered by Boyne and Sands.
- Mucoperiosteal flaps are raised on both sides of the cleft on the buccal and palatal sides (Fig. 7.6).
- Reconstruction of nasal layer and create a nasal seal.
- Nasal dissection superiorly up to the piriform rim and nasal floor.
- Some place collagen membrane below the nasal layer to improve the nasal seal.
- Bone is packed into the space between the nasal layer and oral layer bridging the alveolar segments, and should extend posteriorly into the palatal cleft, superiorly to the nasal floor, and laterally to the paranasal region.
- Defect should be over-filled as resorption of up to 30% may occur.
- Oral closure is effected by advancing the lateral buccal mucoperiosteal flap medially to create an oral seal.
- Lateral buccal flap advancement will leave exposed alveolar bone laterally, which will heal by secondary intention without complication.
- Post-surgical orthodontics follows to provide stability, while bone graft is incorporated and heals.

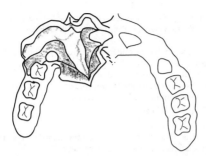

Fig. 7.6 Alveolar bone graft—flaps raised and nasal layer closed.

Outcome assessment of alveolar bone

Outcome assessment of grafting is based on:

- Success of fistula closure.
- Eruption of canine and bony support for adjacent teeth.
- Objective radiographic measurement using panoramic and occlusal radiographs to assess bone height, and more recently conventional or CBCT to assess bone height and width.
- Common rating scales include the Bergland, Kindelan, and Chelsea (Witherow) scales.
- Bergland scale compares the level of the inter-dental septum on the grafted side to the normal side and the aim is to achieve grade I or II:
  - *grade I*—normal height;
  - *grade II*—>75% normal height;
  - *grade III*—50–75% normal height;
  - *grade IV*—< 50%.

Timing

Primary bone grafting (at time of lip repair 3–6 months of age)

- Began in the 1950s.
- Carried out at same time as lip repair with wide dissection and bone (split rib) used to bridge gap.
- Abandoned by all in original form as shown to severely inhibit maxillary growth.
- Primary grafting still part of the treatment protocol in some units in the USA, but in a modified form.

Gingivoperiosteoplasty

- Increasing support in recent times in some US and European centres.
- Requires pre-surgical orthopaedics to bring alveolar segments into near contact.
- Gingival flaps adjacent to the cleft are raised, taking care not to damage underlying tooth germs, and sutured together.
- Evidence that GPP decreases the need for alveolar bone grafting later.

- If alveolar bone grafting is needed later, there is limited evidence to suggest that those patients initially treated with GPP have a better outcome.
- Others have shown that secondary bone grafting is superior to GPP and counsel against GPP.
- GPP still not universally supported because of:
  - lack of long-term maxillary growth studies;
  - lack of consistent results between centres;
  - burden of care for parents.

Early secondary (2–5 years)
- May improve periodontal support for central incisor on the cleft side and facilitate lateral incisor eruption if present.
- Early post-grafting orthodontics to correct incisor crossbite at this age may improve horizontal maxillary hypoplasia.
- Disadvantages include orthodontic compliance and prolonged orthodontic treatment.
- Not widely practised as there is a lack of long-term maxillary growth outcome data.

Secondary (6–13 years): in the mixed dentition
- Most commonly applied technique in UK.
- Timing determined by development of the canine tooth on the cleft side.
- Grafting is carried out when the canine root is half to two-thirds formed.
- Allows eruption of the canine into the newly grafted zone.
- Established technique with long-term growth and dental outcomes.

Late (>13 years): in the permanent dentition
- This results in poor outcome with:
  - compromised periodontium;
  - ↑ tooth loss adjacent to cleft;
  - more need for prosthodontic rehabilitation;
  - higher fistula rate;
  - poor alar base support.
- Not recommended in the UK for planned care.

At time of Le Fort I maxillary osteotomy
Not recommended as maxillary segments are not in continuity and it is easier to complete osteotomy if the maxilla is in one piece.

Donor site (for secondary alveolar bone grafting)
- Grafting material for alveolar bone grafting may be autogenous, xenogenic, allogenic, or alloplastic.
- Particulate bone grafts are superior to block cortical or corticocancellous grafts because they are more readily incorporated into the alveolus with the capacity for post-operative remodelling.
- Several autogenous donor sites have been used for alveolar bone grafting including iliac crest, rib, calvarium, tibia, and mandibular symphysis.

Iliac crest
- Regarded as the gold standard for alveolar bone grafting.
- **Advantages:**
  - rich in osteogenic cells;
  - rapidly transformed into alveolar bone;
  - substantial amounts of cancellous bone can be easily obtained;
  - two-team operating shortens procedure time;
  - excellent long-term outcomes reported.
- **Disadvantages** relate to donor site morbidity:
  - prolonged post-operative pain;
  - gait disturbances;
  - long hospital stay;
  - unsightly scars;
  - sensory disturbance (neuropraxia of lateral cutaneous nerve of thigh).
- Immediate post-operative pain control using infusion techniques and minimally invasive harvesting techniques with trephines have reduced morbidity significantly.

Calvarial bone
- **Advantages:**
  - minimal scarring;
  - minimal post-operative pain;
  - mesenchymal bone.
- **Disadvantages:**
  - cortical bone with minimal cancellous bone;
  - small volumes;
  - dural tears and infections;
  - osteogenic potential of graft affected by technique used;
  - single-team operating.
- Results not as good as iliac crest.

Tibia
- **Advantages:**
  - ease of harvest;
  - minimal morbidity (pain, infections);
  - good long-term outcomes;
  - two-team operating.
- **Disadvantages:**
  - scarring;
  - limited volume of bone;
  - tibial plateau fractures in up to 3% of cases.

Mandibular symphysis
- Method of choice in some European centres.
- **Advantages:**
  - mesenchymal bone;
  - no visible scar;
  - minimal pain and shortened hospital stay;
  - satisfactory long-term outcomes.

- Disadvantages:
  - single-team operating;
  - technically difficult with significant learning curve;
  - damage to the mandibular permanent tooth germs with subsequent tooth loss;
  - limited amount of bone.

Rib
- Now abandoned as:
  - significant resorption.
  - poor long-term outcome.

Bone substitutes
- **Advantages:** no donor site morbidity.
- **Disadvantages:**
  - slower graft revascularization;
  - long-term results equivocal;
  - unpredictable bone formation;
  - unpredictable resorption.

The use of bone substitutes is still not recommended in children.

Bone morphogenic proteins
- Have shown promise in a number of animal models.
- May replace autogenous grafting in the future, but a suitable carrier in humans still to be found.

Revision procedures

Lip

- Residual imperfections and imbalances may occur following primary repair as a result of:
  - poor alignment at the time of surgery;
  - distortion during growth;
  - scar contracture;
  - closure under tension in wide clefts;
  - poor muscle reconstruction.
- Lip distortions should be evaluated together with the nose, bony skeleton, and dentition.
- Underlying skeletal imbalance will be reflected in the soft tissue drape and should be considered when planning lip revision (especially in the older child and adolescent).
- Lip revision is indicated for:
  - lip length discrepancies;
  - vermillion deformities;
  - mucosal excess or deficiency;
  - inadequate muscle reconstruction;
  - poor cutaneous scars.
- Each deformity should be considered on its own merits.
- Mucosal and vermillion deformities can often be treated using:
  - local flaps;
  - Z-plasties;
  - V–Y advancements.
- Lip length discrepancies, poor cutaneous scarring, and inadequate muscle reconstruction usually requires formal revision of the entire lip rather than an attempt to improve the deformities with limited intervention.
- Timing of lip revision may vary and the decision to treat is taken together with parents and child (older children and adolescents will often make their own decisions).
- Obvious deformity should, where possible, be treated before the child starts school to facilitate integration and avoid stigmatization.
- In uncertainty or parental conflict a clinical psychologist should be involved.

Palate

Revisional surgery of the palate is indicated for two main reasons:
- Velopharyngeal incompetence (VPI) secondary to physical inadequacy of the velopharyngeal mechanism.
- Repair of oronasal fistulae.

Surgery for VPI

Philosophies vary from unit to unit regarding optimizing palatal function as identified by video fluoroscopy vs obturating the velopharyngeal gap identified on naso-endoscopy.

Assessment
- Speech.
- Clinical examination.
- Lateral videofluoroscopy.
- Nasendoscopy.

Surgical options based on fluoroscopy include:
- Palatal re-repair to posteriorly reposition levator palatini in the velum and utilize full length of the palate.
- Oral Z-plasty to gain length together with levator palatini repositioning surgery (Furlow's reverse Z-plasty).
- Hyne's pharyngoplasty.
- Coleman fat transfer.
- Buccal interpositional flaps.
- Z-plasty of the oral layer.
- Speech prosthesis.
- Superiorly-based pharyngeal flap.

In summary, the aim of this philosophy of treatment is to provide an optimally-functioning palate in the first instance and to address the anatomical abnormalities that exist thereafter, without creating permanent airway obstruction.

Nasendoscopic diagnosis is useful:
- In those with a coronal closing pattern and a velopharyngeal gap laterally—the aim of surgery is close the lateral gaps (most commonly carried out with an Orticochea or Jackson sphincter pharyngoplasty).
- In those with a lateral 'sphincteric' closing pattern with a gap in the midline—the aim of surgery is to close the midline gap with a midline pharyngeal flap pedicled either superiorly or inferiorly and tailored to the size of the gap.

These surgical options will tether the velum, narrow the velopharyngeal airway, and create a permanent obstruction with potential obstructive sequelae.

Speech in cleft patients has a tendency to deteriorate with age because of the relative increase in pharyngeal size due to growth, adenoid lymphoid tissue involution, and pharyngeal shape change. This means long-term follow-up into adulthood.

Surgery for oro-nasal fistulae
- Common sequelae of cleft palate repair.
- May represent a failure in technique or a problem in wound healing which is often a result of excessive tension.
- Reported incidence varies widely (0–34%).
- Incidence is related to the extent of clefting and surgical technique, but not age at the time of palatoplasty or gender.
- Symptoms associated with oro-nasal fistulae include:
  - audible nasal air escape during speech;
  - hypernasality;
  - food regurgitation into nose.

- Not all fistulae are symptomatic and therefore not all require intervention.
- The decision to treat fistulae is determined on an individual basis, and is guided by speech assessment and patient morbidity.
- Successful fistula repair improves symptoms directly associated with the fistula and velopharyngeal function, therefore existing symptomatic fistula should be repaired before embarking on formal velopharyngeal management.

Fistula repair is often technically challenging because of:
- Excessive scarring.
- Lack of virgin local tissue.
- Ease of access.

No single technique is consistently satisfactory and reported rate of successful closure varies from 33–90%. Many different techniques for closure have been described. Broadly divided into:
- Local soft tissue flaps (turnover flaps, rotation flaps, island flaps).
- Local soft tissue flaps with inter-positional grafts (conchal cartilage, alloplastic materials such as PDS or collagen membranes).
- Regional intra-oral (tongue flaps, buccal flaps, facial artery myomucosal flaps).
- Extra-oral (naso-labial).
- Free tissue transfer (radial forearm, fibula flaps for composite reconstruction).

The technique chosen is based upon:
- Position and size of the fistula.
- Nature and number of previous attempted repairs.

The basic fundamental principle in repairing oro-nasal fistulae is to repair the defect in layers (especially ensuring adequate repair of the nasal layer). The addition of conchal cartilage or alloplastic interpositional grafting has improved success rates.

Management of nose

Primary

- Primary repair carried out at the time as primary lip repair.
- Historically it was believed that primary surgery to the nose would compromise nasal growth and was therefore discouraged.
- Long-term outcomes of a consecutive series of unilateral and bilateral cases showed that primary rhinoplasty does not compromise nasal growth and paved the way for a more aggressive approach to the nose at the time of primary lip repair.
- Various techniques to maintain cartilage repositioning following surgery include:
  - external and internal suspensory sutures;
  - temporary tie-over splints;
  - longer-term internal and external silicone splints.

Secondary

The nose, despite improved results following primary rhinoplasty at the time of lip repair, often requires adjustment on more than one occasion.

Early secondary rhinoplasty

- Age 3 to adolescence, but often prior to school attendance.
- Carried out to improve appearance of the nose to avoid peer ridicule and specifically to address:
  - obvious deformities of the tip, lower lateral cartilage, and alar base in UCLP patients;
  - shortened columella, tip deformities, and widened alar bases in BCLP patients.
- Access to the nose may be via a rim incision in milder cases or more commonly through a trans-columella open tip approach.

Complete septorhinoplasty

- Vomer osteotomies and grafting where necessary.
- Delayed until skeletal maturation is complete.
- Should also only be carried out after orthognathic surgery has been undertaken.
- Cleft nose deformity complex—usual multiple interventions increases the difficulty of the surgery.
- Unless only very minor adjustments are indicated, complete cleft septorhinoplasties should be carried out as open procedures.
- Important to try to address the patient's concerns and wishes as long as these are realistic.
- Patients benefit from at least one session with the team psychologist to:
  - help them articulate their concerns;
  - gauge their expectations;
  - prepare them for surgery.

Orthognathic surgery

- Need for orthognathic surgery varies according to cleft type.
- Lack of maxillary growth may be inherent, but is probably a consequence of soft tissue scarring following primary surgery.
- Improved primary surgical technique means that maxillary growth is compromised less.
- Commonly the maxilla is hypoplastic in all three planes of space resulting in:
  - skeletal Class III jaw relationship;
  - maxillary narrowing (maxillary transverse discrepancy);
  - ↓ facial height.
- Bi-maxillary surgery is commonly indicated, and may include all or a combination of the following:
  - maxillary advancement;
  - maxillary down-grafting;
  - segmental maxillary surgery;
  - mandibular setback;
  - genioplasty.

Traditional orthognathic surgery

Challenging because:
- Large movements often required.
- Extensive scarring from previous surgery makes mobilization and retention of final position difficult.
- Presence of a pharyngeal flap.
- Abnormal bony anatomy with potential to compromise the blood supply to the premaxilla in bilateral cleft cases.
- ↑ tendency to relapse.
- Despite all of these points relapse can be overcome by:
  - aggressive mobilization;
  - adjunctive bone grafting;
  - rigid fixation.
- There is recent evidence to show that rate of relapse in traditional orthognathic surgery is comparable to distraction osteogenesis regardless of the distance moved.
- Traditional orthognathic surgery has the following advantages:
  - more cost-effective than distraction;
  - patient only needs one procedure;
  - patient does not have the burden of prolonged treatment with unsightly distractors.

Distraction osteogenesis

Provides alternative to traditional orthognathic surgery especially in cases that require large movements.

Use external or internal distractors.

Advance 1mm/day after carrying out Le Fort 1 cuts.

Advantages:
- in some series evidence that there may be less relapse especially after large advancements when distraction is used (not replicated in all studies);
- may affect speech less;
- able to adjust if speech becomes compromised.

Disadvantages:
- need to wear unsightly frame for 6–8 weeks if using external distraction with negative psychological consequences;
- expensive equipment;
- extensive work-up if internal distraction is planned;
- need for more than one surgical procedure.

Effect of orthognathic surgery/distraction on speech

- It is important to be aware that maxillary advancement may compromise VPI function and speech.
- Pre-operative speech assessment will give an indication of the risk of developing VPI, but there is no method that will reliably predict which patients will develop it. This is partly because:
  - it is not possible to adequately assess palatal functional reserve;
  - development of VPI after maxillary advancement is not always related to the distance moved.
- Pre-orthognathic/distraction speech investigations include:
  - speech and language therapy assessment;
  - lateral videofluoroscopy;
  - nasendoscopy.
- The chances of VPI developing can be minimized by:
  - careful planning and pre-operative assessment;
  - bi-maxillary surgery to minimize maxillary movement;
  - possibly by utilizing distraction techniques.

Speech

- Development of speech is lengthy and complex, and usually proceeds through a number of stages.
- Process is dependent on a number of factors, including the ability to hear and the presence of an intact velopharyngeal mechanism. Cleft patients may be compromised on both of these fronts.
- The palate separates the oral and nasal cavity with the soft palate permitting two-way air flow at the velopharyngeal orifice.
- In the normal patient, the soft palate is able to close off the nasal airway during speech. This enables the voice to be shaped by the mouth or oropharynx, and is therefore critical for the production of oral sounds.
- English speakers need to produce oral pressures to make all sounds apart from 'm', 'n', and 'ng'.
- Elevation of the soft palate during swallowing prevents food/fluids passing into the naso-pharynx.
- The presence of a cleft palate results in deviant and restricted sound development, and influences pre-speech development in cleft children. This continues to have an influence on speech development post-palate repair even in those children with competent velopharyngeal mechanisms.
- Early babble patterns are indicative of how later speech may develop and this has influenced the timing of palatal repair.
- Speech therapists encourage surgeons to repair the palate at least by the age of 1 year and in many cases earlier.
- In the normal palate the levator veli palatini muscles run transversely across the central 40–50% of the palate and on contraction the palate is lifted to close the velopharynx.
- In CP and submucous CP the levator veli palatini muscle insertions are abnormal:
  - in CP they insert into the side of the cleft;
  - in submucous CP they are discontinuous and variably anteriorly displaced.
- The consequence of poor palatal function is poor speech, which influences social integration.
- The aim of palatal surgery in general and of soft palate surgery in particular is to provide the patient with an adequately functioning velopharyngeal sphincter.
- VPI in cleft patients may result from:
  - poor palatal function post-surgical repair;
  - undiagnosed submucous clefts of the palate;
  - palatal-pharyngeal disproportion;
  - neuromuscular dysfunction.
- Characteristics of cleft speech maybe divided into:
  - resonance/airflow errors;
  - hypernasality;
  - hyponasality;
  - mixed resonance;
  - nasal emission;
  - nasal turbulence;
  - nasal facial grimace.

- Cleft-type speech characteristics:
  - palatal realization;
  - lateral realization;
  - non-oral articulations;
  - nasal realizations.
- These speech problems are related to the abnormal oral and/or nasal structure associated with cleft patients including:
  - VPI;
  - nasal obstruction;
  - oro-nasal fistulae;
  - dental malocclusions;
  - skeletal abnormalities.
- Cleft speech is therefore complex, and requires assessment and treatment by speech and language therapists specifically trained in and dedicated to cleft patients.

Speech assessment

The role of the speech and language therapist is to:
- Assess speech.
- Determine the relationship between speech and structure.
- Devise appropriate treatment strategies.

Speech assessment can be divided into:
- Perceptual listening.
- Clinical examination.
- Use of adjunctive investigations.

Role of speech therapy

Speech therapy can be divided into:
- **Articulation therapy:**
  - the bulk of speech therapy focuses on articulation therapy, which has been shown to result in overall speech improvement;
  - focus of treatment is to modify place of articulation to more anterior positions consistent with normal speech;
  - even in patients with hypernasality improvement in placement of consonant articulation will have a positive effect on intelligibility;
  - patient outcome is improved if therapy is offered on a frequent basis (more than weekly).
- **Resonance therapy:** there is little support in the literature for therapy to modify hypernasality, although more recently there are some who believe that therapy might reduce it, but the evidence for treatment success is still awaited.
- **Behavioural therapy:**
  - feedback therapy may be successful in certain selected cases and has the advantage that the patient, and the therapist are able to monitor the outcome of the intervention and in so doing change speech behaviour;
  - disadvantages of biofeedback include the need for expensive equipment, as well as patient dedication and compliance.
- **Voice therapy:** the abnormalities of voice seen in cleft patients are often a response to velopharyngeal dysfunction and these needs to be addressed accordingly.

Hearing

- Normal hearing is necessary for speech development.
- Eustachian tube (EUT) dysfunction with permanent hearing loss is common in CP.
- Impaired active dilatation and EUT dysfunction has been found in 100% of non-operated CP patients.
- The pathophysiology of EUT dysfunction is related to:
  - muscle pull;
  - oro-nasal reflux, which causes mucosal irritation, oedema, and tubal occlusion (all of which contribute to hearing loss).
- Functional palatal surgery improves velopharyngeal closure preventing reflux and allows tubal oedema to resolve.
- Air insufflation, viewed as an index of EUT function, has shown improvement in passive opening of the EUT following CP repair, but no difference in active opening due to muscular contraction.
- A high percentage of patients with CP will develop otitis media with effusion (OME) despite functional palatal surgery and all of these patients therefore require careful ENT and audiological surveillance throughout their childhood within the MDT setting.
- Some teams opt for aggressive short-term ventilation based on the finding that OME is almost universal in the CP population.
- Others will only place ventilation tubes if there is OME with significant hearing loss (>55dB HL on auditory-evoked brain stem response in the better ear).
- The NICE review on the current evidence on OME in children with CP concluded that there is a lack of evidence on the optimal treatment.
- Treatment should, therefore, be based on the needs of the individual child.
- Insertion of ventilation tubes at the time of primary lip or palate closure should only be carried out after careful otological and audiological assessment, and not inserted routinely.
- There is some case-review evidence for the effectiveness of hearing aids in these children and the alternative of early aiding should therefore be considered.
- NICE recommend the insertion of ventilation tubes as an alternative to hearing aids in children with CP who have persistent bilateral OME, and a hearing level in the better ear of 25–30dB HL or worse confirmed over 3 months.
- Some clinicians involved in the management of CP are concerned that the hearing level of 25–30dB HL recommended by NICE may precipitate an increase in the number of children undergoing ventilation tube insertion with their attendant complications.

Orthodontics

The role of the orthodontist is central to the care of patients with cleft lip and palate characterized by involvement throughout their development, beginning soon after birth and continuing through to the end of growth.

- In the early stages the orthodontist may be involved in pre-surgical orthopaedics.
- In the mixed dentition the orthodontist prepares the patient for secondary alveolar bone grafting.
- In the adolescent the orthodontist will carry out definitive orthodontic treatment separately or as part of a combined surgical orthodontic (orthognathic) treatment plan.

Pre-lip surgery

Orthodontic involvement may include:
- Primary impressions.
- Fabrication of:
  - feeding plates (now felt to be ineffectual);
  - plates to protect the vomer from ulceration;
  - plates to prevent tongue displacement into the palatal cleft in patients with Pierre Robin sequence.
- Pre-surgical orthopaedics (PSO) with or without naso-alveolar moulding (NAM).

Pre-alveolar bone graft

Primary dentition

Orthodontics in the primary dentition is rare and is limited to treatment of anterior crossbites.

Mixed dentition

- Orthodontics in the mixed dentition is mainly carried out to prepare the maxillary arches for bone grafting.
- The timing of therapy is based upon the development of the canine tooth in most units in the UK with the aim being to carry out grafting when the canine root is half to two-thirds formed, as stability of the bone graft is dependent on the presence of teeth within the area of the graft.
- Pre-alveolar bone grafting orthodontics is carried out to:
  - approximate alveolar segments;
  - move adjacent teeth into ideal positions (to enable adequate soft tissue coverage of the graft).
- Preparation for alveolar bone grafting in UCLP and BCLP cases may involve some or all of the following depending on individual need:
  - palatal expansion;
  - correction of anterior crossbite;
  - tipping of teeth;
  - removal of supernumary teeth that may compromise soft tissue closure.

- BCLP cases are complicated by the position of the pre-maxilla, which may need one or a combination of the following:
  - retraction;
  - intrusion;
  - protrusion;
  - osteotomy at the time of grafting to aid positioning.
- It is important to approximate the pre-maxilla and lateral alveolar segments to facilitate soft tissue closure.
- Post-operatively orthodontic appliances are left *in situ* for stability until healing of the bone graft has occurred.

Adolescent

- Therapy is usually accomplished with fixed appliances and treatment time is similar to non-cleft cases.
- Cleft patients, however, pose unique problems, including:
  - missing and malformed teeth, especially lateral incisors;
  - unusual dental positions such as canine impactions;
  - arch collapse with crowding;
  - anterior and posterior crossbites;
  - associated skeletal abnormalities;
  - ↓ facial height;
  - maxillary hypoplasia in all three planes of space (AP, vertical, and transverse).
- Where there is an underlying associated skeletal deformity the need for a combined orthodontic-orthognathic approach should be discussed early on in treatment.
- Attempts should be made to retain the lateral incisor if present.
- If the lateral incisor is missing then a decision needs to be made regarding its replacement either by:
  - closing the space and disguising the canine into the lateral incisor;
  - maintaining the space for prosthetic replacement.
- Following completion of orthodontics these patients need to continue wearing retainers to maintain the final occlusion.
- Final prosthodontic rehabilitation to replace the missing lateral incisor, where indicated will take place after completion of orthodontic treatment.
- If osseointegrated implants are planned then placement should only take place after growth is complete, meaning that a period of temporization may be necessary if orthodontics is completed early in adolescence.

Psychology

- Children pass through a number of developmental stages during which time certain tasks are mastered.
- Healthy psychosocial adjustment depends on the child's ability to successfully pass through each stage.
- This cannot be accomplished alone and depends upon the interaction of the child with the systems within which they function including:
  - family;
  - educational;
  - social;
  - medical.
- The child is at ↑ risk of psychosocial maladjustment during transitional points throughout development.
- Individuals with CLP have the potential for healthy psychosocial adjustment comparable to their peers, but they are at risk of:
  - cognitive;
  - behavioural;
  - emotional;
  - social difficulties.

The clinical psychologist

- Raises team members' awareness of important transitional points.
- Helps identify individuals at risk of psychosocial maladjustment who may benefit from psychological intervention to improve their psychosocial well-being.
- The role of the psychologist changes as the child passes through the various developmental stages on the way to adulthood.

Research has shown that adults with repaired CLP at are ↑ risk of psychosocial adjustment problems relating to:

- Psychological well-being (anxiety and depression).
- Reduced social contacts.
- Delays in marriage and having children.
- Clinical psychology intervention therefore explores:
  - underlying causes of psychosocial maladjustment;
  - promoting self-acceptance;
  - discussing treatment options in collaboration with the team.

Chapter 8

Aesthetics

Introduction

Definition

Aesthetic surgery can be defined as surgery carried out in an attempt to increase an individual's beauty. The term is used interchangeably with cosmetic surgery. It is surgery performed on normal individuals purely to improve appearance and, as such, implies that there is no functional or direct health-benefit gain. Congenitally normal but unaesthetic features, such as a disproportionately large nose, or features that are the result of normal or premature aging may be treated.

Facial age changes

All tissues of the face undergo changes with age. These, combined with gravity and environmental factors such as sun exposure and smoking, produce the characteristic changes in appearance associated with ageing:

- Skin becomes thinner due to ↓ collagen formation and less elastic. Static wrinkles form.
- Loss of subcutaneous fat results in loss of soft tissue volume.
- Muscle tone decreases and bone resorption around the piriform aperture results in loss of soft tissue support. As a result the tip of the nose descends and the nose lengthens.
- Occlusal tooth wear leads to a decrease in lower face height due to anti-clockwise rotation of the mandible. The chin becomes more prominent.
- Dynamic wrinkles due to underlying muscle action become established.
- The combined effects of gravity and weakening ligamentous support cause descent of facial fat pads and skin.
- Weakening of the orbital septum allows herniation of orbital fat resulting in eye bags. Inferior movement of the malar fat pad lengthens the lower eyelid and deepens the naso-labial grooves.
- Descent of buccal soft tissues leads to the formation of marionette lines and jowls over the mandible.
- Soft tissue laxity in the neck results in the characteristic neck 'wattle' and loss of the mandibular cervical angle.

Patient assessment and patient selection

History

- A full medical, psychiatric, social, and drug history should be obtained.
- Many patients take low-dose aspirin prophylactically and often do not volunteer this information unless asked. Aspirin significantly increases intra-operative bleeding and post-operative morbidity, and should be stopped at least 10 days before surgery.
- Smoking significantly decreases skin vascularity and is therefore an important consideration in facelift surgery.

- It is vital to determine precisely what concerns the patient, what their motivation for seeking surgery is, and to be clear what end result they want to achieve. Equally it is important that the clinician explains to the patient in terms that they understand what is realistically possible. Unrealistic expectations usually lead to an unhappy patient. Matching patient expectation to what can be delivered is one of the challenges of aesthetic surgery. If there is any suggestion of the patient being psychologically unsuitable for surgery, treatment should be avoided or a psychological assessment requested.

Examination

In addition to examining the specific feature that the patient is concerned about, the general facial morphology should be assessed and documented:

- Skin type and quality, facial proportions and asymmetries, and facial nerve function should be recorded.
- Standardized photographic records for record and treatment planning purposes are mandatory.

Non-surgical aesthetic techniques

Botulinum toxin

Botulinum toxin is a neurotoxic protein produced by the bacterium *Clostridium botulinum*. It is one of the most poisonous naturally occurring substances. Although highly toxic it can be used in minute therapeutic doses to treat painful muscle spasms and as a cosmetic treatment to relax muscles causing wrinkles. Chemically, there are seven serologically distinct toxin types designated A–G. The toxin is a two-chain polypeptide with a heavy chain linked by a disulphide bond to a light chain. This light chain is an enzyme that attacks a protein at the neuromuscular junction, preventing vesicles from anchoring to the membrane to release acetylcholine. By inhibiting acetylcholine release at the neuromuscular junction the toxin interferes with transmission of nerve impulses and causes flaccid muscular paralysis.

Botulinum toxin type A is marketed under the brand names Botox®, Vistabel®, Dysport®, and Xeomin®.

Botox® injection is the most commonly performed cosmetic procedure worldwide. In the USA, treatments ↑ by over 3000% between 1997 and 2003. In 2004, almost 3 million Botox® procedures were carried out.

Cosmetic use aims to decrease dynamic skin creases by paralysis of the underlying muscles, thereby producing a rejuvenating effect on the facial skin. Sites and muscles targeted include:

- Glabella (frown lines) by injection of the procerus and corrugator supercilii muscles (Fig. 8.1).
- Forehead: frontalis.
- Peri-orbital (crow's feet): orbicularis oculi (Fig. 8.2).

Less commonly, and more subtly, due to functional considerations:

- Oral commissures to correct a downturned mouth: depressor anguli oris.
- Chin: mentalis.
- Naso-labial folds: levator labii alaeque nasi.
- Lips: orbicularis oris.
- Neck bands: platysma.
- Decolletage: platysma.
- 'Gummy smile': to upper lip at base of nose.

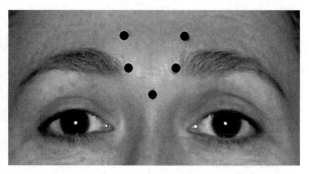

Fig. 8.1 Injection sites for glabellar lines.

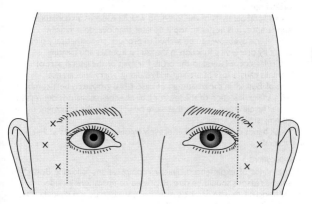

Fig. 8.2 Injection sites for crow's feet.

Practical considerations
- Use of topical anaesthesia and a fine gauge needle (30G, yellow) decreases patient discomfort. Use a 1mL syringe.
- 3 units of Dysport® are equivalent to 1 unit of Botox® or Vistabel®. Dysport® has a quicker onset and diffuses more than Botox®—efficacy is equivalent. Each injection can diffuse 2–3cm radially.
- May take up to 7–14 days to have its effect.
- Length of action is between 4 and 6 months.
- Dilute 100 or 50 units Botox® into saline for injection.
- 100 units in 5mL gives 2 units in 0.1mL; 100 units in 2mL gives 5 units in 0.1mL. Use small volumes and doses at each site—the greater the dilution the greater the diffusion.
- Common doses are:
  - glabella 5–8 units in 5 sites;
  - forehead 3–6 units in 6–10 sites (stay medially to preserve eyebrow arching—2 rows may be needed in a high forehead).
- To avoid extra-ocular muscle compromise—inject well away from orbital rim.
- Avoid total paralysis of the forehead which produces an unnatural appearance. It is better to top it up later than overdo it initially.
- The lateral eyebrow can be arched to produce an aesthetically pleasing result by preserving function in the lateral frontalis and treating orbicularis oculi lateral to the orbit. Paralysis of the lateral part of frontalis causes loss of arching and resulting 'angry appearance'.
- Use of Botox® in the treatment of naso-labial grooves is best combined with a filler. Injection of the levator labii alaeque nasi causes depressed upper lip elevation and can therefore be utilized in the treatment of the gummy smile.
- Neck bands can be treated effectively by injecting 3–5 units at 1–1.5cm intervals.

Complications
In the hands of experienced clinicians complications following Botox® for cosmetic reasons should be rare. Reported complications include:
- Extra-ocular muscle paralysis resulting in strabismus and diplopia. This normally corrects after ~6 weeks.
- Ptosis of the upper eyelid and brow.
- Asymmetrical muscle paralysis.
- Bruising.
- Haematoma.

Contraindications
Botulinum toxin should be avoided in patients suffering from neuropathic/neurological disorders. Injection into an infected site should be avoided.

Fillers

Dermal fillers are injectable substances used to augment the skin. They are used in the cosmetic treatment of static and dynamic wrinkles, as well as deep grooves such as naso-labial folds and marionette lines. They are also used in the treatment of depressed scars. Lips can be augmented with certain fillers.

For many years, the most commonly used agent was collagen. The major drawback with collagen is the possibility of allergy. Skin testing is therefore required prior to treatment. The most commonly used fillers in use at the present include the following:

- Restylane® and Perlane® are both made from hyaluronic acid, a natural carbohydrate polymer found in the ground substance of connective tissue. They last up to 6 months.
- Hylaform® is also a hyaluronate-based filler.
- Sculptra® is polylactic acid which stimulates production of autogenous collagen. The effect is therefore delayed and several treatments are often required to achieve the desired result. It lasts 18–24 months and is used extensively to treat facial lipoatrophy in AIDS patients. It is described as a volumizer rather than a filler.
- Radiesse® is a combination of calcium hydroxyapatite microspheres in a polysaccharide gel. It lasts about 2 years and stimulates collagen formation.
- Evolence® is a porcine collagen derivative with good handling properties and effects that can last more than a year.
- Artifill® is made of synthetic microspheres suspended in a bovine collagen gel. Its effects are claimed to be permanent.

Fillers are injected intradermally or subcutaneously in order to plump out the overlying soft tissues and smooth out wrinkles. Injection technique is key to achieving good results—along the length of fine lines (linear threading technique) or injected in a fan-shaped manner from several directions to fill deeper grooves. Even injection is required to avoid subcutaneous lumps. Injection sites should be massaged to encourage even distribution.

Complications

Include haematoma formation and infection. Uneven injection can lead to subcutaneous lumps, which may be visible as well as palpable.

Resurfacing techniques

- Dermabrasion.
- Microdermabrasion.
- Laser resurfacing.
- Chemical peels.

Dermabrasion

- Involves the use of a rotary hand engine with a diamond wheel or wire brush to abrade the skin.
- Is usually carried out under local or topical anaesthesia and is used for the treatment of age changes, scarring, or photodamage.
- Is commonly used to treat acne scarring, naevi, cloasma, and facial wrinkles.
- In skilled hands it is an extremely effective technique.
- Its main advantage is that the depth of injury can be directly controlled:
  - superficial dermabrasion is sufficient to treat fine wrinkles;
  - deeper treatment into the papillary or reticular dermis may be necessary in the treatment of deep scarring.

- Contraindications include keloid or hypertrophic scar formation, and a history of herpes simplex infections.
- Complications include keloid or hypertrophic scarring, hyper- or hypo-pigmentation, infections, persistent erythema, and oedema. Full-thickness injury to the skin results in healing by secondary intention and consequent scarring.

Microdermabrasion

This non-invasive technique involves the use of aluminium oxide particles to 'sandblast' the skin. This removes the superficial skin layer and produces mild oedema resulting in temporary reduction in fine wrinkles. It may have a rejuvenating effect by stimulating new collagen formation.

Laser resurfacing

Laser resurfacing using a CO_2 or erbium laser is used for similar indications to chemical peels and dermabrasion. Thermal injury to the skin results in removal of surface layers, contraction of collagen, and new rejuvenated collagen formation. The depth of injury produced is controllable with less risk of inadvertent over-treatment than with a chemical peel. It is particularly effective in the treatment of fine, non-dynamic lines and changes produced by photo-ageing. Erythematous scars can be improved and stepped scars may be treated by 'shoulder resurfacing'.

CO_2 treatment to the eyelids to produce skin contraction can be combined with transconjunctival orbital fat removal in cosmetic blepharoplasty.

Other lasers producing light of different wavelengths target various chromopores within the skin and are therefore used to treat varying conditions (Table 8.1).

Table 8.1 Lasers producing light of different wavelengths and their targets

Laser	Wave length (nm)	Skin chromophore
Argon	193	Melanin, blood
KTP	532	Melanin, blood
Krypton	531.7–647	Melanin, blood
Copper vapour	511	Melanin, blood
Dye laser	585	Melanin, blood
Ruby	694.7	Melanin
Alexandrite	755	Melanin
Nd:Yag	1064	Melanin, blood
Holmium:Yag	2100	Water
Erbium:Yag	2940	Water
Carbon dioxide	10,600	Water

Depending on the characteristics of the laser used, pigmented lesions including tattoos and vascular lesions may be treated.

- **Laser safety:** operating room personnel and patients should be protected from inadvertent ocular injury and the ETT from damage. The presence of bacterial and viral DNA has been demonstrated in the CO_2 laser plume. Special masks that filter such partials have been developed and should be worn.
- **Complications include:**
  - ocular damage;
  - full-thickness burn;
  - ectropion following laser blepharoplasty;
  - prolonged erythema;
  - milia;
  - skin irritation;
  - herpes simplex reactivation;
  - bacterial and fungal infections;
  - hyperpigmentation;
  - hypopigmentation;
  - hypertrophic scarring.

Chemical peels

A chemical peel is the application of a chemical agent that causes controlled destruction of the superficial layers of the skin. The superficial damage to the skin causes exfoliation and wound healing.

- **Peels reduce:**
  - fine wrinkles;
  - acne and other scars;
  - pigmentation abnormalities;
  - actinic keratoses;
  - lentigines (solar-induced freckles).
- **Common agents:**
  - glycolic acid;
  - trichloroacetic acid (TCA);
  - TCA with blue glycerine (a blue peel);
  - phenol (carbolic acid).

The effect is modulated by the strength of the solution used and the number of applications, which are determined by the lesion being treated and the skin type of the patient. Care must be taken when treating the eyelids where the skin is thinnest.

- **Complications:**
  - more likely with deeper peels and when using phenol;
  - hyperpigmentation;
  - persistent erythema;
  - reactivation of herpes simplex infection;
  - hypertrophic scarring.

Surgical techniques

Blepharoplasty

This is a procedure used to shape or modify the appearance of the eyelids. The word was first used by Von Graefe in 1818 to describe a procedure for repairing defects in the eyelids secondary to tumour excision.

The eyelids are one of the first structures of the face to develop permanent structural changes due to ageing.

- Changes in elasticity of:
  - orbital septum;
  - tarsus;
  - orbicularis muscle;
  - orbital septum.
- Result in:
  - excess skin;
  - wrinkles;
  - pseudoherniation of orbital fat;
  - baggy, tired looking eyes.

Blepharoplasty will not on its own treat malar bags or the tear-trough deformity.

Aesthetic goals

The perceived aesthetic ideals of the Caucasian eye are shown in Fig. 8.3. It is important to recognize the racial variations.

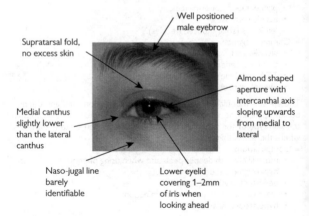

Well positioned male eyebrow

Supratarsal fold, no excess skin

Almond shaped aperture with intercanthal axis sloping upwards from medial to lateral

Medial canthus slightly lower than the lateral canthus

Naso-jugal line barely identifiable

Lower eyelid covering 1–2mm of iris when looking ahead

Fig. 8.3 Perceived aesthetic ideals of the Caucasian eye.

Assessment/history

As with all aesthetic patients:

- What patient perceives to be the problem.
- What are their expectations?
- Why do they want the surgery?
- Previous surgery.
- Dry eyes.
- Contact lenses.
- Diplopia.

The following areas should be assessed:

- Position of the eyebrow (sometimes a brow-lift is required).
- Amount of redundant skin.
- Symmetry, position, and relative excess of the fat pads.
- Ability to close the eyes easily.
- Position of the eyelids relative to the eyes.

Specific tests

- **Snap test:** examination for lower eyelid laxity. The lower eyelid is pulled down gently—it should snap back within 1s. With low elasticity this may only happen on blinking.
- **Distraction test:** is positive if the lower lid can be pulled down >7mm from the globe (indicates laxity of the lower lid). In these patients blepharoplasty without a lower lid tightening procedure may lead to ectropion and scleral show (the appearance of sclera below the iris when the patient looks ahead).
- **Examine for compensated brow ptosis:** look for descent of the eyebrows when the eye closes. This demonstrates that the brow is ptotic. In these patients frontalis activity keeps the eyebrows elevated when the eyes are open. This indicates that a brow lift may be required. Blepharoplasty in such patients may result in a worsening of their appearance.
- **Location of site of herniation of fat pads:** gently press on the globes and observe the areas of fat prolapse.
- **Presence of Bell's phenomenon:** usually on eyelid closure the globes rotate upwards and the cornea is protected. If absent there is risk of damage to corneas after blepharoplasty.
- **Ophthalmology assessment:**
  - should include visual fields and acuity;
  - if the patient has symptoms or signs of dry eyes then a Schirmer test is indicated;
  - take good standardized photographs.

Techniques of blepharoplasty

Upper

The eyelids are marked with the patient sitting up. The lower incision is marked so as to place the surgical scar within the supratarsal fold. The surgeon then pinches the excess tissue with blunt forceps until the lids separate slightly. This continues across the eyelid. Care is taken not to extend too far medially or laterally, as these areas produce visible scars. A strip of tissue including skin and orbicularis muscle is excised. If protruding fat needs to be excised from the medial and lateral upper fat pads this is achieved through small stab incision in the orbital septum. Beware a herniating lacrimal gland and the levator aponeurosis. Meticulous haemostasis is essential.

Lower

Great care must be taken with lower blepharoplasty as it is easy to excise excess tissue and in so doing produce an ectropion or scleral show. The incision is made just below the lower lash line (subciliary). Either a skin only, or skin and muscle flap is raised. With the mouth open (puts tension on the lower lid) the flap is elevated and the excess tissue marked and removed. The excised tissue is triangular in shape with the maximal vertical dimension beneath the lateral canthus. Fat removal, if required from the three compartments, is achieved by small incisions through the orbital septum. Care should be taken to ensure excess fat is not removed as this can cause an undesirable sunken appearance.

- **Lower lid transconjunctival blepharoplasty**—this technique enables fat from the three fat pads to be removed via an incision on the inside of the lower eyelid thus avoiding any external scars. However excess eyelid skin and orbicularis muscle cannot be removed.
- **Fat preservation techniques**—the grooves between the lower eyelid and the cheek skin are known as the tear-trough deformities. Correction of this defect can be achieved by transposition of orbital fat into the area (Loeb's/Hamra's technique) or placement of a Flower's tear-trough implant.

Other techniques involve tightening of the stretched orbital septum which replaces the orbital fat within the orbit.

Upper-eyelid fold reconstruction

This technique involves suturing the superficial layers of the eyelid to the deeper structures thus reconstructing the supratarsal fold.

Lateral canthopexy

Repositioning of the lateral canthus superiorly can improve lower eyelid position and reduce the possible complications of scleral show with lower lid blepharoplasties. Wedge resections of the lower eyelid may be necessary with very lax lower eyelids.

Complications of blepharoplasty

- Ocular damage.
- **Corneal abrasion and ulceration** can occur. Prevention by meticulous protection of the eye is important.
- **Dry eyes:** this is common in the immediate post-operative period and is due to oedema. A good pre-operative history is important to identify patients with a pre-existing history of dry eyes. Patients with persistent dry eyes should be referred to an ophthalmologist and prescribed artificial tears.
- **Haematoma:** meticulous haemostasis is essential during the procedure. If recognized in the immediate post-operative period should be evacuated.

- **Loss of eyelashes:** caused by diathermy or incision too close to the hair follicles.
- **Lower eyelid complications**, e.g. ectropion leading to epiphora.
- **Scleral show:** the lower lid should cover ~1mm of the limbus when the patients looks directly ahead.
- **Diplopia:** usually temporary following fat repositioning techniques due to the change in orbital volume. Can be due to damage to the inferior oblique muscle situated just within the margin of the bony orbit lying between the medial and middle fat compartments. Leads to double vision looking up and laterally.
- **Blindness:** this is the most devastating complication:
  - risk as reported by DeMere is ~0.04%;
  - the usual cause is retrobulbar haemorrhage within the immediate post-operative period;
  - ↑ pressure leads to retinal artery occlusion and ischaemia of the optic nerve;
  - it is essential to inform the patients of this risk and tell them to return if any severe pain occurs behind the eye, the eye becomes proptosed, or the visual acuity reduced;
  - emergency treatment is by lateral canthotomy and cantholysis, and then surgical decompression (see ➜ Initial management of ocular injuries, p. 16).
- Other complications such as infection are possible but rare due to the excellent blood supply to the area.
- **Asymmetry:** caused by over-resection of skin or fat.

Brow lift

- Consideration of the position of the brow is essential when assessing a patient who is requesting a blepharoplasty.
- If the brow position is too low then an upper blepharoplasty will make the aperture smaller and the patient will look worse.
- Surgical brow lifting can be performed either with open or closed (endoscopic) techniques.
- Minor elevation of the brow can be achieved with botulinum toxin when injected into the depressors (corrugator, procerus, and the superior lateral part of orbicularis oculis).
- An attractive brow should angle upwards in its medial half and drop down slightly or remain horizontal for the rest of the lateral brow. The female brow arches more and is slightly higher laterally compared with the male brow. The brow skin is thicker than the eyelid skin and it is important that this thicker skin should not occupy the normal position of the thinner eyelid, otherwise the patient will appear tired or cross.
- There is no agreed measurement to diagnose brow ptosis. Patients should bring photographs of themselves when younger to compare eyebrow level. However, a useful measurement is the distance between the inferior limbus of the cornea to the centre of the brow. If this is <22mm there is likely to be brow ptosis.

Techniques

- **Direct brow lift:** this is the oldest and simplest technique. There is little risk of damage to the facial nerve. It is suitable for patients with mild ptosis and bushy eyebrows. However, it leaves a visible scar above the eyebrows (Fig. 8.4).
- **Mid-forehead brow lift:** the incision line should be within a prominent horizontal skin crease. Transverse incisions are made in the galea centrally to avoid damaging the supraorbital nerves. Procerus and corrugator are divided. The galea is shortened as much as is required and the excess cutaneous tissue excised. Careful repair in layers is essential to avoid scarring.
- **Coronal forehead lift:** traditionally open but now almost exclusively endoscopic (Fig. 8.4).
- **Endoscopic brow lift:**
  - this technique uses 3–5 incisions placed within the hairy scalp anteriorly and laterally;
  - dissection centrally is in a subperiosteal plane, but lateral to the anterior temporal line the dissection should be below the temporoparietal fascia on the surface of the deep temporal fascia;
  - dissection continues over the lateral orbital walls and to the superior orbital rim;
  - supraorbital and supra-trochlear nerves are identified and protected;
  - an up-cutting periosteal elevator is used to divide the pericranium horizontally at a number of levels;
  - centrally over the glabella region the pericranium is divided and the corrugator supercilii and procerus exposed;
  - the brow is then lifted and suspended using a number of different techniques, e.g. screws, clips, or resorbable implants.

The endoscopic brow lift produces less loss of hair, paraesthesia, and scarring than coronal techniques. The procedure should not be used in patients with high hairlines as, after surgery, the hairline will be higher. In patients with high hair line and brow ptosis, a coronal approach at the hairline is indicated.

- **Complications of brow lifts:** include infection, haematoma, neurological damage, brow asymmetry, lagophthalmos (inability to close eyes) and hair loss.

Otoplasty

This is the surgical technique designed to correct congenitally prominent ears. Cosmetic otoplasty was first performed in 1881 (Fig. 8.5).

The auricle is a fibroelastic cartilage structure medially covered by connective tissue and skin. The arterial supply is from the posterior auricular and superficial temporal arteries. Sensory innervation is from the auricultemporal (V3) and great auricular (C3) nerves, Arnold's nerve (X), and branches from the facial nerve.

The auricle is fully formed at birth. It reaches 85% of its final size by the age of 3 years and is virtually adult size by 6 years. Elongation of the lobule in the older patient gives the appearance of continued ear growth.

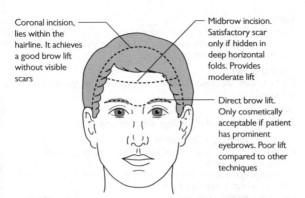

Coronal incision, lies within the hairline. It achieves a good brow lift without visible scars

Midbrow incision. Satisfactory scar only if hidden in deep horizontal folds. Provides moderate lift

Direct brow lift. Only cosmetically acceptable if patient has prominent eyebrows. Poor lift compared to other techniques

Fig. 8.4 Access for brow lift.

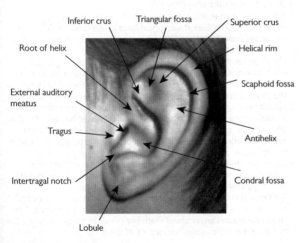

Inferior crus

Triangular fossa

Superior crus

Root of helix

Helical rim

Scaphoid fossa

External auditory meatus

Tragus

Antihelix

Intertragal notch

Condral fossa

Lobule

Fig. 8.5 Surface anatomy of the ear.

Aetiology of the prominent ear
- Excessively deep concha.
- Failure of an anti-helical fold to develop.
- A combination of these.

Other ear abnormalities include the 'constricted' ear, cryptotia (root of the helix is buried in the temporal skin), cup ear, shell ear, Stahl's ear, bat ear, Machiavellian ear, and lop ear.

Assessment

A full medical history is essential, including history of poor scars and keloid formation, together with assessment of patient's expectations, physical examination, and photographic records.

Timing of surgery

Ideally before the child becomes self-conscious of the problem (age 5–6 years).

Techniques

Techniques fall into either cartilage cutting or cartilage sparing.

Methods for correcting a deep concha

- **Suturing:** the concha is sutured down to the underlying mastoid fascia with mattress sutures.
- **Cartilage excision:** the concha is reduced in height by removing a full thickness crescent of cartilage from the conchal cup.
- **Cartilage scoring technique:** the anterior surface of the rim of the conchal cup reduces the conchal prominence.

Methods to reduce the anti-helical fold

- **Suturing technique:** Mustarde introduced a technique whereby sutures are placed from the scaphoid fossa to the concha to develop a new anti-helical fold. It has the advantage that, with no incisions, the anti-helical fold is smooth.
- **Cartilage scoring technique:** a number of different techniques have been developed to score partially through the anterior surface of the cartilage in the region of where the anti-helical fold should be. Relies on the physical properties of the cartilage, such that any physical alteration (incising or scoring) will cause the cartilage to deform away from the incised surface (Gibson principle). A tunnel is created between the skin and cartilage anteriorly. The cartilage is either abraded or scored (a simple and effective technique involves bending the tip of a 22G needle to right angles and using this to score the cartilage).
- **Posterior anti-helical fold weakening:** this technique weakens the posterior aspect of the anti-helical fold so that, when combined with suturing techniques, it will allow the cartilage to bend.
- **Incisional techniques:** Luckett described a technique whereby a single incision through the anti-helical line allows the fold to be created. The technique creates an unnatural sharp line (a pair of parallel incisions produces a more rounded appearance of the fold).

Post-operative care

- The ears should be dressed carefully. Jelonet® and cotton wool in proflavine allows gentle packing to maintain shape and support the healing cartilage.
- The ear is then covered anteriorly and posteriorly with gauze and cotton wool, and a light head bandage applied.
- It is essential that any complaints of pain be treated seriously. Haematoma beneath the skin can result in necrosis of the cartilage and distortion of the ear, as can too tight a bandage.

- The dressing is usually taken down on the first post-operative day and checked for any haematoma. The patient then has the head band replaced for a further week or wears a light sports band at night for a further 6 weeks.

Complications
- Haematoma.
- Loss of cartilage and resultant deformity.
- Asymmetry.
- Over- and under-correction.
- Keloid scars.
- Infection.

Facelift (rhytidectomy)

The effect of ageing and gravity on the face affects the skin and the deep structures leading to:
- Brow ptosis.
- Prominent naso-labial grooves.
- Marionette lines.
- Hollowing in the infraorbital regions.
- Jowls.
- Loose submental skin.
- Less elastic skin.
- Wrinkles.

Assessment of the patient
This involves a thorough past medical history and psychological profile. Any predisposing factors for infection or haematoma formation must be identified. Smoking should stop and aspirin should be discontinued at least 10 days prior to surgery.

Facelift anatomy
The facelift anatomy consists of a number of layers:
- Skin.
- Subcutaneous fat.
- Superficial musculo-aponeurotic system (SMAS).
- Muscles of facial expression.
- Thin layer of fascia.
- Facial nerve.

SMAS
- A layer of fascia continuous with the frontalis muscle, galea aponeurotica, temporoparietal fascia and platysma muscle.
- Is tightly bound to the zygoma.
- Is less distinct anteriorly at the level of the naso-labial fold.
- Sensory nerves lie superficial to the SMAS and most of the branches of the facial nerve lie deep to it.

There are a number of ligaments that secure the superficial structures to the bone (the retaining ligaments of the face):
- **Osseocutaneous ligaments**: i.e. over the zygoma (McGregor's patch) and anterior part of the mandible.
- **Musculocutaneous ligaments**: these are thickenings of the fascia between the muscle and the skin. They occur at the parotid and masseter.

Malar fat pad

This is a structure below the skin (second layer of the face). It is superficial to the SMAS. Different techniques have been described to elevate this structure, usually with the skin dissection to allow repositioning of the fat pad cranially.

Platysma

This is part of the SMAS/muscle layer in the cervical area. The medial aspects of the muscle become stretched with age giving the appearance of bands in the neck. Special treatment of the platysma is often necessary.

Nerves

The frontal branch of the facial nerve can be at risk during the facelift. It lies in the temporoparietal fascia and runs along Pitanguy's line (0.5cm below the tragus to 1.5cm above the eye brow laterally). The great auricular nerve that supplies sensation to the ear is susceptible to damage where it crosses the sternocleidomastoid muscle (Erb's point is where it crosses the posterior border).

Skin-only facelift

In this technique, the skin is undermined and any excess removed. It has the highest relapse rate and can look somewhat unnatural. Access is via pre-auricular (tragal) incisions with temporal and post-auricular extensions (hidden in the hair line).

SMAS/platysma facelift

- Access: as for skin-only facelift.
- Skin is undermined as far forward as the naso-labial fold and then the SMAS layer is elevated.
- The dissection layer must be changed when the zygomaticus muscle is reached, so that the dissection is superficial to the muscle to avoid damaging branches of the facial nerve.
- The SMAS can be tightened and the excess excised or plicated (and used to augment the zygoma).
- As the platysma and the SMAS are continuous, tightening the SMAS in a cephalad direction will also elevate the platysma.
- The changes in the cervical region depend on the structure of the bony mandible, position of the hyoid bone, anatomy of the muscles, and quantity of adipose tissue.
- The skin is draped over the tightened SMAS, analogous to clothes over a tight corset.
- Additional procedures on the platysma include platysmal plication medially, excision of part of the muscle, and resuturing. This gives a more enduring and natural appearance.

Mask/subperiosteal facelift

- Coronal and intra-oral incisions.
- Dissection is subperiosteally over the forehead, superficial to the deep temporal fascia to reach the zygomatic bone.
- Attachments to the zygoma are released.
- Intra-orally dissection proceeds subperiosteally over mid-face.
- Soft tissues are suspended.

- Technique allows changes to be made to the skeletal base, e.g. widening of the orbital aperture, reduction of the heavy supraorbital bone and augmentation of the malar region.
- Allows radical changes to the face, but recovery time is longer (several months).

Minimal-access cranial suspension (MACS lift)

- Benefits from shorted scar.
- SMAS suspended with non-absorbable sutures.
- Can be compared with the 'S' lift (mini facelift).
- Benefits from reduced recovery time.

Endoscopic facelift

The face can be dissected subperiosteally using a number of small incisions. This technique is indicated where there is little redundant skin.

Complications of facelifts

- Haematoma and secondary skin necrosis.
- Neurological injury (particularly the facial nerve).
- Loss of hair.
- Infection.
- Changes in skin pigmentation.
- Asymmetry.
- Pixie ears.
- Hypertrophic scars.

Liposuction

This is a technique for aspirating subcutaneous fat. Fat may be either in:

- Superficial compartments: contains many fibrous strands which are responsible for the skin dimpling in 'cellulite'.
- Deep compartments: fat in the deeper layers is less compact.
- Compartments are divided by the superficial fascia.

Once fat cells have been removed they cannot be replaced. However, the remaining ones can hypertrophy. Liposuction in the maxillofacial region is usually confined to the submental/cervical region, or is used to aspirate fat from the umbilical regions or inner aspect of the knee to augment other areas within the face.

Dry liposuction

This is a historical technique. Fat is aspirated without prior infiltration of tumescent solution. This method was associated with high blood loss. It has no place in the head and neck region.

Wet liposuction

Tumescent solution (Hartman's solution with added adrenaline, hyalase, LA, and steroids) aids liposuction and reduces haemorrhage infiltrated prior to the liposuction. The fat is aspirated using one of the many cannulae available. It is important that, when aspirating the fat, the tip of the cannula stops short of the skin as otherwise dimpling can occur.

Complications
- Damage to other structures.
- Paraesthesia.
- Haemorrhage.
- Infection.
- Contour irregularities.

Colman fat technique
- Described by Colman.
- Fat is aspirated, centrifuged, and serum removed.
- Purified fat re-injected using small cannulae and multiple passes through the tissues at different levels.
- It is reported that, using this technique, the fat cells remain viable and resorption of the fat is low.

Implants

In facial cosmetic surgical practice implant materials can be used to augment various anatomical sites. The most common sites are the nose, cheekbones, and chin.

The ideal implant material is:
- Inexpensive.
- Biocompatible.
- Inert.
- Free from the risk of transmitted infection.
- Dimensionally stable.
- Easily available avoiding a second surgical donor site.

Implant materials can be classified as:
- Autogenous grafts (from the same individual).
- Homografts (from the same species).
- Allografts (same species, non-identical).
- Isografts (same species, genetically identical).
- Xenograft (different species).
- Alloplast (implanted inorganic material).
- Autogenous implant materials include bone, cartilage, fat, and dermatofat grafts.
- Homografts and xenografts (bovine or porcine) include cadaveric lyophilized bone and cartilage.

Autogenous grafts

Bone and cartilage grafts are used to fill contour defects on the facial skeleton or for augmentation of normal structures. The nasal dorsum is commonly grafted with autogenous calvarial bone. All bone grafts are subject to resorption to a greater or lesser extent and, therefore, cannot be regarded as structurally stable. There is a common misconception that bone, which ossifies intra-membranously (e.g. calvarial), resorbs less than that which has an endochondral origin.

Cartilage is more dimensionally stable than bone. It may be harvested from the ear (conchal cartilage) or nasal septum. Larger amounts may be taken from the costal cartilages.

Alloplastic implants
- **Pre-formed alloplastic implants:** Medpor® (polyethylene), Proplast®, or silicone. Available in various sizes. Used extensively to augment:
  - chin;
  - mandibular angles;
  - zygomas;
  - fixed in position by screw fixation to the underlying bone.
- **Custom-made titanium implants:** can be used at various sites including calvarium, zygoma, and mandible. A 3D CT scan is required from which appropriate software allows a model to be milled by CAD/CAM technology or produced by stereolithography. An implant can be made as the mirror image of the normal side.

Rhinoplasty

Definitions

Rhinoplasty describes a range of surgical procedures that may be used to reshape the nose:
- **Primary rhinoplasty:** operation on a nose that has not had previous surgery.
- **Secondary or revision rhinoplasty:** surgery on a nose that has had one or more previous operations that have not produced the desired change.
- **Aesthetic or cosmetic rhinoplasty:** aimed at improving the appearance of the nose.
- **Functional rhinoplasty:** surgery aimed at relieving nasal obstruction.
- Aesthetic and functional rhinoplasties are frequently combined.
- **Closed rhinoplasty:** access to the nasal bones and cartilages is via incisions within the nose.
- **Open rhinoplasty** involves a trans-columellar incision, which is then extended along the vestibular surface of the columella to expose the lower lateral cartilages.

Anatomy
- The vault of the nose is formed by the nasal bones, the upper lateral cartilages, and the lower lateral cartilages (from above downwards).
- The lower lateral cartilages have medial and lateral crura.
- The nasal bones join the frontal bones at the radix and the nasal tip is attached to the upper lip by the columella.
- The nasal septum is made up of the septal cartilage, nasal crest of the maxilla, vomer, and perpendicular plate of the ethmoid bone.
- The skin lined entrance to the nose is called the vestibule. Hair growing in the vestibule are the vibrissae and the part of the vestibule immediately beneath the tip is the dome.

Planning

A thorough history and examination is required to ascertain precisely what result the patient wishes. Unrealistic expectations should be addressed at this stage and the achievable result discussed frankly. Computer programs that allow post-operative result prediction should be used with caution. Photographic records are essential.

Whilst some surgeons carry out analysis of facial morphology, measuring fronto-nasal, naso-labial angles, and the angular relationship of the nose to other facial features, most rely on clinical assessment alone.

Closed rhinoplasty access
- An inter-cartilaginous incision is made though the membrane between the upper and lower lateral cartilages.
- If joined to a cruciate incision through the membranous septum, access to the dorsum of the nose and caudal septum is achieved.
- A cartilage splitting incision achieves similar access and can be used when resection of the lower lateral cartilage is required.
- A rim incision is an incision along the inferior border of the lower lateral cartilage. If combined with an inter-cartilaginous incision, the lower lateral cartilage can be dissected and exteriorized to allow resection under direct vision.
- Bony osteotomies can be carried out either via the closed approach or with the aid of transcutaneous stab incisions.

Open rhinoplasty access
- Allows superior access to the nasal tip and is used when complicated adjustments to the nasal tip are required, e.g. in treatment of the cleft nose deformity.
- The nasal tip may be refined by resection of the cephalic border of the lower lateral cartilages and can be narrowed by approximation of the lower lateral cartilages.

The many techniques described for rhinoplasty, which can be used alone or in combination, allow both radical and subtle changes in shape to be achieved.

Reduction rhinoplasty
- Usually involves resection of the dorsum of the nose to reduce a nasal hump. This produces an 'open roof deformity', which is then corrected by lateral nasal osteotomies and in-fracture of the nasal bones.
- The nose can be narrowed by rasping or in-fracture.

Augmentation rhinoplasty
- Augmentation of the nasal dorsum involves placement of a graft to increase projection.
- Augmentation materials include:
  - autogenous/lyophilized (dried by freezing in a high vacuum) cartilage or bone;
  - alloplastic material, such as Medpore®.
- Spreader grafts between the septum and upper lateral cartilages widen the nose.

Rhinoplasty can be carried out with either local (± sedation) or general anaesthesia. Nasal splints placed during nasal bone fracture remain in place for 1 week. Recovery time to allow bruising to resolve is usually 2 weeks.

Complications
- Bleeding.
- Infection.
- Distorted sense of smell.
- Sinusitis.
- Septal perforation.
- Sensory disturbance (nose or upper anterior teeth).
- In the long term, changes due to scarring may distort the nose necessitating revision.

Cheiloplasty
- Cheiloplasty is the technical term for surgery which changes the size or shape of the lip.
- Lip reduction: the process of surgically reducing the size of the lip or lips in order to reduce the appearance of abnormally large or protruding lips.
- Lip enhancement for those who wish to make their lips larger.

Abnormally large or protuberant lips may be congenital (e.g. ethnic variations or the double lip deformity) or acquired (e.g. orofacial granulomatosis). Lip reduction surgery involves excision of an ellipse of mucosa, submucosa, and occasionally orbicularis oris muscle, extending from oral commissure to oral commissure. The anterior aspect of the incision is placed posterior to the lip seal and wet line so the scar is hidden.

Lip enhancement
Can be achieved using various materials:
- An injectable filler such as Restylane® (allows enhancement of the white roll of the lip and philtrum, as well as augmentation of the vermillion portion of the lip).
- More permanent results can be achieved using autogenous fascial grafts or an alloplastic material such as Gortex®.

Other considerations

Medicolegal matters

Cosmetic surgical practice is potentially a medicolegal minefield. Patients may have unrealistic expectations regarding outcomes. Narcissistic individuals can be impossible to satisfy and litigation is common. Thorough pre-operative assessment to determine the patient's wishes and frank discussion about what surgery can achieve and possible complications are imperative to avoid future unhappiness with outcomes. Detailed contemporaneous notes should be kept and a 'cooling down' period (2 weeks minimum) allowed between consultation and treatment.

Ideally patients should be seen twice for consultation before surgery. The patient should be written to after each consultation with a summary of the discussion. Where necessary, a witness should be present if a consultation is likely to be contentious. Increasingly cosmetic practitioners are videoing consultations. Finally, the cost of treatment and who will pay for treatment of complications should be discussed prior to surgery so there can be no doubt about the patient's financial liability.

Regulation of cosmetic practice

A review of the regulation of cosmetic treatment in the UK was recently published by the Department of Health in response to the PIP breast implant incident. The key recommendations of the committee, chaired by the Chief Medical Officer, Sir Bruce Keogh are:

- The scope of the EU Medical Devices Directive should be extended to include all cosmetic implants including dermal fillers. UK legislation should be introduced to enact the changes sooner. Legislation should be introduced to classify fillers as a prescription-only medical device.
- The Royal College of Surgeons (RCS) should establish an Interspecialty Committee on Cosmetic Surgery, made up of representatives of all the relevant specialty and professional associations. The purpose of this group is to set standards for cosmetic surgery practice and training, and make arrangements for formal certification of all surgeons regarded as competent to undertake cosmetic procedures, taking account of training and experience.
- All those performing cosmetic interventions must be registered. The Health Education England (HEE) mandate should include the development of appropriate accredited qualifications for providers of non-surgical interventions and it should determine accreditation requirements for the various professional groups. This work should be completed in 2013.
- Surgical providers should provide both the person undergoing a procedure and their GP with proper records.
- The RCS Interspecialty Committee on Cosmetic Surgery should develop and describe a multistage consent process for operations. Consent must be taken by the surgeon performing the operation to ensure that the patient and practitioner have a shared understanding of the desired outcome and the limitations, implications, and risks of the procedure.

- Evidence-based standardized patient information should be developed by the RCS Interspecialty Committee on Cosmetic Surgery, with input from patient organizations.
- For non-surgical procedures a record of consent must be held by the provider.
- Existing advertising recommendations and restrictions should be updated and better enforced.
- The use of financial inducements and time-limited deals to promote cosmetic interventions should be prohibited to avoid inappropriate influencing of vulnerable consumers.
- Accessible resolution and redress—the remit of the Parliamentary and Health Service Ombudsman (PHSO) should be extended to cover the whole private healthcare sector. This will de facto include cosmetic procedures of all kinds.
- All individuals performing cosmetic procedures must possess adequate professional indemnity cover that is commensurate with the type of operations being performed. For surgeons working in this country, but who are insured abroad, indemnity insurance must be commensurate with similar UK policies.
- The Review Committee supports the future development of insurance products such as risk pool arrangements to cover product failure and certain complications of surgery.

Training in cosmetic surgery in the UK

Until recently there was no formal training pathway for cosmetic surgery in the UK. Moreover although the terms cosmetic and plastic surgery are often used interchangeably by the public, surgeons from other specialities other than plastic surgery also undertake cosmetic procedures. In 2007 interface fellowships open to plastic, maxillofacial, ENT, ophthalmic, breast surgeons, and dermatologists where established under the auspices of the CST. Eighteen fellowships are available each year, are awarded by competitive interview, are fully funded, and last for 4 months.

The temporomandibular joint

Anatomy

Bones

- A synovial joint between the mandibular condyle and the glenoid fossa of the temporal bone.
- The lateral pole of the condyle lies 1–1.5cm deep to the skin surface.
- The condyle is narrower antero-posteriorly compared to mesiodistally.
- The glenoid fossa is bounded anteriorly by the articular eminence, limiting the anterior movement of the mandibular condyle.

Disc

- The fibrocartilaginous articular disc has a thickened periphery—the annulus—and a central depression.
- The disc is tightly bound to the medial and lateral pole of the condyle by the capsular ligament.
- In the sagittal section the disc is biconcave in shape with a posterior bilaminar zone enclosing neurovascular tissue.
- The articular disc divides the joint into upper and lower joint compartments.
- The upper joint cavity contains 1.2mL and the lower contains 0.9mL of synovial fluid.
- Normally moves anteriorly with the head of the condyle on mouth opening.
- Shows excellent healing ability.

Ligaments

- **Lateral (temporomandibular) ligament:** is attached to the articular tubercle above and extends below at 45° to be attached to the posterior and lateral border of the condyle. It prevents posterior displacement of mandibular condyle.
- **The stylomandibular ligament:** thickened band of deep cervical fascia from the styloid process of the temporal bone to the angle of the mandible.
- **The sphenomandibular ligament:** long membranous band that lies medial to the joint running from the spine of the sphenoid bone to the lingula on the medial aspect of the mandible.

Muscles of mastication

- Supplied by motor division of V3.
- **Elevators:** temporalis, masseter, and medial pterygoid.
- **Protrusion:** lateral and medial pterygoids.
- **Depression:** lateral pterygoid, infra- and supra-hyoid muscles.
- **Lateral excursion:** contralateral pterygoids and ipsilateral temporalis.

Nerve supply

- Branches of V3 via auriculotemporal, masseteric, and posterior deep temporal nerves.
- The articular tissues and central disc contain no nerves.
- The capsule, disc periphery, and retrodiscal bilaminar zone contain pain and proprioception fibres.

Disorders

Developmental

- Aplasia/hypoplasia of the joint/condyle—may be part of hemifacial microsomia.
- Condylar hyperplasia.

Acquired

- Autoimmune or inflammatory: rheumatoid/psoriatic arthropathy, ankylosing spondylitis.
- Neurological—TMJDS/myofascial.
- Metabolic—gout.
- Degenerative—osteoarthritis.
- Idiopathic—idiopathic condylar resorption (ICR) (Fig. 9.1).
- Traumatic:
  - fracture;
  - effusion;
  - subluxation/dislocation.
- Infective: septic arthritis, untreated otitis media may lead to ankylosis.
- Neoplastic:
  - benign;
  - malignant.

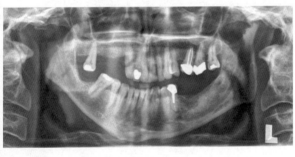

Fig. 9.1 OPT showing idiopathic condylar resorption.

Trismus

- Classically, an inability to open mouth due to muscular spasm, but commonly used to refer to limited mouth opening.
- Normal inter-incisal mouth opening is 35–45mm.
- Extra-articular causes:
  - odontogenic infection;
  - facial trauma including dento-alveolar surgery;
  - myofascial pain/TMJDS;
  - following ID LA block;
  - depressed fractured zygoma/arch;
  - radiation fibrosis;
  - tetanus;
  - quinsy;
  - local malignancy;
  - submucous fibrosis;
  - coronoid hyperplasia;
  - malignant hyperpyrexia.
- Intra-articular causes:
  - ankylosis—bony/fibrous;
  - facial trauma—effusion, fracture;
  - meniscus displacement;
  - osteophyte formation;
  - septic arthritis.

Myofascial pain

- **Synonyms:** myofacial pain/facial arthromyalgia.
- Spectrum of facial pain disorders secondary to parafunctional habits, without signs and symptoms of TMJ internal derangement.

Temporomandibular joint dysfunction

- Most common non-infective pain disorder of the oro-facial region.
- Meta-analysis show that the overall prevalence of TMJDS in population studies ranges from 30–45%.
- More common in ♀; ♂:♀ ratio of 1:3.
- Mean age is between 30 and 40 years.
- Pain is typically diffuse, cyclical and distributed in multiple sites, especially the muscles of mastication; it is frequently worse in the morning.
- Related to stress and parafunctional habits.
- **Associations:** depression, back pain, tension headaches, migraine, irritable bowel syndrome, fibromyalgia.

Features
- Pain.
- Clicking.
- Locking.
- Crepitus.
- Trismus.

Clinical findings
- Tenderness of the pre-auricular region and muscles of mastication.
- Clicking, usually with abnormal path of opening.
- Evidence of parafunctional activity—such as clenching causing dental attrition, linea alba affecting the buccal mucosa, scalloped tongue, masseteric hypertrophy, and biting of finger nails.

Internal derangement
- Occurs where the articular disc within the joint interferes with smooth functioning of the joint.
- Clicking usually indicates reducible displacement of the disc.
- Clicking is usually related to abnormal paths of opening, with protrusion and/or lateral deviation.
- Some patients will go on to develop locking.
- **Closed lock:** mouth cannot open beyond around 25mm as the head of the condyle impinges on an anteriorly displaced disc.
- **Open lock:** patient unable to close the mouth without manipulation, since condyle is trapped in front of posteriorly displaced disc.
- Locks may be reducible (patient can manipulate the jaw to regain mobility) or irreducible.
- Disc may perforate (associated with joint crepitus and the development of osteoarthritis).

Investigations
- Routine radiography does not change management in classical TMJDS.
- An OPT may eliminate dental pathology radiating to the ear in a non-classical pain pattern.

- Radiographic features of OA:
  - narrowing of joint space;
  - bone cyst (geode) formation;
  - remodelling;
  - osteophyte formation.
- MRI is the gold standard imaging for the TMJs. It can be useful in the assessment of patients with trismus where a closed lock (or other pathology) is suspected (Fig. 9.2).
- Approximately a third of asymptomatic patients have anterior displacement of their discs on MRI scan.
- CT scanning is superior for assessing bone detail.

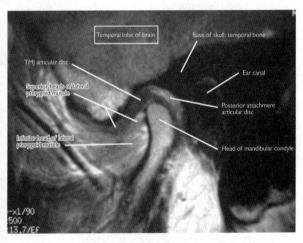

Fig. 9.2 MRI of the right temporomandibular joint.

Management/treatment

- Reassurance and explanation.
- Education regarding parafunctional habits.
- Jaw exercises, e.g. straight line to eliminate click.
- Physiotherapy.
- Analgesia.
- Heat.
- Rest/soft diet/relaxation.
- Splints/bite guards/bite raising appliances:
  - variety of materials, designs, and for either jaw;
  - possible mechanisms of action include reduction of bruxism and other parafunctional habits, production of a gap between the condyle and fossa to free the disc, and possible placebo effect.

Other interventions

Tricyclic antidepressants
- Have analgesic and muscle relaxant effects independent of their antidepressant action.
- No RCTs show efficacy in TMJDS.

Occlusal rehabilitation
- Most patients with abnormal occlusions do not suffer TMJ pain.
- No evidence of benefit.
- Orthodontic treatment or orthognathic surgery is not a treatment for TMJDS.

Arthrocentesis and manipulation
- To treat anteriorly displaced disc/closed lock unresponsive to conservative measures.
- Studies show 83% success rate in treating closed lock with arthrocentesis.
- LA or GA.
- Joint is washed out and adhesions freed (lysis and lavage).
- Medicaments placed:
  - **triamcinolone**—for pain and arthritic change; overuse of steroids may cause condylar resorption;
  - **bupivacaine, morphine**—for pain;
  - **hyaluronic acid**—to aid in closed lock.

Arthroscopy
- For diagnosis ± treatment.
- Performed under GA.
- Allows lysis and lavage.
- Other suggested procedures and benefits:
  - surgical freeing of adhesions;
  - fixation of retrodiscal tissues to eliminate anterior dislocation;
  - meniscopexy (fixing the disc into a posterior position);
  - eminoplasty for treatment of recurrent dislocation.
- Complications (greater than for arthrocentesis):
  - perforation of middle cranial fossa, EAM, tympanic membrane, or middle ear;
  - bleeding into EAM;
  - haemarthrosis;
  - auriculotemporal and facial nerve injuries.
- Direct comparison studies between arthrocentesis and arthroscopy have shown arthroscopy to be slightly more effective than arthrocentesis in improving maximal incisal opening.
- Arthroscopy allows intra-articular pathology to be observed and treated.

Open procedures
- Meniscopexy.
- Menisectomy.
- Condylar shaves.
- Eminectomy.

Surgical approach to the TMJ

Skin incision: tragal or pre-tragal with temporal extension (Bramley/Al-Kayat is one modification).

Dissection at cephalad aspect to temporalis fascia.

At caudal aspect along the avascular plane anterior to the cartilaginous tragus.

Join up cephalad and caudal aspects posterior to the parotid until root of zygomatic arch can be palpated.

Incise superficial layer of temporalis fascia to expose superficial temporal fat pad layer.

Incise periosteum over the arch reflecting the parotid anteriorly along with frontal branch of VII (runs just deep to the superficial temporalis fascia).

Expose TMJ capsule (+eminence if required).

Meniscopexy

Indicated in closed lock, which has not responded to conservative measures.

Incise capsule.

Explore upper and lower joint spaces.

Identify and mobilize disc by freeing the adhesions.

Fix disc posteriorly either by suturing to the periosteum of the zygomatic arch with non-resorbable suture or using a Mitek/Arthrex anchor embedded in the posterior aspect of the condylar head.

Menisectomy

May be indicated in significant disc degeneration or perforation.

Dissection should ensure complete disc removal (medial aspect may be difficult to access).

Some advocate interpositional pedicled temporalis fascia over condylar head.

Condylar shave

High condylar shave usually used to treat degenerative disorders such as OA.

The procedure helps recreate a smooth articular surface by removal of the osteophytes in OA.

Eminectomy

May be of benefit in a closed lock and avoids entering the joint space.

Also used by some in recurrent dislocation.

Temporomandibular joint replacement

Indications
- End stage degenerative disease: osteoarthritis (OA) or rheumatoid arthritis (RA).
- Adult ankylosis.
- Loss of vertical mandibular height and/or occlusal relationship secondary to bone resorption—ICR, trauma, and developmental anomalies.
- Neoplastic processes requiring condylar resection.
- Revision procedures where other treatments have failed.
- Avascular necrosis.

See Fig. 9.3.

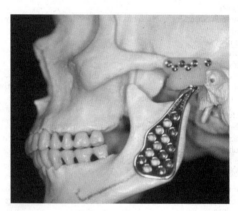

Fig. 9.3 Biomet total joint replacement.

Contraindications
- Active infection.
- Insufficient local bone.
- Known allergic reaction to implant materials, e.g. nickel.
- Severe parafunctional habits (e.g. bruxism).
- Inability to undergo rehabilitation.
- Patients who are still growing.

Options
- Pre-formed.
- Custom-made.

Complications
- Loosening or displacement.
- Infection.
- Dislocation.
- Foreign body or allergic reaction to implant components.
- Wearing through of the fossa material.
- Facial nerve damage.
- Malocclusion.
- Hearing complaints.

Ankylosis

Definition
- Fusion of the joint with reduced or absent movement.
- Usually intra-articular (**true ankylosis**).
- Extra-articular (**false ankylosis**) may occur with fusion between the zygoma and the coronoid process following trauma. Treated with coronoidectomy.
- Other extra-articular causes—include haematoma, CVA, hysterical trismus, bony exostoses, fibrous adhesions, and tumours (Fig. 9.4).

Causes
- Adults: usually trauma.
- Childhood: trauma (intra-capsular fracture) or infection (usually middle ear/mastoid).
- Bilateral early childhood or congenital ankylosis results in micrognathia, and a bird-face deformity.
- Unilateral growth impairment from ankylosis results in secondary changes in the occlusal plane and facial asymmetry.

Investigation
CT ± 3D CAD/CAM or stereolithographic modelling.

Special considerations
Difficult intubation—awake fibre-optic or tracheostomy.

Approach
- Upper as per surgical approach to TMJ.
- Lower approach also required if joint replacement planned (retromandibular approach).
- Facial nerve trunk passes in the bridge of tissue between.
- Ankylotic mass exposed.
- Condylar neck is mainly resected with a burr or piezo knife and the deepest aspect completed by fracturing the remaining cortex.
- The ankylotic mass is removed by dissection or by bony sculpturing of a new fossa.
- Beware:
  • intracranial proximity;
  • proximity to the ear canal;
  • maxillary/middle meningeal arteries (Fig. 9.5);
  • pterygoid venous plexus.
- Gap arthroplasty:
  • creates false joint at the condylar neck;
  • interpostion of local tissue or alloplastic material.
- Partial joint replacement: costochondral graft, but growth unpredictable in children.
- Prosthetic total joint replacement in adults (see ➡ Temporomandibular joint replacement, p. 364).

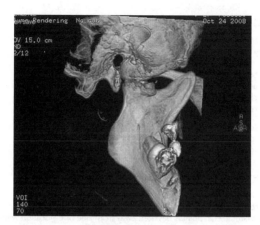

Fig. 9.4 Reformatted CT showing bony ankylosis.

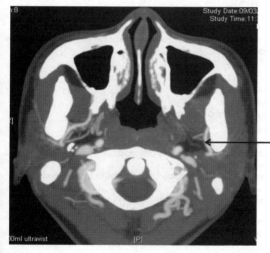

Fig. 9.5 Proximity of the maxillary artery (arrow) on a CT angiogram.

Dislocation

- Occurs where the condyle lies irreducibly anterior to the eminence.
- May be:
  - unilateral;
  - bilateral;
  - acute;
  - chronic (>3 months);
  - recurrent.

Causes
- Wide opening/yawning.
- Lax ligaments.
- Trauma.
- Oro-facial dystonias, e.g. antipsychotic medication side effect.

Clinical findings
- Anterior open bite with hollowing in pre-auricular region.
- If unilateral, chin point is deviated away from side of dislocation with a lateral open bite on the ipsilateral side.
- Radiography not necessary unless history of trauma.

Management
Acute
- Stimulation of the gag reflex suggested, but not predictable.
- Manipulation via sustained pressure on the posterior teeth to overcome masseteric spasm.
- LA, IVS, or GA.

Chronic
- Condylotomy.
- Condylectomy.
- Osteotomy and gap arthroplasty.

Recurrent
- Non-surgical:
  - Botulinum toxin injection into pterygoid muscles;
  - Neck collar/bandage;
  - Injection of autologous blood to induce haemarthrosis and scarring.
- Surgical:
  - Augment eminence, e.g. downfracture of zygomatic arch (Dautrey procedure, rarely used nowadays), bone graft;
  - Remove eminence—eminectomy;
  - Capsulorrhaphy—electrothermal capsulorrhaphy can be performed along with arthroscopy using laser to treat recurrent dislocations.

Rare disorders

Septic arthritis

- Rare.
- Usually in adults.
- May develop from odontogenic focus/otitis media.

Neoplastic

Benign

- Osteochondroma.
- Osteomas.
- Synovial chondromatosis:
  - multiple nodules of cartilage formed as loose bodies in joint space;
  - treatment with removal and synovectomy;
  - recurrence common.

Malignant

- Secondary deposits (breast, bronchus, kidney, thyroid, or prostate).
- Osteosarcoma.
- Invasion from local malignancy: parotid, oral SCC, cutaneous malignancy.

Inflammatory

- RA and psoriatic arthropathy frequently show radiographic features without symptoms.
- Inflammatory arthropathies show radiographic features of erosions and resorption.
- May cause progressive anterior open bite. Should be stable prior to definitive orthognathic intervention.

Idiopathic condylar resorption—ICR

- ICR is a progressive alteration in condylar shape and change in condylar mass (Fig. 9.6).
- Majority are asymptomatic with progressive decrease in posterior facial height, retrognathism, and the development of an AOB with clockwise rotation of the mandible.
- Has been associated with RA, SLE, scleroderma, and neoplasia. Steroid use is also a predisposing factor, but in majority no predisposing cause is found, hence the term idiopathic condylar resorption.
- Treatment includes total joint replacement ± orthognathic surgery to correct the secondary deformity (Fig. 9.7).

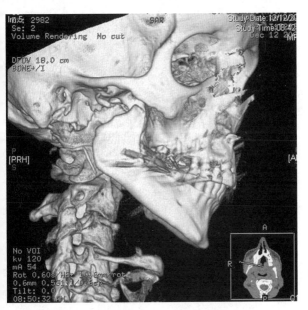

Fig. 9.6 Reformatted CT showing ICR.

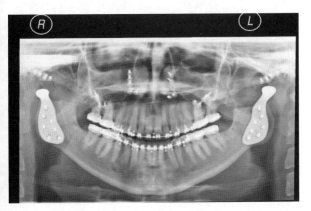

Fig. 9.7 Bilateral total joint replacement in a patient with ICR.

Surgical principles and oral surgery

General surgical principles

Informed consent

- Should be obtained by a clinician who is capable of performing the procedure, or who has been trained to obtain consent for that specific procedure (GMC guidelines).
- A patient must have capacity to give consent.
- An adult (age 16) should be assumed have capacity.
- Adequate information should be available about the risks and benefits, including those of no treatment.
- Fraser competency applies to a child under 16 who has capacity to give consent to an intervention.
- The law where a child with capacity disagrees with their parents is complex and differs within the UK. Legal advice may need to be sought.
- The Mental Capacity Act 2005 gave legal status to advance directives (living wills) and to an appointed advocate.

Preventing thromboembolic disease (NICE, 2010)

- Assess patients for risk factors pre-operatively.
- Advise stopping combined oral contraceptive pill (OCP) 4 weeks before surgery.
- Discuss risks and benefits of prophylaxis with patients.
- Discuss signs and symptoms to look for following discharge.
- Advise to seek advice on flying in the post-operative period.

Risk factors

- Age >60.
- Bed or chair bound >3 days before surgery, including ICU.
- Dehydration.
- Surgery >1h.
- Acute cancer.
- Acute cardiac or respiratory failure.
- Previous DVT or pulmonary embolus (PE) in self or close relative.
- OCP or HRT.
- Inherited thrombophilias.
- Anti-phospholipid syndrome.
- Pregnancy.
- Myeloproliferative disease.
- Nephrotic syndrome.
- Varicose veins with phlebitis.
- Obesity (BMI >30).

Prophylaxis includes:

- Graduated compression—use thromboembolic deterrent (TED) stockings.
- Intermittent pneumatic compression or foot impulse devices intra-operatively.
- Low-molecular-weight heparin (LMWH).
- Maintenance of hydration.
- Encouraging early mobilization.

Preventing surgical infections

Healthcare associated infections (HAIs) (NICE, 2008) include:

- Surgical site infection.
- Respiratory and urinary tract infection.
- Bacteraemias, including methicillin-resistant *Staphylococcus aureus* (MRSA).
- Antibiotic associated diarrhoeas, including *Clostridium difficile*.

Surgical site infection
- Occurs in 5% of all operations.
- Comprises 20% of HAIs.

Reduction in surgical site infections:
- **Pre-operatively:**
  - avoid routine hair removal;
  - if hair has to be removed, use electric clippers with a single-use head on the day of surgery (do not use razors);
  - give antibiotic prophylaxis to patients before clean surgery involving the placement of a prosthesis or implant, clean-contaminated surgery, or contaminated surgery;
  - do not use antibiotic prophylaxis for clean, non-prosthetic surgery;
  - use local antibiotic formulary and always consider potential adverse effects when choosing specific antibiotics for prophylaxis;
  - consider giving a single dose of antibiotic prophylaxis intravenously at start of anaesthesia;
  - give a repeat dose of antibiotic prophylaxis when the length of the operation exceeds the half-life of the antibiotic;
  - give antibiotic treatment (in addition to prophylaxis) to patients having surgery on a dirty or infected wound.
- **Intra-operatively:**
  - avoid diathermy for surgical skin incisions;
  - maintain sterile operating conditions;
  - maintain patient homeostasis;
  - cover surgical incisions with an appropriate interactive dressing at the end of the operation.
- **Post-operative phase:**
  - use an aseptic non-touch technique for changing or removing surgical wound dressings;
  - use sterile saline for wound cleansing up to 48h after surgery;
  - advise patients that they may shower safely 48h after surgery;
  - do not use topical antimicrobial agents for surgical wounds that are healing by primary intention to reduce the risk of surgical site infection;
  - refer to a tissue viability nurse (or another healthcare professional with suitable expertise) for advice on appropriate dressings for the management of surgical wounds that are healing by secondary intention.

Anaesthesia

The choice of anaesthesia includes local anaesthesia (LA), local anaesthesia and sedation (IV or oral), and general anaesthesia (GA).

The choice of anaesthesia is governed by:
- Patient acceptance.
- Patient suitability.
- Degree of difficulty of the procedure.
- Likely length of procedure.

Local anaesthesia

Topical anaesthetics
- Lignocaine paste (5%) or spray (10%) for oral mucosa.
- Tetracaine, lignocaine, or amethocaine for conjunctiva.
- Cocaine 4% for nasal mucosa.
- Eutectic mix of local anaesthetics (EMLA) lignocaine and prilocaine for skin—effective to 5mm depth.
- Ametop®: topical amethocaine.

Injected LA
- Lignocaine 2% with 1 in 80,000 adrenaline: commonest for intra-oral and skin surgery. Not contraindicated on ears and noses.
- Maximum safe dose of lignocaine is 7mg/kg (with adrenaline) and 3.5mg/kg (without adrenaline).
- 1mL of 2% lignocaine contains 20mg.
- Maximum number of 2.2mL cartridges of 2% lignocaine with 1 in 80,000 adrenaline equals 1 cartridge to 1 stone in weight.
- Prilocaine 3% with octapressin—less vasoconstriction than adrenaline.
- Maximum safe dose of prilocaine is 4mg/kg.
- Articaine 4% with 1 in 100,000 adrenaline. Popular in dental practice due to fast action. Use for ID blocks not recommended following several reported cases of long-term sensory impairment.
- Bupivacaine 0.25 or 0.5% ± adrenaline. Long-acting but 30min onset of action.
- Maximum safe dose of bupivacaine is 2mg/kg.
- Levobupivacaine has similar properties to bupivacaine, but lower toxicity.

LA injection techniques
- Block of named nerve, e.g. ID, lingual, infraorbital.
- Block of anatomical structure: diamond-shaped infiltration around nose/ear.
- Infiltration: dental, skin.
- Intra-ligamentary.

Complications of LA
- Failure:
  - poor technique—not enough or wrong place;
  - local infection;
  - unusual anatomy.

- Intravascular injection:
  - ischaemic area on face;
  - haematoma;
  - mild transient palpitations.
- Rarely:
  - facial palsy;
  - needle tract infection;
  - soft tissue trauma.

Sedation

- Inhalation:
  - common in dental practice;
  - safe;
  - relative analgesia—involves inhalation of a mix of nitrous oxide (NO) and O_2 with patient management techniques;
  - useful in children—gives sedation and analgesia;
  - quick onset and recovery;
  - contraindicated in pregnancy.
- Oral:
  - temazepam 10–30mg taken 1h pre-operatively;
  - diazepam 5–15mg;
  - oral sedation is unpredictable in its effects;
  - consent the patient before administration.
- Intravenous (IVS):
  - benzodiazepines cause hypnosis, sedation, and amnesia;
  - the elderly and children are very sensitive—children may become hyperstimulated rather than sedated;
  - single drug sedation is safe—the Poswillo recommendations regulate the use of sedation for those on the GDC register in the UK;
  - midazolam is the drug of choice for IVS—it has a short half-life, good amnesic properties, and fast recovery; the dose should be titrated to the patient's response—5mL ampoules containing 5mg of drug recommended;
  - oxygen saturation and BP should be monitored—suitable resuscitation facilities and trained staff should be available;
  - multiple drug sedation techniques should only be carried out by trained anaesthetists;
  - flumazenil is a specific antagonist to benzodiazepines—due to a short half-life more than one dose may be required (dose 200 micrograms plus 100 micrograms/min until reversal);
  - propofol sedation increasingly popular—rapid onset, short acting, amnesic, usually anaesthetist delivered.
- Intranasal:
  - unpredictable absorption.
- Rectal:
  - unpredictable absorption.

General anaesthesia

Regulations from the General Dental Council

The Poswillo Committee recommendations (1990) effectively removed the use of GA and regulated the use of sedation in general dental practice. The 2001 GDC recommendations added to these and failure to comply risks charge of serious professional misconduct for those regulated by the GDC.

GA for dental procedures should be available only where appropriate facilities exist—in effect in a hospital setting. The referring practitioner must:

• Take a full medical history, explain the risks and alternatives to a GA.
• Justify the referral for GA in the referral letter.
• Retain a copy of the letter.

Fitness for anaesthesia

The American Society of Anaesthesiologists (ASA) classification is widely used:

• ASA grading:
  • 1: normal healthy patient;
  • 2: patient with mild systemic disease;
  • 3: patient with severe systemic disease;
  • 4: patient with severe systemic disease that is a constant threat to life;
  • 5: moribund patient not expected to survive without surgery;
  • 6: brain-dead declared patient undergoing organ retrieval.
• The risk of complications following a GA correlates well with the ASA grouping.

Pre-operative assessment

Includes:

• History of presenting problem, medical history (MH), and systemic inquiry.
• Examination of presenting problem and cardiovascular system/ respiratory system (CVS/RS).
• Investigations to assess suitability for GA:
  • BP;
  • pulse;
  • urinalysis;
  • haematological/biochemical investigations as indicated;
  • group and save/cross-match as per local blood ordering policies;
  • ECG if indicated;
  • CXR if indicated (Royal College of Radiologists guidelines).
• Special investigations, e.g. echocardiogram, lung function tests.

Principles of general anaesthesia

Anaesthesia is the combination of analgesia, hypnosis, and muscle relaxation. Induction and maintenance of anaesthesia may be performed by intravenous or inhalation agents.

- Intravenous agents:
  - propofol;
  - thiopentone;
  - etomidate.
- Inhalation agents:
  - NO;
  - sevoflurane;
  - isoflurane;
  - halothane (rarely used).
- Muscle relaxants:
  - used to aid intubation and mechanical ventilation;
  - depolarizing agents, e.g. suxamethonium (short-acting, not used commonly, but still drug of choice in rapid sequence induction);
  - non-depolarizing agents, e.g. rocuronium, vecuronium, atracurium, pancuronium (reversible with neostigmine).
- Analgesics (opioids):
  - used to supplement anaesthesia, e.g. remifentanil (by continuous infusion) and alfentanil (as aid to induction);
  - used for analgesia, e.g. morphine, fentanyl.

Airway control

Basic airway management techniques to maintain, but not secure the airway include:

- Suction/removal of debris and foreign bodies.
- Chin lift.
- Jaw thrust.
- Oral (Guedel) airway.
- Nasopharyngeal airway.

In practice, a combination of these is often required, particularly in the trauma situation.

Definitive airway management skills for oral and maxillofacial surgery include:

- Laryngeal mask airway (LMA).
- Endotracheal intubation (oral, nasal)—may require blind or fibre-optic techniques.
- Surgical airways.

The laryngeal mask airway

The LMA is commonly used in dento-alveolar surgery and other less major procedures. LMAs are single use. Reinforced masks are used in intra-oral surgery. Paralysis is not necessary and patients breathe spontaneously. Care must be taken not to dislodge the mask and lose the airway when manipulating the mandible. Good communication with the anaesthetist is essential.

Endotracheal intubation

Intubation requires neuromuscular relaxation to enable passage of the tube through the cords. This may be carried out under direct vision with the use of a laryngoscope. Where there is trismus or potential difficulty in viewing the cords intubation may be carried out 'blind' or with the aid of a fibre-optic endoscope. The airway is protected by a sub-glottic inflatable cuff. Be aware if a throat pack is placed (see NPSA Guidance 2009).

Surgical airways

Indication—actual or anticipated failure to secure the airway in any other manner:

- Needle cricothyroidotomy.
- Surgical cricothyroidotomy.
- Surgical or percutaneous tracheostomy.

GA in oral and maxillofacial surgery has special features requiring sharing of the upper airway.

Potential upper airway obstruction in oncology/trauma/cervicofacial infections

- Summon senior anaesthetic help early.
- Discussion of potential problem with whole team—what do you and the anaesthetist plan in case of failed intubation?
- Consider not attempting GA.
- Consider awake/fibre-optic, or blind intubation.
- Difficult airway trolley should be available and familiar to you.
- Consider surgical airway under LA and then GA when airway secure.
- Failed intubation in a difficult airway—communication and preparation between surgeon and anaesthetist are essential. Options:
  - wake the patient up if non-emergency surgery;
  - LMA and surgical airway if other indications;
  - emergency cricothyroidotomy is rarely indicated, but a safer first step than emergency tracheostomy in a dire situation.

Other anaesthetic considerations in major maxillofacial surgery

Hypotensive anaesthesia

- Remifentanil infusion or vasodilator agents, such as labetalol.
- Commonly used in orthognathic surgery, this has revolutionized the morbidity of these procedures.
- Less profound hypotensive anaesthesia is used in major head and neck oncology cases, although is less well tolerated in this group who are often arteriopaths.
- Let anaesthetist know when you are due to start wound closure, so that the BP can come up to ensure adequate haemostasis.
- Beware post-operative rebound hypertension and bleeding.

Management of head and neck oncology cases

- Elective tracheostomy policy.
- Practice varies widely between units, and both conservative and more aggressive approaches to elective tracheostomy in head and neck surgery have pros and cons:
- **Conservative approach**: elective tracheostomy in only:
  - bilateral neck dissection;
  - posterior tumours;
  - mandibulotomy cases;
  - those with co-morbidity, such as chest disease;
  - previous radiotherapy to head and neck;
  - in other cases, patient remains intubated overnight—some may require later tracheostomy due to failure to extubate.

- **Aggressive approach:**
  - higher rate of elective tracheostomy is practised in some units, often with the patient returning to a high dependency area of the head and neck ward;
  - some cases will have tracheostomy-related complications.
- No adequate RCTs have compared approaches.

Management of the medically compromised patient

- Steroid therapy.
- Those at risk of endocarditis.
- Anti-coagulant/anti-platelet therapy.
- Bisphosphonates.
- Osteoradionecrosis.

Readers are referred to other texts for the management of other medical conditions.

Steroids

Those on exogenous steroids develop hypothalamic-adrenocortical suppression. At times of stress the normal physiological response is for the adrenal medulla to secrete catecholamines. These bind to vascular alpha and beta adrenoreceptors to divert blood flow as may be required in a 'fight and flight' response. Receptor response to catecholamines is dependent on the presence of corticosteroids, which are usually simultaneously secreted at times of stress from the adrenal cortex. In the absence of steroids, the net result of the catecholamine surge on the CVS can be a precipitous fall in BP—this is the basis of a steroid crisis. There are no recorded cases of steroid crisis in oral and maxillofacial surgery (two reported cases were not worked up for other causes of post-operative hypotension), and there are a maximum of six cases in the English-speaking literature related to trauma and other surgical procedures where the diagnosis is likely.

Historically, patients having surgery have been managed by variably increasing the steroid dose, e.g. doubling the oral dose or giving IV supplementation.

Current thinking as follows:

LA

- Patients on <7.5mg prednisolone/day do not require cover.
- Those on higher doses can double the dose on the day of surgery only.

GA

- *Minor surgery*—100mg hydrocortisone IV pre-operatively (IM absorption unpredictable).
- *Major surgery*—100mg hydrocortisone IV pre-operatively and 50mg 8h for 48h.
- Dose and management varies with steroid dose and severity of surgery.

Patients at risk of infective endocarditis

There is no good evidence that antibiotic prophylaxis reduces the risk of infective endocarditis (IE) in susceptible patients. Current guidelines (NICE, 2008) have ruled that antibiotic prophylaxis for infective endocarditis should no longer be given.

Anti-coagulants/anti-platelets

- Warfarin—inhibits the production of vitamin K dependent clotting factors II, VII, IX, and X.
- Aspirin irreversibly inhibits the thromboxane A2 stage of the COX pathway responsible for degranulation of platelets.
- Clopidogrel irreversibly blockades the ADP receptor on platelets inhibiting aggregation. Has synergistic effect with aspirin.
- Platelet half-life = 5–7 days, so it takes 7–10 days for adequate numbers of functional platelets to reach the circulation following stopping aspirin or clopidogrel.

Warfarin

- Check the patient's INR card at the first appointment to assess control and target.
- Dento-alveolar surgery is safe up to international normalized ratio (INR) of 4.0—result within the preceding 24h (use carboxymethylcellulose packs and suturing of sockets routinely).
- Major surgery:
  - **emergency**—consider use of prothrombin complex concentrate (this has superseded FFP) and/or vitamin K with haematology advice, see BNF for details;
  - **elective**—discontinue warfarin 3 days pre-operatively covering those with prosthetic cardiac valves with LMWH. Restart warfarin on day of surgery and continue LMWH until INR in target range.

Aspirin

Does not usually require discontinuation but is often stopped in some aspects of aesthetic facial surgery.

Clopidogrel

- Manufacturers'/BNF advice: discontinue 7 days before major surgery.
- Continue for dento-alveolar surgery (carboxymethylcellulose packs and suturing).

Post-operative bleeding

- Primary: immediate bleeding that occurs at the at time of surgery.
- Reactionary occurs within 48h of surgery due to opening of small blood vessels, disturbance to a blood clot, or wearing off of the effect of a vasoconstrictor.
- Secondary: occurs after 48h, often 1 week post-operatively. Usually result of an infection, which destroys the clot or damages blood vessels in the base of the wound.

Bisphosphonates

- Potent inhibitors of osteoclastic activity—increasing usage in medicine.
- Used IV (pamidronate, zoledronate) in hypercalcaemia, secondary to:
  - bony metastases, e.g. breast cancer;
  - myeloma;
  - Paget's disease.
- Used orally to treat and prevent osteoporosis (alendronate).
- Effects last ?decades.
- Bisphosphonate-related osteonecrosis of the jaws (BRONJ) first described in 2003.
- Only affects the jaws, overall incidence 10 patients /year/per million population.
- Risk much higher with IV preparations—oral risk low 1/1000–1/10,000, IV 1:10–1:100 (Faculty of General Dental Practice (FGDP)/British Association of Oral and Maxillofacial Surgeons (BAOMS), 2012).

ONJ presents:

- As non-healing socket with exposed bone or sequestra.
- Usually due to extractions, but can be spontaneous/due to denture trauma.
- Rarely with pathological fracture.
- ♀♂.
- Mandible > maxilla.
- **Stage 1:** asymptomatic bone exposure/necrosis.
- **Stage 2:** symptomatic bone exposure/necrosis.
- **Stage 3:** as for stage 2, but includes extra-oral sinus/pathological fracture/osteolysis to lower border.

Prevention

- Ensuring dental health before starting therapy—referral from GMP or oncologist to GDP.
- Avoidance of extractions once on bisphosphonates.
- Regular dental care.
- No evidence that stopping bisphosphonates decreases risk or aids management of BRONJ.
- If extractions are required ADA and BDA do not recommend cover with peri-operative prophylactic antibiotics, although it is commonly employed.

Management of BRONJ

- Should be conservative—further intervention risks further necrosis.
- Any debridement should be minimal.
- Biopsy may be necessary to rule out malignancy—submit tissue for microbiology also.
- Antibiotics if symptomatic, guided by C&S.
- Progression of necrosis is frequent and may result in pathological fracture—mandibular resection ± reconstruction may be indicated.

Osteoradionecrosis

Definition

Osteoradionecrosis (ORN) is a condition of non-vital bone in a site of radiation injury characterized by:
- Hypovascularity.
- Hypocellularity.
- Hypoxia.

± Injury leads to three grades of disease:
- **Grade I**: most common, exposed alveolar bone.
- **Grade II**: ORN that does not respond to hyperbaric oxygen (HBO) therapy and requires sequestrectomy/saucerization.
- **Grade III**: demonstrated by full-thickness involvement and/or pathological fracture.

Cause

- Rare in patients who receive <60Gy radiation therapy.
- Incidence decreased over the last 3 decades.
- Incidence is increased in patients who receive combined chemo-radiation.
- Injury:
  - none;
  - tooth extraction;
  - related cancer surgery;
  - biopsy;
  - denture irritation;
  - exposure of the irradiated bone under soft tissue necrosis;
  - implant placement (success in irradiated bone 60 vs 95% in non-irradiated).

Clinical symptoms/signs

- Pain.
- Swelling.
- Trismus.
- Exposed bone.
- Pathological fracture.
- Malocclusion.
- Oro-cutaneous fistula.

Prevention

- Dental assessment and extractions before cancer surgery, and at least 2 weeks before RT (head and neck cancer MDT should have restorative dentist as a core member).
- Maintenance of dental health post-treatment of patients who have had RT to the jaws.
- Extractions after RT—wait until mucositis has subsided.
- ORN risk is greater beyond 18 months after finishing RT.
- Mandible > maxilla.
- Suggested ways to reduce risk of ORN in extractions in irradiated bone:
  - pre-operative HBO?
  - avoid LA with adrenaline;

- atraumatic technique;
- antibiotic prophylaxis;
- pentoxifylline?

Management of ORN

- Oral hygiene/chlorhexidine.
- Antibiotics guided by C&S.
- Minimal intervention/sequestrectomy.
- Vascularized free tissue transfer in Stage III disease:
  - composite flap to replace irradiated bone and mucosa;
  - higher flap failure and complications than non-irradiated recipient site.
- HBO in ORN remains controversial. Marx reported high success with HBO in treating established ORN (Marx protocols), but these results have not been reproduced in subsequent studies.
- Small early studies of pentoxfylline and tocopherol (vitamin E) with clodronate show promise.

Dento-alveolar surgery

Third molars/impacted wisdom teeth

- Commonest missing tooth—25% of all third molars missing.
- Eruption average age 16–25 years.
- May remain unerupted.
- Commonly become impacted.
- Impaction—soft tissue only or bony.
- Bony impaction:
  - vertical 38%;
  - mesio-angular 44%;
  - disto-angular 6%;
  - horizontal 3%.
- Still in top 15 NHS UK surgical procedures.

Removal of symptomatic wisdom teeth (see NICE guidance, ➲ NICE guidelines regarding wisdom teeth (2000), p. 390) is justified, with benefits outweighing risks of removal. No RCTs compare the long-term outcome of early removal with retention of pathology free third molars.

Possible consequences of retention

- Removal when older with ↑ surgical and general complications.
- Dentigerous cyst formation (rare).
- Caries in distal aspect of second molar.
- No evidence of association with lower incisor crowding.

Possible consequences of removal

- Nerve damage lingual/ID.
- Dry socket (3–35%).
- Infection.
- Bleeding.
- Swelling.
- Trismus.
- Rarely iatrogenic # of mandible.
- Oro-antral fistula.
- Displacement of upper third molar into maxillary sinus or infra-temporal fossa.
- Displacement of lower third molar into sub-lingual or sub-mandibular space.
- Damage to second molar restoration.
- TMJDS.

Controversies in wisdom tooth removal techniques

- Flap design: triangular, envelope.
- Lingual flap retraction ± nerve protection.
- Bone removal:
  - site: buccal approach vs lingual split;
  - method: drill vs chisels.
- Tooth division: drill vs osteotome.
- LA vs GA: bilateral lower wisdom tooth removal under LA has been shown to be a safe technique.

BMJ Clinical Evidence (web publication May 2008) has looked at the evidence for different surgical methods of removing wisdom teeth. Despite much well-known work in the field of lingual nerve injury following wisdom tooth removal, there is no good quality evidence to support the practice or not of retraction. Some studies have shown a higher incidence of lingual nerve damage (up to 9.1%) when a retractor is used, but there is some suggestion that this is operator dependant. In skilled hands, careful lingual nerve protection when the retractor has been correctly inserted puts the nerve at less risk from bur/chisel trauma.

Lingual nerve damage
- Incidence varies widely between studies: 0–22%.
- Permanent disturbance 0–2%.
- Causes:
  - damage by retractor;
  - damage by bur/chisel.

ID nerve damage
- Temporary up to 5% (more related to anatomy). One RCT demonstrated up to 19% incidence in high-risk cases where coronectomy may have been indicated.
- Permanent 0.2–1%.

Nerve damage in wisdom tooth removal
Seddon's classification of nerve injury:
- Neuropraxia: physiological disruption, but anatomy intact.
- Axonotmesis: axons disrupted, epi- and peri-neurium preserved.
- Neurotmesis: severed nerve.

In theory, neurotmesis has a greater chance of recovery if the severance has occurred in a bony canal, rather than in soft tissue (ID vs lingual).

After peripheral nerve injury, proximal axons suffer retrograde degeneration, which may extend as far as the cell body (trigeminal ganglion for ID and lingual). The distal axonal segments undergo Wallerian degeneration with loss of the myelin sheath. Axonal regrowth occurs at up to 2mm/day.

Definitions of altered sensation
- Hypoaesthesia: ↓ sensation.
- Paraesthesia: altered sensation.
- Dysaesthesia: unpleasant sensation.
- Anaesthesia: no sensation.

Factors predictive of difficulty in wisdom teeth removal
Winter's lines are described historically, but are rarely used in practice.
- Type of impaction.
- Depth of application point.
- Density of bone (age, ethnicity).
- Surgical access (trismus, obesity).
- Root morphology.
- Proximity to inferior dental bundle (IDB).
- Associated pathology.

Radiographic signs of close involvement with inferior dental bundle
- Narrowing of canal.
- Loss of lamina dura.
- Change in direction of canal.

If involvement is suspected:

Cone beam CT scan
- Consider tooth division.
- Consider coronectomy (one RCT has shown 0% ID damage vs 19% where root removal completed in high-risk cases). However, coronectomy failed in 38%, i.e. roots were dislodged. Follow-up was 2 years and thus fate of retained roots undetermined.

IDN injury
- If noted at time of surgery immediate repair should be undertaken, but technically challenging.
- If noted at review monitor with light touch perception/sharp and blunt discrimination ± two point discrimination. If no improvement, consider referral to specialist unit.

Management of lingual nerve injuries following wisdom tooth removal
- Recovery not guided by bony canal.
- Heterogeny of fibre types vs IDB makes regeneration back to correct receptors less likely.
- Exploration and repair indicated at 3 months if no recovery.
- Success variable: consider referral to specialist unit.

NICE guidelines regarding wisdom teeth (2000)
Prophylactic removal of wisdom tooth is no longer indicated. Removal of wisdom teeth should be limited to patients with evidence of pathology:
- Severe or recurrent pericoronitis.
- Unrestorable caries/distal caries in adjacent molar.
- Non-treatable pulpal and/or peri-apical pathology.
- Cellulitis.
- Abscess and osteomyelitis.
- Internal/external resorption of tooth/adjacent teeth.
- Fracture of tooth.
- Disease of follicle including cyst/tumour.
- Tooth/teeth impeding surgery or reconstructive jaw surgery.
- Tooth involved in/within field of tumour resection.

In Scotland the SIGN guidelines apply.

Apicectomy and RRF

Indications
- Failure of orthograde approach where repeat endodontic therapy may be detrimental to tooth or cannot be repeated.
- Post crown on tooth with apical pathology and a good coronal seal, where crown and post removal risks root fracture.
- Inaccessible apical one-third of root, e.g. calcification, curved, or open apex.
- Root perforation (often poor prognosis).

- Fractured and symptomatic apical one-third following trauma.
- Apical pathology requiring biopsy or enucleation of cyst.

Contraindications
- Unrestorable tooth.
- Periodontal disease/perio-endo lesion.
- Furcation involvement.
- Proximity to IDB.

Flap designs
- Edges should be on sound bone.
- Two- or three-sided gingival margin:
  - good access;
  - ↑ recession around crown margins;
  - indicated in ?buccal post perforation;
  - more difficult to suture.
- Luebke–Oschenbein flap is three-sided, but supragingival. Unwise in possible post perforation, but good access and easy to suture.
- Semilunar flap gives reduced access, less easy to suture than Luebke–Oschenbein, wound can dehisce.

Points
- Apical soft tissue should be sent for histology.
- Apical radiolucency over 1cm likely to be radicular cyst, rather than apical granuloma (a collection of granulation tissue, not containing histological granulomata).
- Apex removal resects the apical delta of canals and enables retrograde root-filling to be placed.
- Apicectomy should be close to 90° to reduce surface area of exposure of transected dentinal tubules.
- At least 3mm should be apicected.
- Retrograde cavity preparation with ultrasonic tip is recommended by endodontists.
- Retrograde materials:
  - mineral trioxide aggregate (MTA)/Portland cement;
  - super EBA;
  - glass ionomer;
  - composites for dentine;
  - intermediate restorative material (IRM)—ZnO/Eugenol based;
  - amalgam success rate low and introduces mercury into the tissues—possible toxicity therefore no longer recommended.
- Success rates vary in literature from 30–90% higher on upper anteriors and single-rooted teeth.
- Success rates for repeat repair or pre-existing loss of supporting bone low (<40%).

Dento-alveolar surgery for orthodontics
- Upper labial fraenectomy.
- Impacted canines.
- Exposure of impacted/unerupted teeth.
- Miniscrews for anchorage.

Upper labial fraenectomy
- No adequate RCTs exist comparing no intervention with surgery.
- An upper midline diastema is common in the mixed dentition and often closes with eruption of the permanent canines.
- Fewer carried out than in the past.
- Fraenectomy theoretically only of value in helping to close a midline diastema if traction on it produces movement of the incisive papilla.
- Excision of the fraenum must include that part which passes between the upper incisors.
- Some advocate a bur cut—no studies support this and there is a risk of damage to the roots of the upper central incisors.

Management options for impacted canines
- Keep deciduous canine and leave permanent *in situ*.
- Keep deciduous canine and remove permanent.
- Remove deciduous and permanent canines, and close space/place implant.
- Expose and bond permanent canine. Consider retaining deciduous temporarily if permanent well displaced. May also require removal of adjacent first premolar.
- Transplantation—poor success rate.
- Decision regarding best option result of discussions including patient (± parents) and orthodontist.

Exposure of impacted/unerupted teeth
- Aim to remove bone/mucosa preventing eruption, and enable orthodontic bonding and traction to align the tooth.
- Commonly upper canine teeth, occasionally upper incisors (often following previous supernumery removal or trauma), lower premolars.
- Association between ectopic teeth and missing teeth.
- If canines are not buccally palpable at age 10 consider palatal position.
- Extraction of deciduous canines at age of 10 years will allow spontaneous alignment of 75% of ectopic permanent canines.

Procedure
- Palatal canines:
  - exposed through a palatal flap (usually under GA);
  - bone removal to expose tip and maximum convexity of crown;
  - options: bonding a bracket and chain ± re-covering: excision of overlying palatal mucosa + WHP dressing or cover plate;
  - Cochrane review 2008: no evidence to support one surgical technique over another.
- Buccal teeth: exposure with an apically repositioned flap ± bonding of bracket at surgery or later.

Miniscrews/plates
- Provide bony anchorage.
- Increasingly popular.
- NICE guidance advises use should be audited.

Odontogenic infections

- Infections associated with teeth.
- Definitive treatment is drainage of the infection/pus and/or removal of the offending tooth/pulp.
- Infections are bacterial—arising from necrotic pulp, pericorontitis, and periodontal pockets.

Severe infections

- Can be life-threatening emergencies as they spread into the potential fascial spaces within the head and neck.
- Can track into the cavernous sinus or mediastinum.
- Pus in the potential spaces in the head and neck is a serious hazard to the airway and requires urgent management.
- Severity depends upon:
  - local anatomy;
  - virulence of the organisms;
  - host resistance.

Microbiology

- Mixed infection: *Bacteroides* (anaerobic) and *Streptococcus* (aerobic and anaerobic).
- Usually sensitive to penicillins.
- Resistance rare.

Fascial tissue spaces

These are potential spaces between tissue planes which can fill up with pus—the opening of planes aided by enzymatic tissue lysis caused by pathogenic bacteria.

- Buccal space:
  - commonest space to be affected by a dental abscess, both from upper and lower teeth;
  - bounded by buccinator attachment;
  - contains the buccal fat pad;
  - can usually be drained intra-orally.
- Masticator space:
  - involved in molar teeth abscesses, lower more than upper;
  - bounded by muscles of mastication.
- Deep masticator space:
  - lies between the pterygoid muscles and mandibular ramus;
  - superficial masticator space lies laterally to the ramus and comprises the submasseteric space below the superficial temporal space;
  - infection gaining access to the pterygoid space can potentially spread intra-cranially;
  - deep masticator space gives access to the parapharyngeal space that, in turn, contains the carotid sheath giving potential access for pus to track to the mediastinum.
- Parotid space lies within the parotid fascia.

- Sublingual space:
  - lies between the floor of the mouth and mylohyoid muscle;
  - communicates around its free posterior edge with the submandibular space in the neck.
- Ludwig's angina is defined as bilateral cellulitis of the submandibular and sublingual spaces.
- Canine fossa:
  - bound by the peri-oral muscles of facial expression;
  - infection can spread via the ophthalmic veins to the intracranial circulation.

Diagnosis
- Severe pain.
- Swelling.
- Discharge.
- Swinging pyrexia.
- Tachycardia.
- Raised white cell count.
- Later:
  - drooling;
  - difficulty breathing or speaking;
  - severe trismus;
  - stridor (inspiratory wheeze).
- Death by septicaemia/respiratory arrest/intra-cranial or intra-thoracic complications.

Treatment
- Involve senior anaesthetic help early.
- Fibre-optic intubation and/or a surgical airway may be indicated.
- Urgent incision, drainage, and exploration of fascial spaces, multiple drain insertion + extraction of offending tooth.
- High-dose antibiotics (triple therapy—amoxicillin/gentamicin/metronidazole) ± steroids.
- Mortality of Ludwig's angina is 5%.

Necrotizing fasciitis
- Rare.
- High mortality.
- Polymicrobial *Streptococcus/Staphylococcus/Bacteroides/Clostridia*.
- Monomicrobial: group A streps or MRSA.
- Usually in occurs in the immunocompromised.
- Treatment is wide surgical debridement and IV antibiotics.

Osteomyelitis
- Rare—acute or chronic.
- Secondary to immunosuppression/diabetes in developed world.
- Common in developing world secondary to odontogenic infection/fracture.

Microbiology
- *Bacteroides* spp.
- *Staph. aureus.*
- *Klebsiella.*
- *Proteus.*

Signs/symptoms
- Pain.
- Trismus.
- Tooth mobility.
- Mental nerve paraesthesia.
- Pyrexia.
- Necrosis of bone, leading to sequestration.

Investigation
- Pulpal vitality.
- Radiography: moth-eaten bone, sub-periosteal bone deposition.
- Pus for C&S.
- Management:
  - removal of non-vital teeth;
  - penicillin/metronidazole or clindamycin with microbiological advice;
  - removal of sequestra;
  - submission of tissue for microbiology and histology.

Other odontogenic infections

Apical dental abscess
Secondary to pulp necrosis.

Pericoronitis
Acute inflammation ± pus formation around the crown of a tooth.

Periodontal abscess
Arises in a periodontal pocket.

Dry socket
- Localized osteitis (bony inflammation) after extraction. Associated with:
  - smoking;
  - difficult extraction (more common in mandible);
  - OCP;
  - LA.
- Prophylactic pre-operative antibiotics have been shown in some studies to reduce the incidence of dry socket in third molar surgery.

Non-odontogenic infections

Actinomycosis
- Persistent low-grade infection associated with multiple sinuses.
- *Actinomyces israelii* and others/commensals in tonsil.
- Cervicofacial infection follows extraction or fracture.
- Tx: drainage and long-term penicillin V (at least 6 weeks).

Cat scratch disease
- Common cause of cervical lymphadenopathy in children.
- Causative organism *Bartonella henselae*.
- Diagnosis—antibodies to *Bartonella*.
- Histology of an excised lymph node shows granulomas, but is not pathognomonic.
- Treatment is symptomatic.

Staphylococcal lymphadenitis
- Seen mainly in children following minor breach in skin or mucosa.
- May result from nose picking.
- Flucloxacillin is antibiotic of choice.
- Suppurative lymphadenitis may need drainage of pus.

Mycobacterial lymphadenitis
- Typical or atypical: former is rare in the UK except amongst immigrant populations.
- Presentation: lymphadenitis ± suppuration.
- Diagnosis: acid-fast bacilli (AFB) may be seen on ZN staining. Culture may be needed for up to 12 weeks.
- Treatment:
  - surgical debridement;
  - typical TB—anti-tuberculous therapy;
  - atypical mycobacterial lymphadenitis—clarithromycin;
  - involve the paediatric team in definitive management.

Biopsy

A biopsy is a sample of tissue taken from a patient for histopathological examination to provide a diagnosis.

Types
- **Incisional:** removes a sample of the lesion for diagnosis:
  - needle (FNA for cytology, core biopsy, or Tru-cut);
  - punch biopsy;
  - scalpel.
- **Excisional:** removes whole lesion.

Lesions warranting biopsy
- All excised lesions should be submitted for histological evaluation.
- Soft tissue lesions, which cannot be accurately diagnosed clinically, should warrant biopsy, particularly white and red patches.
- Frozen sections:
  - intra-operative biopsy specimens taken during major surgery in order to verify clearance at the surgical margins;
  - in oral SCC surgery—highly sensitive and specific but cannot predict close (<5mm) margins;
  - laboratory requires frozen sections to be booked prior to theatre.
- Specimens should be covered in 10× their volume of 10% formalin.
- Fresh tissue may need to be submitted discuss with pathologists.
- Tissue may need to be sent for microbiological analysis/culture, e.g. TB.
- Tissue for immunofluorescence (vesiculobullous) disorders can be transported in normal saline, FSS (frozen section substitute) or liquid nitrogen. Discuss with laboratory.

Sentinel node biopsy
See Sentinel node biopsy, p. 91.

Cysts

Definition

Cysts are pathological cavities that are usually lined by epithelium and contain fluid. Most jaw cysts arise from odontogenic epithelium and grow by a variety of mechanisms, e.g. inflammation causing epithelial proliferation, bone resorption secondary to pressure/prostaglandins, and alterations in cystic osmotic pressure.

Odontogenic cysts

Diagnosis

- Often present as asymptomatic radiolucencies.
- May present with infection/pathological fracture.
- Vitality testing of associated teeth.
- Aspiration of the cyst contents is sometimes useful and can differentiate a maxillary cyst from the maxillary sinus.

Treatment options

- Observation may be appropriate, e.g. following endodontic therapy or, in an older patient, with an asymptomatic static radiolucency.
- Enucleation of the cyst together with any associated pathology and primary closure—peri-operative antibiotics will reduce the chance of the bony blood-filled cavity becoming infected and, thus, allow organization of the clot to bone.
- Enucleation and packing with, e.g. WHP (condemns the patient to pack changes and rarely indicated).
- Marsupialization:
  - opening and biopsy of cyst and suturing of lining to oral mucosa;
  - healing is slow;
  - can be useful in children to enable tooth eruption or when GA for enucleation is contraindicated.

Radicular dental cysts

- Secondary to a necrosis of pulp.
- Described as a residual cyst if left following tooth removal.
- Derived from epithelial cell rests of Malassez, which are stimulated to proliferate in an infected peri-apical granuloma.
- Straw-coloured fluid containing cholesterol crystals with protein content >5g/dL.
- Tx = orthograde endodontic treatment—small (<1cm) radicular cysts may heal spontaneously.
- Enucleation ± apicectomy/orthograde endodontic treatment/ extraction.

Dentigerous cysts

- Form around crown of unerupted permanent teeth (usually wisdom teeth or canines).
- Arise from reduced enamel epithelium.
- Tx: enucleation or marsupialization ± removal of the unerupted tooth.

Keratocysts
- Renamed WHO classification as keratinizing odontogenic tumours.
- Commonest site—angle of the mandible.
- Radiographically usually multilocular.
- 40% in a 'dentigerous' position.
- Lined by ortho- (10 %) or para-keratinized (83%) epithelium (7% have both)—fluid has protein content <4g/dL.
- Aspiration may be helpful for protein content (biochemistry) and keratinization (cytology).
- Histologically high mitotic activity: growth is neoplastic with invasion of the medulla and not by bony expansion.
- Tx = enucleation ± Carnoy's solution (decreases recurrence).
- Satellite cysts or daughter cysts increase the likelihood of recurrence, as does an association with Gorlin–Goltz syndrome.
- Orthokeratinizing keratocysts are much less aggressive. Review for recurrence (up to 60%) particularly in Gorlin–Goltz syndrome.

Gorlin–Golz syndrome
(See ● Basal cell carcinoma, p. 154.)
- Rare.
- Autosomal dominant.
- Multiple basal cell carcinoma lesions on the skin aggressive, should not treated with RT (poor response rate, predisposes to new lesions).
- Palmar pits.
- Keratinizing odontogenic cysts in the jaws.
- Fused or bifid ribs.
- Calcification of the falx cerebri.
- Cataracts.

Calcifying epithelial odontogenic cysts
- Rare.
- Areas of calcification and 'ghost cells' on histology.
- Tx = enucleation.

Non-odontogenic cysts

Stafne bone cyst
- Not a true cyst but a developmental inclusion of salivary tissue in the mandible.
- Usually incidental finding on X-ray (radiolucency below the ID canal).
- Well corticated.
- Sialography via the submandibular duct is diagnostic.

Aneurysmal bone cysts
- Slowly expand.
- Vascular bone.
- No epithelial lining.
- Symptomless, unless traumatized.
- Soap bubble appearance on X-ray.
- Tx = enucleation.
- Excision is usually curative.

Solitary bone cysts (traumatic bone cysts)
- Have no epithelial lining.
- Usually found as an incidental finding on X-ray.
- Found above ID canal in body of mandible.
- Characterized by a scalloped upper border passing up between the teeth roots.
- Commonest in young men.
- Tx = enucleation/curettage (probably heal spontaneously on simply opening the cavity to confirm the diagnosis).

Fissural cysts
- Arise from embryonic junctional epithelium at sites of embryological fusions.
- Rare in the mouth, e.g. incisive canal or nasopalatine cysts (heart-shaped radiolucency in premaxilla >6mm in diameter), incisive papilla cysts and nasolabial cysts (arise in soft tissue).
- Tx = enucleation.

Intra-oral benign tumours

Odontogenic tumours

Only the commonest will be discussed.

Odontomes
- Malformations of dental hard tissue.
- Not true neoplasms but hamartomas.
- Compound odontomes have multiple primitive small teeth in fibrous sac.
- Complex odontomes are an irregular (disorganized) mass of dental hard tissue.

Cementomas
- Part of the spectrum of cemento-osseous dysplasias.
- Three types:
  - periapical cemental dysplasia (common in those of African origin);
  - focal cemento-osseous dysplasia (Caucasians);
  - florid cemento-osseous dysplasia (common in those of African origin).

Ameloblastoma
- Probably arise from odontogenic epithelium.
- Locally invasive.
- Commonest in posterior mandible (75% in ascending ramus), in men and those of African origin.
- Can become huge if neglected.
- Three clinical variants:
  - unicystic is the least aggressive type and expands into the surrounding bone. Radiographically it is unilocular and may be mistaken for an odontogenic cyst;
  - polycystic: multiloculated appearance on X-ray, resorption of teeth roots;
  - peripheral: occurring in soft tissue.
- Histologically two main types:
  - plexiform (cord-like structures);
  - follicular (columnar ameloblast-like cells).
- Treatment:
  - unicystic—conservative/enucleation;
  - polycystic—excision with a margin ± reconstruction.
- Recurrence after enucleation >50%.
- Careful follow-up required; recurrent ameloblastoma, which escapes to the skull base is potentially fatal.
- Malignant ameloblastoma:
  - rare;
  - well-differentiated/benign histology, but metastasis usually to lung (theory of inhalation).
- Ameloblastic carcinoma is described in the literature as showing histologically malignant features.

Adenoameloblastoma/adenomatoid odontogenic tumour
- Anterior maxilla in ♀.
- Often associated with an unerupted tooth.
- Radiographically resembles a dentigerous cyst, which extends beyond the ACJ and may show flecks of calcification.
- Tx = excision, recurrence is rare.

Calcifying epithelial otodontogenic tumour (CEOT or Pindborg tumour)
- Rare.
- X-ray shows a radiolucency with scattered opacities.
- Tx = excision with margin.

Odontogenic myxoma
- Odontogenic mesenchyme origin.
- Affects the bone of young adults and can invade extensively.
- Multilocular radiolucency.
- Histologically 'myxoid tissue' is cell poor and rich in mucopolysaccharide with spindle cells.
- Tx = excision with margin.

Ameloblastic fibroma
- Very rare, seen in teenagers.
- Painless expansion.
- Unilocular radiolucency on X-ray, often in posterior mandible.
- Tx = enucleation.
- Recurrence up to 15%.
- Sarcomatous change of fibrous tissue is a rare complication.

Non-odontogenic tumours
- **Epithelial:** squamous cell papilloma ?secondary to HPV infection.
- **Connective tissue:**
  - fibroma;
  - lipoma;
  - osteoma (can be associated with Gardener syndrome).
- **Neurofibroma:**
  - rare tumour of fibroblasts affecting a peripheral nerve;
  - tongue most often site affected;
  - may be associated with Von Recklinghausen syndrome.
- **Granular cell myoblastoma:**
  - rare;
  - originates from histiocytes;
  - arises as nodule often on tongue;
  - excision is curative.
- **Ossifying fibroma:**
  - clearly defined fibro-osseous lesion of the jaws;
  - presents as a painless, slow growing swelling;
  - can expand buccal and lingual plates;
  - radiolucent area surrounded by radio-opaque margin on X-ray;
  - histology similar to fibrous dysplasia.

Bone disorders: neoplastic

Malignant tumours of the facial bones

- Primary: rare:
  - osteosarcoma;
  - multiple myeloma;
  - primary intra-osseous carcinoma.
- Secondary:
  - by local extension, e.g. SCC of floor of mouth, malignancy of the paranasal sinuses (SCC > adenocarcinoma > ACC);
  - Metastasis from distant site—breast, lung, thyroid, kidney, prostate.

Bone disorders: non-neoplastic

Fibrous dysplasia

- Monostotic (one bone affected).
- Polyostotic (multiple bones affected).
- Albrights's syndrome (polyostotic FD with skin pigmentation and precocious puberty).
- Presentation in adolescents and young adults with painless rounded bony swelling in maxilla, which can disturb occlusion or function.
- X-ray initially radiolucent lesions, eventually radio-opaque or sclerotic-ground glass appearance.
- Histology shows bone replaced by fibrous tissues, woven bone, and giant cells.
- Prognosis good when growth ceases (but may progress after completion of growth).
- Tx = cosmetic or functional.

Cherubism (familial fibrous dysplasia)

- Autosomal dominant.
- Rare.
- Symmetrical.
- Multicystic.
- May regress with maturity or continue progression.

Hyperparathyroidism

- Primary (hypersecretion of parathyroid hormone (PTH) by parathyroid adenoma).
- Secondary (usually caused by renal failure leading to parathyroid hyperplasia).
- Tertiary hyperparathyroidism (where parathyroid over-activity becomes autonomous, even when cause of secondary problem is treated).
- Histology of bone lesions shows osteoclastic giant cells.
- Multilocular cysts on X-ray, i.e. osteitis fibrosa cystica (Von Recklinghausen's disease of bone). Indistinguishable histologically from central giant cell granuloma.
- Primary: ↑ Ca^{2+}, ↓, or normal phosphate, ↑ alkaline phosphatase (ALP), and ↑ PTH. Removal of parathyroid tumour leads to resolution of bone lesions.
- Secondary: normal Ca^{2+}, ↑ ALP, ↑ PTH, and ↑ phosphate.
- Tertiary: ↑ Ca^{2+}, ↑ ALP, and ↑ PTH.

Paget's disease (osteitis deformans)

- Polyostotic disease, rarely leading to clinical symptoms.
- Disorder of bone turnover, commonly affecting pelvis, calvarium of skull and limbs, occasionally maxilla and mandible.
- Initially osteolytic vascularity ↑ with bleeding, rarely high output cardiac failure.
- Later osteosclerotic with ↑ ALP.
- X-rays show radiolucency, loss of trabeculation and lamina dura, followed by radio-opacity (cotton-wool areas) and hypercementosis.
- Histology disorganized bone with reversal lines forming a mosaic pattern.
- Disorganized thicker bones are weaker predisposing to pathological fracture.
- 2–5% risk of osteosarcoma.

Classic radiographic appearances of jaw lesions

Multilocular radiolucencies

- Keratocyst.
- Ameloblastoma.
- Osteitis fibrosa cystica (Brown tumour of HPT).
- Central giant cell lesion.
- Cherubism.
- Odontogenic myxoma.
- Aneurysmal bone cyst.

Radiolucencies at the angle of the mandible

- Dentigerous cyst.
- Keratocyst.
- Ameloblastoma.

Radiopacities

- Chronic apical infection.
- Odontoma.
- Osteoma.

Mixed

- Osteomyelitis.
- CEOT.
- Cemento-osseous dysplasia.
- Osteosarcoma.

Neck lumps

Cervical lymph nodes

General
- Lymphadenitis = inflammation of a node.
- Lymphadenopathy = disease in a node.
- Lymph nodes in health are not normally palpable.
- A node is usually palpable only once size exceeds 1cm.
- Nodes that become inflamed can heal by resolution or with scarring, and remain palpable.
- Most palpable nodes in children are infective/reactive.
- Most palpable nodes over age 50 are metastatic aerodigestive SCC.

Anatomy
The following division of the neck nodes into regions as described at Memorial Sloan-Kettering is accepted universally:
- **Level I:** contains the submental and submandibular nodes.
- **Level II:** upper third of the jugular nodes medial to the SCM, inferior boundary is the plane of the hyoid bone (clinical) or the bifurcation of the carotid artery (surgical).
- **Level III:** middle jugular nodes bounded inferiorly by the plane of the cricoid cartilage (clinical) or the omohyoid (surgical).
- **Level IV:** defined superiorly by the omohyoid muscle and inferiorly by the clavicle.
- **Level V:** contains the posterior cervical triangle nodes.
- **Level VI:** includes the paratracheal and pretracheal nodes.
- **Level VII:** retropharyngeal nodes.
- The submental nodes (submental triangle):
  - drains the medial cheek;
  - lower lip and chin;
  - lower anterior teeth;
  - tip of tongue and anterior floor of mouth.
- The submandibular nodes between the anterior and posterior bellies of digastric muscle, outside capsule of submandibular salivary gland:
  - drains ipsilateral oral cavity including teeth;
  - lower eyelid;
  - cheek;
  - nasal mucosa and skin.
- The facial node (anterior border of masseter on course of facial vein) drains facial skin, palate, upper teeth, and buccal mucosa.
- The parotid nodes (intra- or extra-glandular part of the parotid) drain forehead, scalp, auricle, EAM, eardrum, and EUT.
- The retropharyngeal nodes (posterior to the pharyngeal wall, between the prevertebral fascia and the pharyngeal wall) drain posterior nasal cavity, palate, nasopharynx, and EUT.
- Upper jugular nodes drain the larynx, upper trachea, and oesophagus.
- The jugulo-digastric node drains the posterior tongue, pharynx and tonsil.

- The spinal accessory node is located along the SAN, and receives afferent flow from the occipital, mastoid, and maxillary sinus.
- The supraclavicular node is located at the jugulosubclavian junction and receives afferent flow from the spinal accessory, lower neck, upper chest, lung, and GIT.
- The internal jugular node is located along the internal jugular chain and receives afferent flow from the superior nodal group, mucosal sites in the head and neck, and thoracic and axillary nodes.

Causes of lymphadenopathy

Infective
- Local bacterial:
  - teeth;
  - skin;
  - tonsils.
- Local viral:
  - URTI;
  - primary HSV.
- General bacterial:
  - TB;
  - cat scratch disease;
  - secondary syphilis.
- General viral:
  - HIV;
  - CMV;
  - EBV;
  - Rubella (occipital nodes, other causes are HIV and lice).

Neoplastic
- Local metastatic:
  - aerodigestive tract mucosal SCC;
  - other head and neck malignancy (skin, salivary, thyroid, paranasal sinuses);
  - breast;
  - stomach.
- General:
  - lymphoma;
  - leukaemia.

Other
- drugs (allopurinol, penicillin, cephalosporins, atenolol, captopril, phenytoin, etc.);
- sarcoidosis.

Management of cervical lymphadenopathy
- History.
- Examination.

Investigations may include:
- OPT;
- USS;
- FNAC;

- MRI;
- FBC, ESR, serology for CMV, HSV, monospot, LDH, ACE;
- Biopsy may be indicated.

Lymphoma

- May be nodal or extra-nodal.
- Diagnosis usually requires histology rather than cytology; i.e. biopsy.
- Hodgkin (Reed–Sternberg cells)/non-Hodgkin lymphoma (NHL).
- Staging requires bloods (FBC, LDH, ESR), as well as CT (chest, abdomen, and pelvis):
  - *Stage I*—confined to single nodal region;
  - *Stage II*—two or more regions on same side of diaphragm;
  - *Stage III*—involvement of nodes on both sides of diaphragm;
  - *Stage IV*—spread beyond lymph nodes;
  - ± A (no systemic symptoms) or B (weight loss >10%, unexplained fever or night sweats).
- Treatment:
  - IA and IIA—RT;
  - IIB to IVB—chemotherapy.
- 5-year survival >90% IA, <40% IVB.
- Classification constantly changing and complex.

Midline neck swellings

- Thyroglossal duct cyst:
  - moves up on tongue protrusion;
  - may present with infection;
  - removal to include midline of hyoid (Sistrunck's procedure) to reduce recurrence rate.
- Sub-lingual dermoid cyst: lies in between bellies of genioglossus deep to mylohyoid and, thus, can be removed intra-orally.
- Thyroid swellings.

Lateral swellings

- Branchial (lympho-epithelial) cyst:
  - commonly arises from proliferation of residual remnants of second branchial cleft;
  - alternative theories of origin include proliferation of lymphoid tissue associated with epithelial remnants.
- Tumour in tail of parotid.
- Carotid body tumour:
  - lie at site of bifurcation;
  - of chemoreceptor origin;
  - compressible;
  - bruit on auscultation;
  - other parapharyngeal space tumours include schwannomas and neurilemmomas.
- Cervical rib: may have associated thoracic outlet syndrome.

- Cystic hygroma (see ➋ Vascular malformations of the head and neck, p. 290).
- Pharyngeal pouch:
  - presents in posterior triangle behind SCM;
  - may fill after meal and empty on lying down;
  - endoscopic-stapling treatment of choice.

Facial palsy

Aetiology

Central
- Vascular.
- Central nervous system (CNS) degenerative disease.
- Trauma.
- Tumours.
- Congenital (Mobius syndrome).

Temporal
- Bacterial/viral infections.
- Trauma.
- Tumours.
- Cholesteatoma.
- Iatrogenic.

Parotid
- Tumours.
- Trauma.
- Iatrogenic.
- Idiopathic.

UMN vs LMN lesions
- Nuclei of lower motor neurones lie in motor nucleus of VII in the pons.
- Lesions including and distal to motor nucleus cause LMN palsy.
- Bell's (LMN) palsy is a diagnosis by exclusion, caused by ?herpes simplex virus. Aciclovir and prednisolone decrease the incidence of permanent paralysis.
- UMN lesions spare the frontal region due to bicortical innervation of the VII nerve motor nuclei to the upper face. Some movement is preserved in emotion.
- Bilateral LMN palsy—consider Lyme disease (*Borrelia bergdorfi*) or Guillain–Barré syndrome.

Diagnosis
- History.
- Examination to include:
  - upper vs lower motor lesion;
  - House–Brackmann score (I–VI) grades degree of nerve damage;
  - hearing;
  - stapes reflex;
  - tearing test;
  - taste;
  - submandibular salivary flow.
- Investigations:
  - neurophysiology;
  - plain films;
  - MRI/CT;
  - USS.

Goals of reconstruction

- Normal appearance at rest.
- Sphincter control.
- Symmetry with voluntary and involuntary movement.

Reconstructive options

- **Direct repair:** requires healthy nerve and healthy muscle.
- **Interpositional nerve graft:**
  - donor—sural, greater auricular, cervical plexus (C3, C4);
  - connect stump to zygomatic and/or buccal branches;
  - recovery takes 6–18 months;
  - mass movement, dyskinesia, and synkinesia common.
- **Myoneurotization:** motor nerve and end-plate transplanted.
- **Cross-facial nerve graft:**
  - *stage 1*—pass nerve graft from buccal branch on normal side to affected side (monitor with Tinel testing);
  - *stage 2*—harvest functional muscle (gracilis, pectoralis minor) for free microneurovascular transfer to affected side and re-innervate with cross-facial nerve graft.
- **Nerve transfer:** phrenic or hypoglossal nerve transferred to distal facial nerve. Produces synkinesis, rather than spontaneous expression.
- **Dynamic muscle transposition:** temporalis (fold-over or direct), masseter, SCM, platysma, or anterior belly of digastric.
- **Static procedures:** e.g. brow lift, gold weights into eyelid, selective balancing neurectomy, facelift.

The paranasal sinuses

- Sinus is a Latin word meaning fold or pocket.
- Sinuses in the skull are the parasanal sinuses and the mastoid air cells in the temporal bone.
- Possible biological roles:
  - lightening the skull;
  - adding resonance to the voice;
  - humidification and warming of inhaled air.
- Parasanal sinuses are vestigial at birth.

Drainage

- Maxillary sinuses drain into middle meatus.
- Ethmoidal cells: anterior, middle (both drain to middle meatus), and posterior (drain to superior meatus).
- Frontal sinus drains into the middle meatus.
- Sphenoidal sinus drains into the spheno-ethmoidal recess above the superior concha.
- Nasolacrimal ducts drain to the inferior meati.

Maxillary sinus (antrum)

Largest of the four paired parasanal air sinuses. The alveolus lies inferiorly, orbits superiorly, and nasal cavity medially.

Acute maxillary sinusitis

- Often follows viral URTI.
- Bacterial infection (anaerobes, *Haemophilus*, *Staph.*, and *Strep.*).
- May be difficult to distinguish from toothache (upper second premolars and beyond often have roots projecting into sinus).
- Pain over maxillae worse on bending head forwards.
- Nasal obstruction or discharge.
- Tenderness in the canine fossa.
- Maxillary teeth TTP.
- Post-nasal drip, pyrexia may also be present.
- X-rays—OM view may show antral opacities (polyps or mucosal swelling) or fluid levels.
- Tx = antibiotics (doxycycline or amoxicillin) and decongestants (oxymetazoline or xylometazoline) ± analgesics.

Chronic maxillary sinusitis

- Can follow acute sinusitis.
- Mucosal lining hypertrophies and can form polyps contributing to obstruction of the ostia.
- Post-nasal drip is often present.
- Tx aimed at reventilation of sinus.
- FB if present (e.g. tooth root) needs removal (incision in the canine fossa and bony window into the antrum by Caldwell–Luc approach or by FESS).
- Re-ventilation takes place by:
  - endoscopic enlargement of the ostium ± drainage of other affected sinuses;
  - FESS 'turns a hall connected to a series of small rooms into a gymnasium'.

Extractions and the antrum
- Displacement of teeth and/or roots into the sinus during extractions most often the straight conical palatal root of first molar.
- Two X-ray views required to localize (or CBCT).
- Removal under GA:
  - via socket;
  - Caldwell–Luc;
  - FESS;
  - concurrent repair of any oro-antral communication fistula (OAC).

Oro-antral fistula
- A fistula is an abnormal permanent passageway between two body surfaces.
- An acute oro-antral communication commonly occurs following extraction:
  - may heal spontaneously;
  - may subsequently fistulate.
- An OAF is an epithelial lined tract between mouth and maxillary sinus. Can follow extraction of maxillary molar or premolar teeth.
- Diagnosis: air bubbles through the tract when the patient attempts to blow out against a closed nose.
- Antral mucosa/polyp may prolapse through the extraction socket.
- OAF may be presentation of antral carcinoma.

Management
If small and suspected at time of extraction avoid nose blowing, suture socket, ± antibiotics.

Buccal advancement flap
- Excise fistula (and submit for histology) or use as superior layer by placing a purse string suture), and raise a wide-based buccal flap over bone. Incise the periosteum along the length of the flap to allow the mucosa to advance over the socket.
- Close over bone without tension and suture to palatal mucosa.
- Mattress sutures can be helpful.
- Prescribe antibiotics post-operatively.
- Flap reduces the depth of the sulcus at this point.

± buccal fat pad flap
- When performing a buccal advancement flap, the buccal pad of fat is often exposed.
- Mobilize the fat and use it to provide a two-layered closure (improves security of repair and rarely fails).

Palatal advancement flap
- Excise fistula (use as stated if possible) and raise a full-thickness mucoperiosteal palatal flap based on the palatine artery—rotate over the socket and suture.
- Bare bone in the palate left to granulate under a cover plate.
- Problem: distortion/shortening of the flap as it is rotated.
- May be required when buccal advancement has failed.

Dental osseointegrated implants

Introduction
- Osseointegration described by Professor P-I Brånemark in 1960s.
- Osseointegration = direct structural and functional connection between the implant surface and bone.
- Requires minimally traumatic placement of a biocompatible implant into bone, achieving primary stability.
- Healing period shortened (<6 weeks) with rougher, chemically treated surfaces.
- Immediate loading possible in some sites.
- Shorter implants demonstrate high long-term success rates.
- Long 'zygomaticus' implants developed to engage distant bone of malar prominence.

Implant tissue interface
- Exact mechanism of osseo-integration unknown.
- Direct bone-implant contact occurs with titanium, Ti alloys, aluminium, cobalt and nickel-based metals.
- Titanium mainly used as it forms an oxide surface layer that is inert and resistant to body fluids, is easily machined, and is strong enough to withstand masticatory load.

Placement of an implant
Results in:
- Bleeding and local inflammatory reaction.
- A blood clot which forms between implant and bone.
- Blood clot organizes into a dense procallus.
- Mesenchymal cell differentiation into osteoblasts and fibroblasts.
- Procallus calcifies with the formation of woven bone at 3 weeks.
- Lamellar bone laid down at 7 weeks.
- Bone at implant interface becomes denser and matures with functional loading.
- Peri-implant sulcus forms lined with non-keratinizing epithelium.
- Connective tissue fibres run parallel to the implant surface forming a tight cuff not a direct attachment.

Anatomical considerations
- Implant success is proportional to bone density.
- Mandibular implants are more successful than maxillary ones.
- The nasal floor, maxillary sinuses, and incisive foramen all affect implant placement.
- With resorption bone stock becomes concentrated between the nasal wall, maxillary sinus, and tuberocity.
- The canine eminence may be the most predictable site for implant placement in the maxilla.
- Bone resorption narrows arch width and increases intermaxillary distance.

- Implants may diverge away from the sagittal plane with greater lateral loading.
- The mandible is predominantly cortical bone, especially at the symphysis.
- The IDN restricts implant length proximal to mental foramen.
- Implants should not be placed within 2mm of the IDN.
- The IDN can be damaged as it loops anterior to mental foramen.

History, examination, investigations → treatment plan

Patient assessed on clinical need and general and local considerations.

General factors include:
- Psychiatric disorders including dysmorphobia.
- Pregnancy in the view of the need for radiographs.
- Immunosuppression (drug or disease).
- Previous radiotherapy ↑ failure rates <50% (role of HBO uncertain).
- Smoking.
- Bisphosphonates (↑ risk BRONJ).
- Poorly-controlled diabetes.

Local factors include:
- Poor oral hygiene.
- Ongoing periodontal disease.
- Dental caries.
- Epithelial or connective tissue disease affecting wound healing (erosive LP, pemphigus).

Investigations and records
E.g. PAs, OPT, CBCT, photographs and study casts.

Treatment plan based on:
- Diagnostic set-up (occlusion, implant position, prosthetic appearance).
- Surgical guide copied from diagnostic set-up or custom-made from CBCT for guided surgery.
- Implant sites and need for grafting determined by prosthesis (fixed or removable) and imaging.

Surgical procedure
- LA, ± sedation, or GA.
- Antibiotic use controversial.
- Precise technique with minimal soft and hard tissue trauma.
- Minimal access using surgical guides, incisions lying over or close to the crest of ridge.
- Guides can be hard or soft tissue born and may be retained with miniscrews.
- In anterior maxilla, crestal incision is palatal to ridge to bring keratinized mucosa to buccal and improve aesthetics.
- Flaps are subperiosteal; any relieving incisions should be remote from implant sites.
- Irrespective of the system used a series of drills is employed to enlarge and deepen the implant site.

- Ideally, 3D implant position should not compromise choice of abutment, emergence profile, or prosthesis.
- Continuous irrigation to avoid thermal bone necrosis.
- Depth is pre-planned and assessed using manufacturers' gauges.
- Intra-operative radiographs may be used to avoid damage to vital structures.
- Dense bone is tapped to ease insertion of threaded implants.
- Once completed, implant site should be irrigated to clear any debris.
- Implants can be submerged or transmucosal; increasingly used as:
  - single-stage procedure;
  - allows continuous assessment during healing;
  - soft tissues mature as bone heals.
- Meticulous wound closure, avoiding tension.
- Care with provisional prosthesis to avoid direct pressure on site.
- Buried implants uncovered after 3–4 months.

Advanced techniques

Patients who most benefit from implants often have least bone. Methods devised to overcome these difficulties include:

- Ridge expansion in the maxilla using osteotomes to compact the central cancellous bone against the buccal and palatal walls. This corrects width but not height.
- Bone grafting of smaller sites using autogenous bone (external oblique ridge, chin), osteoconductive alloplasts (tri-calcium phosphate, hydroxyapatite), xenografts (bovine, equine, porcine), or osteo-inductive materials (e.g. bone morphogenic proteins in a carrier graft).
- Larger onlay grafts (iliac crest, calvarium).
- Sinus floor elevation lifts the sinus lining creating space for a graft ± implant.
- Distraction osteogenesis (demanding of patient and surgeon).
- Free tissue transfer, for larger defects usual following ablative surgery.
- Augmentation of the soft tissue envelope with free connective tissue grafts from palate, or xenograft collagen sheets.
- Guided tissue regeneration using a membrane to exclude gingival tissues from the wound allowing bone or periodontal ligament progenitor cell migration into the area.

Online resources

Clinical Evidence website. Available at: ✆ http://clinicalevidence.bmj.com

GMC. *Consent guidance: patients and doctors making decisions together.* Available at: ✆ http://www.gmc-uk.org/guidance/ethical_guidance/consent_guidance/index.asp

Hospital Episode Statistics. Available at: ✆ http://www.hesonline.nhs.uk

NICE website. Available at: ✆ http://www.nice.org.uk

SIGN website. Available at: ✆ http://www.sign.ac.uk

Oral medicine

Introduction

This chapter covers a disparate group of conditions that may present within the oral cavity. Some are manifestations of systemic disease; others are localized to the head and neck region. An overview of the common infective conditions is included. Finally, conditions causing facial pain are considered; this section should be read in conjunction with Chapter 9 on temporomandibular joint disorders.

Oral ulceration

Definition

Defect in the continuity of oral epithelium where the underlying connective tissue is exposed. Causes include:

- Traumatic:
  - physical;
  - chemical;
  - burns.
- Infective: bacterial or viral.
- Idiopathic: recurrent oral ulceration.
- Iatrogenic: drug induced.
- Mucocutaneous:
  - vesiculobullous disorders;
  - erosive lichen planus.
- Neoplastic: see Chapter 2 topics.
- Systemic disease:
  - haematological disorders;
  - gastrointestinal disease;
  - autoimmune disorders.

Clinical

- Diagnosis based on history: site, shape, size, symptoms including pain, duration, number present.
- History should include questioning about general health especially GI, joint, and eye symptoms as oral ulceration may be a manifestation of systemic disease.
- Investigations should be directed towards suspected condition and include biopsy (mandatory if present for >4 weeks) bloods, immunology, HLA screening.

Treatment

- Dependent on cause.

Recurrent oral ulceration

Up to 25% of the population are reported to suffer from recurrent aphthous ulceration at any one time, usually starting in childhood or adolescence. The underlying disease process is thought to represent a T-cell-mediated immunological reaction. Different subgroups of patients appear to have different predisposing factors for their disease. The following have all been implicated:

- Trauma.
- Genetic:
  - ↑ frequency with HLA-A2, A11, B12, DR2;
  - FH in 40%.
- Nutritional:
  - ↑ in Crohn's/coeliac disease (both associated with certain HLA types) and other inflammatory bowel disorders, ?secondary to malabsorption.

- **Haematological deficiencies**: cause thinning of epithelial barrier.
- **Immunodysregulation**:
  - HIV;
  - chemotherapy;
  - IgA deficiencies.
- **Hormonal**:
  - related to fall in progesterone in luteal phase menstrual cycle;
  - often resolve during pregnancy.
- **Hypersensitivity response**: patients may demonstrate atopy or allergies to food.
- **Stress related**: possibly secondary to effects of stress on the immune system.
- **Drugs**: especially nicorandil, immune-modulating drugs, and NSAIDs.
- **Cessation smoking**.

There are three main types of aphthous ulceration:
- Minor, ~80% of all cases.
- Major (10%).
- Herpetiform (10%).

Minor aphthous ulceration
- More common in ♀.
- Almost exclusively non-keratinized mucosa, especially buccal/labial.
- Often prodromal phase—burning or itching.
- <5mm diameter, usually1–5 at once, extremely painful.
- Ulcer with removable yellow/white membrane and erythematous halo. Last 10–14 days.
- Heal without scarring.
- Episodes vary from every few weeks to every few years.

Major aphthous ulceration
- Usually occur post-puberty.
- Occur on any mucosal surface including attached, although usually affect labial/buccal mucosa and soft palate.
- Up to 3cm diameter.
- Up to 10 present at one time.
- More pronounced erythematous halo than minor.
- Last up to 6 weeks.
- May heal with scarring.

Herpetiform
- Name a misnomer—not caused by herpes virus.
- More common in ♀, occur in adulthood.
- Usually affects non-keratinized mucosa, although any mucosal surface can be affected.
- Up to 100 small (1–3mm) ulcers lasting 7–10 days; may coalesce and resemble primary herpetic stomatitis.
- Frequent recurrences (may be almost continuous for 2–3 years).

Investigations
- Review medical history for evidence of systemic disorders.
- Bloods:
  - *commonly*—FBC, B12, red cell folate, serum ferritin;
  - *others advocate*—B vitamins, auto-antibodies;
  - *more controversial*—zinc, magnesium.
- Consider biopsy if persist.

Treatment
- Chlorhexidine mouthwash has been shown in RCTs to decrease length of ulceration.
- Topical LA.
- Doxycycline mouthwash.
- Topical corticosteroids.
- If very severe consider oral prednisolone.
- Triamcinolone injections for major aphthae (if biopsy negative for malignancy).

Behçet's syndrome

Definition/epidemiology

- Multisystem disorder that classically presents with the triad of oral ulceration, genital ulceration, and uveitis.
- Most common in Turkey; also middle Eastern and Mediterranean population—along the 'Silk Road'.
- Usually young adults, ♂ > ♀, ♂ more severe symptoms.
- In UK, 1–5:100,000 affected.

Cause

- Unknown.
- Strong HLA association, HLA B51, HLA B27—milder symptoms.
- Other genes implicated, e.g. IL10.
- Possible disturbance of T-cell immune regulation.
- Rates tend towards indigenous population after immigration suggesting environmental factors also involved.

Clinical features

Oral

- Oral ulceration often first feature.
- 99% will develop oral ulceration during course of illness.
- Similar to recurrent oral ulceration (ROU), but soft palate and oropharynx involved.
- Often >6 ulcers present, last 10 days.
- All three types of ROU seen but herpetiform rare.

Genital

- Similar appearance to oral ulcers, but may heal with scarring as deeper.
- ♀ vulva, cervix, vagina; ♂ scrotum, although anywhere in groin may be affected.
- Present in 75% patients.

Ocular

- Eye signs more common and more severe in ♂.
- Present in 70–85%.
- Anterior or posterior uveitis, conjunctivitis, corneal ulceration, and retinal vasculitis may all occur.
- May lead to optic atrophy, cataracts, glaucoma, and blindness.
- 1:4 may have some visual loss.

Other systems—secondary to vasculitis

- CNS: stroke, headaches, diplopia, balance disturbances, behavioural changes, bladder/bowel incontinence.
- Skin (50%): erythema nodosum and vasculitic changes usually affecting lower limbs, acne.
- Musculoskeletal (2/3 cases): especially knees, ankles, wrists.
- GIT: vomiting, diarrhoea, symptoms similar to IBS, anorexia.
- CVS: pericarditis—very common, DVT, cerebral venous thrombosis, aneurysms.

Investigations
- No diagnostic test is positive in all cases.
- Skin hyper-reactivity common—1–2 days after injection saline under skin, results in a sterile pustule.
- Raised ESR and IgA.

Treatment—with rheumatologists
- Immunomodulating drugs:
  - steroids—topical, oral, or IV;
  - colchicine—reduces level inflammation of mucosa, effective for oral/genital/skin involvement;
  - thalidomide;
  - mesalazine if GI symptoms;
  - ciclosporin especially if eyes affected;
  - cyclophosphamide IV if vision threatened.
- Analgesics especially NSAIDs.
- Biological therapies, e.g.:
  - infliximab, anti-TNF;
  - interferon alpha;
  - adalimumab, anti-TNF;
  - etanercept.

Prognosis
- Usually relapsing/remitting.
- Highly variable pattern of presentation and outcome.
- Mortality low unless CNS or significant vascular involvement. Leads to CNS/pulmonary haemorrhage or bowel perforation.

Lichen planus

Definition

Immunologically mediated disease of stratified squamous epithelium mucocutaneous tissues. Affects skin, oral mucosa, genitalia (Fig. 11.1 and Fig. 11.2).

Epidemiology

Affects 1% population (2% for oral LP), presents 30–55 years, ♀ >♂ for oral lesions, ♂=♀ for skin lesions.

Cause

Aetiology unknown. ?T-cell-mediated immune response.

Clinical features

Oral
- Most commonly affects buccal/labial mucosa, tongue, gingivae.
- Usually bilateral.
- Often asymptomatic.
- Ulcerated/atrophic areas may become painful.
- Six clinical subtypes identified; more than one type may be evident:
  - *reticular* (70–80%)—raised white lines/striae;
  - *erosive* (9%)—painful, slow healing ulcers/erosions, desquamative (gingivitis);
  - *atrophic*—red atrophic areas, desquamative gingivitis;
  - *popular*—white papules;
  - *plaque-like*—thick white plaques;
  - *bullous.*

Other manifestations
- Violet papules 3–5mm diameter: often with white (Wickham's) striae on flexor surface wrists, ankles.
- May occur in skin creases.
- May get thickened scaly patches especially around ankles—hypertrophic LP.
- Itchy (Koebner phenomenon), but painful when scratched.
- Skin lesions usually resolve in 6–9 months.
- Nail involvement: vertical ridges, occasional destruction of nail.
- Scalp: may develop permanent bald patches.
- Glans penis and vulva: similar appearance to oral lesions.

Diagnosis

Clinical appearance and biopsy of non-ulcerated lesion.

Treatment

- Asymptomatic: reassurance, no active treatment.
- If pain/ulceration: escalating treatment:
  - *topical steroids*—hydrocortisone/betamethasone lozenges, spray, inhalers; prednisolone or betamethasone mouthwash;
  - intralesional triamcinolone for large, non-healing ulcers;
  - 2–3 weeks oral prednisolone.

- Other drugs—usually in tertiary care:
  - azathioprine;
  - ciclosporin;
  - 0.1% tretinoin gel;
  - tacrolimus;
  - cyclophosphamide.

Prognosis

Oral lesions may persist for many years.
  Small risk of malignant change, especially if erosive.

Lichenoid reactions

- Closely resemble lesions of erosive LP but due to drug reactions, e.g. antimalarials or gold injections (hypersensitivity to amalgam, constituents of toothpaste or unknown irritant).
- May closely match pattern of restorations.
- Usually respond to removal of offending agent.
- Patch testing /biopsy may aid diagnosis.

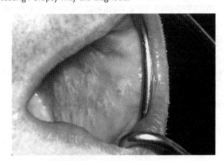

Fig. 11.1 Lichen planus.

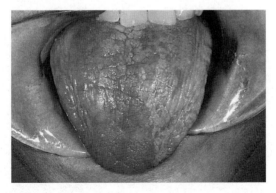

Fig. 11.2 Lichen planus.

Desquamative gingivitis

Descriptive term for chronic mucosal desquamation seen as part of a number of diseases. ♀>♂.

Causes
- LP.
- Vesiculobullous diseases.
- Allergic responses, e.g. toothpaste.
- Psoriasis.
- Drug reactions.

Clinical appearance
- Affects gingival tissues from margin to alveolar mucosa.
- Initially loss of gingival stippling and erythema.
- Vesicles/bullae form: often rupture before presentation.
- Long-term: areas of ulceration/erosion/atrophy.
- Most common anteriorly, rarely affects palatal/lingual mucosa.
- May be asymptomatic or sting/burn, aggravated by certain foods.

Investigation
Biopsy including immunofluorescence, ?patch testing.

Treatment
- Oral hygiene: plaque aggravates condition (gingival LP not seen in edentulous patients).
- Topical steroids.
- Treatment otherwise dependent on underlying condition.

Pemphigus

Definition
Potentially life-threatening vesiculobullous autoimmune disorder affecting skin and mucous membranes.

Epidemiology
Rare, ♂=♀, most commonly presents in middle age. Higher risk groups: Ashkenazi Jews, Mediterranean descent.

Cause
- Autoantibodies directed against components of epithelial desmosome tonofilament, preventing epithelial cell adherence leading to intra-epithelial clefting.
- Rarely drug-induced or paraneoplastic.
- *DR4* and *DRw4* gene mutations common in people with pemphigus; may increase susceptibility to disease.

Subtypes
- Vulgaris and vegetans (vegetans rare, subtype of vulgaris).
- Erythematous and folliaceus: don't usually affect oral cavity.

Clinical: pemphigus vulgaris
- Commonest type.
- Affects skin and any mucous membrane.
- Chronic course.
- Oral lesions precede skin lesions by up to 1 year and may sometimes be the only clinical manifestation.
- Orally, most common on soft/hard palate, buccal mucosa, lips, gingivae (as desquamative gingivitis).
- Fragile, flaccid bullae: rupture easily to form superficial erosions (Fig. 11.3).
- Positive Nikolsky sign (digital sliding pressure causes epithelial separation).
- Eyes: simple conjunctivitis (no scarring/symblepharon formation so no threat to vision).

Investigation
- Biopsy for histology (H&E, specimen into formalin) (intra-epithelial vesicles, 'tombstone' appearance) and immunofluorescence (specimen into frozen section substitute or normal saline and same-day transport to laboratory).
- Intra-epithelial immune deposits (mainly IgG, IgM, and C3) present intra-epithelially on direct immunofluorescence.
- Indirect immunofluorescence positive in 80–90%. Rarely performed.
- Anti-desmosomal antibodies in serum. Levels indicate disease activity.

Treatment

If untreated can rapidly be fatal secondary to superimposed infection, fluid and protein loss from extensive ruptured bullae, or swallowing difficulties if oesophageal involvement. Mortality approaches 10%. Treatment options include:

- Prednisolone: up to 200mg/day (monitor BP, may need anti-hypertensives initially) with PPI ± osteoporosis prophylaxis.
- Once settled reduce to maintenance dose.
- Pulse therapy—high-dose IV prednisolone and cyclophosphamide 3 days/month for at least 6 months.
- Azathioprine, cyclophosphamide, mycophenolate mofetil, and ciclosporin can be used as adjunct to help reduce steroid doses.
- Dapsone or colchicine.
- Tetracycline reduces infection in ruptured bullae.
- Biological agents such as rituximab.

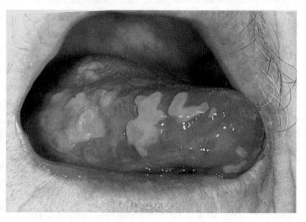

Fig. 11.3 Pemphigus—erosions.

Pemphigoid

Definition

Subepithelial vesiculobullous disorders—autoimmune origin. Two main subtypes affect oral cavity—bullous pemphigoid and benign mucous membrane (often called cicatricial) pemphigoid.

Bullous pemphigoid

Epidemiology

Most common of vesiculobullous autoimmune conditions. Presents age 60–70, ♂=♀.

Cause

Autoantibodies directed against basement membrane cause subepithelial clefting.

Clinical

- Lesions are thick-walled bullae preceded by erythematous rash/pruritis that may last for several weeks.
- Lesions primarily affect skin of limbs/abdomen.
- 30% have oral lesions (tough bullae that rupture to form areas of shallow ulceration). Can be induced by pressure.
- Desquamative gingivitis common.

Investigation

- Biopsy for histology (subepithelial clefting) and immunofluorescence.
- Direct immunofluorescence: linear deposits of IgG at epithelial basement membrane zone.
- Indirect immunofluorescence: positive in 40–70%.

Treatment

Systemic steroids, azathioprine, methotrexate, or dapsone have all been used. Tetracyclines, sometimes combined with nicotinamide, may help reduce infective sequelae

Benign mucous membrane pemphigoid

Epidemiology

Presents on average 10 years earlier than bullous pemphigoid and is rarer. ♀>♂.

Cause

Autoantibodies against one or more components of basement membrane leading to subepithelial clefting.

Clinical

- Affects mucous membranes commonly.
- Skin lesions rarer; same as bullous pemphigoid.

Oral manifestations
- Desquamative gingivitis.
- Bullae/vesicles often seen—thick-walled, therefore less likely to rupture than in pemphigus.
- Form extensive painful ulcers that may take weeks to heal.
- Can affect any part of oral cavity, but tend to recur at the same sites.

Ocular manifestations
- Present in ~25% patients who have oral manifestations.
- Initially, conjunctivitis and erosions as well as subconjunctival scarring.
- Xerophthalmos can occur as lacrimal gland function reduces with scarring. Cornea produces keratin as a protective layer leading to ↓ vision.
- Symblepharons (scarring between lids) further decreases vision.
- Blindness if untreated.

Other manifestations
Can also affect genital, nasal, oesophageal, and laryngeal tissues and skin, lesions similar to those in the oral cavity. Laryngeal involvement can be serious with airway obstruction from large bullae.

Investigation
- Biopsy: normal tissue shows subepithelial clefting.
- Direct immunofluorescence: linear IgG and C3 deposits at basement membrane zone.
- Indirect immunofluorescence: rarely positive (~5% patients).

Treatment
- As for bullous pemphigoid.
- Ocular: all patients require regular ophthalmology review even if no clinically obvious lesions.

Erythema multiforme

Definition
Sudden-onset, immunologically mediated hypersensitivity reaction affecting skin and mucous membranes (Fig. 11.4).

Epidemiology
Uncommon, affects young ♂ aged 20–30 years or children, often +ve FH.

Causes
Aetiology unclear, appears to be acute hypersensitivity reaction. Triggers can be identified in half of cases and include:
- Drugs, e.g. carbamazepine, phenytoin, penicillins, NSAIDs. Classical historical drug causes (barbiturates, sulphonamides) are rarely prescribed these days.
- Infection: classically herpes simplex virus, mycoplasma pneumonia.
- UV light.
- Chemicals, e.g. food colourants, perfumes.
- Pregnancy.
- Malignancy.
- Immune conditions.

Clinical
- Wide spectrum of symptoms from mild to life threatening.
- Prodromal headache, malaise, arthralgia.
- Oral ulceration, haemorrhagic lesions, circumoral crusting.
- Similar lesions may affect genitalia.
- Eye lesions: photophobia, conjunctivitis, symblepharon.
- Skin lesions: target lesions (mainly hands/feet), concentric rings with central papule that becomes ulcerated, surrounded by red and then pale oedematous ring.
- Usually subsides in 2 weeks but can last >6 weeks.
- Recurs in up to 25% cases.
- Stevens–Johnson syndrome: severe form of EM, often drug related, must have either eye or genital involvement. Toxic epidermal necrolysis may be severest part of same spectrum.

Investigation
- Diagnosis is clinical.
- Investigation for underlying trigger may reduce recurrences.

Treatment
- Withdraw triggering factors.
- Supportive therapy: nutrition, IV rehydration, OH.
- Prednisolone or other immunosuppressants if severe.
- Aciclovir if herpes simplex.

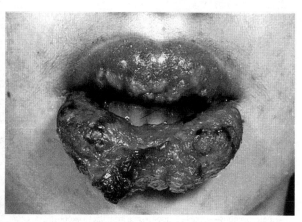

Fig. 11.4 Erythema multiforme.

Leukoplakia

Definition
- WHO: 'white patch/plaque that cannot be characterized clinically or pathologically as any other disease'.
- Diagnosis of exclusion.

Epidemiology
3% white adults, middle aged/elderly, ♂>♀.

Risk factors
- Tobacco.
- Alcohol.
- Betel nut.

Clinical
- Variable appearance:
  - **homogenous**—uniform white plaques, may be widespread (Fig. 11.5);
  - **heterogenous**—variable in appearance from flat to exophytic, often on erythematous background (speckled or erythroleukoplakia) (Fig. 11.6) associated with higher risk malignant transformation.
- Can affect any site: buccal mucosa/vermillion/gingivae most common.
- High-risk sites: floor of mouth/lateral tongue.

Investigation
Biopsy of most irregular site especially if erythroleukoplakia. Histology may show:
- Epithelial atrophy.
- Hyperplasia with/without hyperkeratosis.
- No dysplasia.
- Dysplasia of varying degree—mild/moderate/severe. 3–6% of oral white patches will show SCC. WHO recommends the term 'squamous intraepithelial neoplasia'.

Relationship to oral SCC
- Over 50% oral SCC arises without premalignant stage.
- Only 50% oral leukoplakias show dysplasia.
- The term potentially malignant oral lesions (PMOL) is useful.
- Oral leukoplakia without dysplasia is still a PMOL (in ♀ non-smokers progression to SCC still occurs—?HPV-related).
- No valid markers of progression of PMOL to SCC.
- Studies relate to LOH (loss of heterozygosity), *p53* status.
- *p53* is normal tumour suppressor oncogene.
- Wild or mutant *p53* (detected by IHC) is frequently found in PMOL, which progress to SCC.
- Mild dysplasia often regresses.
- Mild dysplasia < 5% risk of progression.
- Severe dysplasia ?15% risk of progression, but figures vary widely.
- Cochrane Collaboration 2004 reported no RCTs for any intervention in oral leukoplakia which was proven to reduce the risk of development of oral SCC.

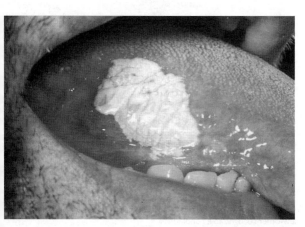

Fig. 11.5 Homogenous plaque of leukoplakia.

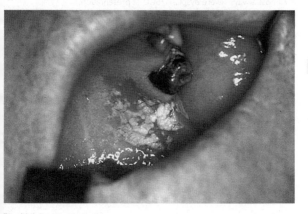

Fig. 11.6 Speckled leukoplakia.

Management
- Patient education regarding risk factors.
- Long-term follow-up, especially if high-risk appearance/high-risk site/ widespread mucosal involvement.
- Clinical photography.
- Excision/ablation if biopsy shows dysplasia.
- See **→** Premalignant conditions, p. 69.

Proliferative verrucous leukoplakia
- Variant with particularly high risk of malignant transformation. Almost all lesions will develop SCC within a decade.
- Initially flat white lesion, develops exophytic/papillomatous appearance.
- ?Associated with papilloma virus.
- Requires excision.

Erythroplakia
WHO definition: 'any lesion of the oral mucosa that presents as bright red velvety plaques, which cannot be characterized clinically or pathologically as any other recognizable condition'.
- Clinically well-demarcated erythematous papule/plaque, often associated with leukoplakia.
- Almost always severe dysplasia/SCC at presentation.
- Very high risk malignant transformation.
- Risk factors as leukoplakia.
- Tends to affect older men.

Aggressive management with low threshold for excision/ablation.

Submucous fibrosis

Definition
Chronic, progressive scarring of the superficial oral connective tissue.

Epidemiology
Adults from Asia and emigrants from this area.

Risk factors
- Paan (areca nut/slaked lime/tobacco): alkaloids trigger hyperplasia of fibroblasts.
- Genetic predisposition, ↑ frequency in HLA-A10, -B7, and -DR3.

Clinical
- Chronic progressive disease.
- Initially stomatitis with ulceration, erythema, and pigmentation.
- Trismus develops secondary to formation of tight vertical bands of buccal mucosa.
- Mucosa appears pale/stiff with areas erythro/leukoplakia and atrophy.
- Burning especially with spicy foods.
- Tongue/soft palate may be affected. Tongue decreases in size, epithelial atrophy with loss of filiform papillae.
- Tonsillar atrophy.
- Dry mouth.
- Late stage:
  - hearing loss due to stenosis Eustachian tubes;
  - nasal tonality to voice;
  - dysphagia if oesophagus affected.

Investigation
- Biopsy.
- Haematinics: often anaemic.

Treatment
- Stop risk factors: will halt but not improve symptoms.
- Surgery: short-term result—fibrous banding recurs even in donor tissue grafted from distant site.
- Intralesional triamcinolone to bands: limited benefit.

Prognosis
Long-term review. Up to 8% will develop oral cancer.

Erythema migrans

Definition
Common, aetiology unknown, also called geographic tongue/benign migratory glossitis.

Epidemiology
Found in 1–3% adults, any age. Familial clusters suggest genetic aetiology, ♂>♀, higher incidence in patients with psoriasis.

Clinical
- Usually asymptomatic; some patients complain of pain with spicy foods.
- Commonly anterior two-thirds tongue but all mucosal surfaces can be involved.
- Initially, raised white lesion that develops central well-demarcated erythematous areas in which atrophy filiform papillae has occurred.
- Change in site, size, and appearance with time.
- More common if fissured tongue.

Investigation
- Diagnosed on clinical appearance.
- Biopsy—similar histologically to psoriasis.
- Consider checking for underlying causes of burning mouth/tongue.

Management
- Reassurance.
- Topical anaesthetic or occasionally topical corticosteroids if pain.

Herpes simplex: oral infection

Definition
- DNA virus only found in humans (all herpes viruses are DNA viruses with the characteristic of latency).
- Oral lesions usually due to HSV-1.
- HSV-2 much less common orally (usually genital infection) but clinically indistinguishable.
- Primary and recurrent infection seen—different clinical presentations.

Epidemiology
- ~60–80% adults in the developed world have antibodies indicating prior infection.
- Higher in developing countries.

Primary HSV (primary gingivostomatitis)
Clinical
- Incubation period 3–9 days.
- Transmitted by direct contact or viral shedding from carrier in saliva or other body fluids.
- Often subclinical, asymptomatic in 80%.
- Malaise, fever, anorexia, tender lymphadenopathy in anterior triangle neck.
- Vesiculobullous eruption mucosal surfaces. Pinhead ulcers fuse to form large painful erosions affecting free and attached mucosa.
- Often diagnostic punched-out lesions at midpoint of gingival margin.
- May also be affect vermillion/peri-oral skin.
- Children—gingivostomatitis, if older—pharyngotonsillitis.
- Lasts 5–10 days.

Diagnosis
- Largely clinical.
- Rising HSV antibody titres, cytology, culture, PCR detection HSV DNA.

Treatment—symptomatic support
- Oral hygiene.
- Fluids.
- Bed rest.
- Antipyrexials/topical LAs.
- Antiviral agents—if immunosuppressed or early presentation.

Recurrent herpes simplex infections
After primary infection, virus remains latent in dorsal root and autonomic/cranial nerve ganglia (trigeminal or geniculate) and can be reactivated. May cause clinical signs but some patients will have asymptomatic shedding of viral particles into saliva and will be infectious at this time.

Incidence
Up to 15% adult population have recurrent infections.

Reactivating factors
- UV light.
- Stress.
- Trauma.
- Febrile illnesses.
- Immunosuppression.

Clinical
- Herpes labialis (cold sores):
  - prodromal burning/tingling;
  - macules → vesicles → pustules → scabbed lesions over 3–4 days;
  - heal without scarring;
  - may also affect nasal mucocutaneous junction.
- Intra-oral herpes:
  - *ulcers*—often multiple, gingiva/hard palate; heal in 1–2 weeks.

Erythema multiforme

Treatment
- Topical antivirals, e.g. 5% aciclovir applied in prodromal period.
- Systemic antivirals indicated if immunosuppressed/frequent recurrences. Must be given early.
- Prophylactic oral antivirals if severe.
- Increasing resistance to antivirals becoming problem in immunosuppressed patients.

Herpes varicella zoster virus

Definition
- Human herpes type 3 virus.
- Primary infection: chickenpox (varicella).
- Viral reactivation: shingles (zoster).

Epidemiology
- Chicken pox mainly affects children with peak age 5–9 years.
- Shingles is a disease of the elderly, immunosuppressed, and alcoholic.

Chicken pox

Clinical
- Droplet spread via mucosa upper respiratory tract.
- Incubation period 14–21 days.
- Prodromal illness with malaise, pharyngitis, rhinitis.
- Oral (buccal mucosa) vesicles and ulceration may precede skin lesions.
- Skin: pruritic erythema → vesicle → pustule → crusted lesion.
- Begins—face/trunk; extremities involved later.
- Contagious until all lesions crusted.

Diagnosis
- Clinical grounds.
- Rising antibody titres.

Management
- Supportive.
- Antivirals if early diagnosis and immunosuppressed.

Shingles

Clinical
- Virus dormant in dorsal/cranial root ganglion after primary infection.
- Reactivates → shingles in one dermatome.
- Prodromal period with neuralgia 1–4 days prior to rash.
- Vesicles → pustules → ulceration → crusting over 7–10 days.
- Pre-herpetic pain may lead to unnecessary extractions.
- Skin may heal with scarring/hypopigmentation.
- If ophthalmic division trigeminal nerve involved → corneal ulceration/visual loss.
- Up to 15% develop post-herpetic neuralgia (PHN).
- Higher incidence with increasing age.
- Responds to gabapentin or anticonvulsants.
- Most cases PHN resolve spontaneously within 1 year.
- HZV infection risk factor for stroke and MI.

Management
- Aciclovir if seen within 3 days of first vesicle: ↓ incidence PHN.
- Ophthalmology opinion essential if ophthalmic branch affected.

Ramsay Hunt syndrome
- Rare syndrome.
- Unilateral VII nerve palsy.
- Herpes zoster vesicles in the EAM and ipsilateral pharynx.
- Vertigo/hearing loss secondary to involvement of CN VIII.

Epstein–Barr virus

Definition
Human herpes type 4 virus implicated in numerous conditions, spread via saliva.

Oral manifestations

Infectious mononucleosis
- Infection often subclinical especially in children.
- Prodromal lethargy.
- Sore throat/tonsillar enlargement, fever, rhinitis, cough.
- Generalized tender lymphadenopathy in >90%.
- Hepatosplenomegaly, rarely splenic rupture.
- Skin rashes (also seen if given amoxicillin).
- Petechiae hard/soft palate.
- ANUG.
- May be protracted recovery over many months.
- Remains latent in pharyngeal/salivary epithelial cells.
- Atypical lymphocytes in peripheral blood, resemble monocytes. Diagnosis confirmed using Paul–Bunnell test for antibodies—positive in 90% adult cases, less useful in children. Treatment is supportive only unless life-threatening airway obstruction secondary to tonsillar enlargement—treat with systemic steroids.

Hairy leukoplakia
(See Fig. 11.7.)
- Hyperkeratosis usually lateral border tongue, may involve any part oral cavity.
- Associated with immunosuppression—seen mainly in transplant and HIV-positive patients.
- Diagnosed by biopsy and identification of EBV.
- No treatment required. May resolve with antivirals but recurs once stopped.
- Indicator for HIV testing in consented patient.

Other possible head and neck associations of EBV
- Nasopharyngeal carcinoma.
- Burkitt's lymphoma.
- Lymphoproliferative disorders.

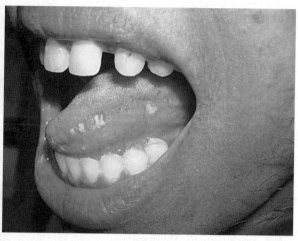

Fig. 11.7 Hairy leukoplakia.

Herpangina

Definition
Coxsackie infection (usually type A) spread by faeco–oral route, commonest <4 years old.

Clinical
- Incubation period 2–6 weeks.
- Periodic epidemics, usually every few years.
- Most cases mild/subclinical infection.
- Fever, general malaise, vomiting, headache.
- 2–4mm vesicular → ulcerative lesions of oropharynx.
- Site pathognomic: affects uvula, palate, fauces.

Treatment
- Supportive only as self-limiting.

Hand, foot, and mouth disease
- Lesions as already described but extending throughout oral cavity.
- Up to1cm diameter.
- Also affects palmar surfaces hands and feet.

Mumps

Definition

RNA paramyxovirus infection, mainly affecting parotid glands.

Epidemiology

Incidence ↑ in UK following ↓ measles, mumps, rubella (MMR) vaccination uptake →↓ herd immunity, especially in young adults.

Clinical

- Spread by droplet/direct contact.
- Incubation period ~16 days.
- 30% subclinical infection.
- Prodromal period with fever, headache, anorexia, myalgia.
- Swelling lower pole parotids, unilateral in ~25%, peaks at 2–3 days (see ➲ Diffuse gland swelling, p. 188).
- Submandibular glands affected ~10%.
- Redness/oedema of Wharton's/Stensen's ducts. In adults involvement of other tissues is much more common.
- Epididymo-orchitis (25%): usually unilateral, infertility rare.
- Oophoritis and mastitis: post-pubertal ♀.
- Pancreatitis.
- Deafness.
- Meningoencephalitis.
- Thyroiditis.

Diagnosis

- Clinical.
- Rise in mumps-specific IgM.

Treatment

- Supportive: analgesics, hydration.
- Hospital admission may be required in adults.

HIV infection

Definition

The human immunodeficiency virus (HIV) is a RNA retrovirus that is able to incorporate its DNA into that of the host. Antibodies develop, but are not protective, leading to lifelong infection. It affects cells with CD4 receptors, mainly T-helper cells, monocytes, and dendritic cells. Damage and decrease in number of these leads to a marked reduction in the CD4 count and thus the T-mediated immune response. Patients are therefore prone to infection with fungi, encapsulated bacteria, and other viruses. Spread is via exchange of infected body fluids including saliva and blood. Worldwide, heterosexual sex is the most common mode of transmission.

Epidemiology

WHO estimated that 34 million worldwide were infected at the end of 2011. Infection rates approach 50% in some sub-Saharan African nations.

Clinical

Acute infection

- Often subclinical, symptoms in 80%.
- Acute self-limiting viral illness clinically similar to infectious mononucleosis (within few weeks of infection).
- Seroconversion occurs within 1–2 months.

Asymptomatic stage

- 8–10 years, increasing with modern treatment →?lifelong asymptomatic infection.
- May have generalized persistent lymphadenopathy (PGL). Biopsy is indicated if persistent raised ESR or LDH or localized, bulky nodes as ↑ incidence of NHL in HIV.

HIV disease

Symptomatic HIV infection, including fungal and viral infections, e.g. *Pneumocystis carinii*, histoplasmosis infections, virally induced malignancies, CNS symptoms including dementia, weight loss, and general deterioration.

AIDS (acquired immunodeficiency syndrome)

Variable presentation, includes CD4 count <200 (poor prognosis).

Oral manifestations of HIV infection

Strongly associated

- Candidosis: often affecting entire oropharynx (Tx—systemic anti-fungals).
- Hairy leukoplakia (EBV).
- HIV periodontal disease:
  - initially linear erythema along gingival margin;
  - ANUG;
  - gross vertical bone loss in presence good oral hygiene;
  - limited response to conventional periodontal treatment—may progress to noma (cancrum oris).

- Kaposi's sarcoma:
  - HHV-8 related;
  - multifocal neoplasm of vascular origin;
  - clinically red/brown, non-blanching lesions;
  - common in oral cavity;
  - treatment only indicated if causing symptoms;
  - RT, intralesional vincristine, local excision—all palliative only.
- Non-Hodgkin lymphoma, often extra-nodal.

Less commonly associated
- Aphthous ulceration, often atypical, but only if had prior to HIV infection.
- Salivary gland disease: HIV associated lympho-epithelial cysts or focal lymphocytic sialadenitis affecting both parotid glands.
- Viral infections other than EBV, e.g. HSV, VZV, CMV, HPV (high incidence dysplasia in oral papilloma caused by HPV). Undertake biopsy if suspicious.
- Idiopathic thrombocytopenic purpura.

Possibly associated with HIV
- Other bacterial/fungal infections.
- Hyperpigmentation.
- Neurological problems, e.g. trigeminal neuralgia, dysaesthesia, palsies.
- SCC oropharynx: same risk factors as general population but develop disease at earlier age.

Diagnosis
- Counselling mandatory prior to testing.
- Blood or saliva can be tested.
- HIV antibodies develop by 3 months (98% sensitivity, may be negative early).
- Antigen testing and/or PCR may detect infection earlier.
- ↓ CD4 counts and CD4/CD8 ratio—used more for disease monitoring—treatment instigated if CD4 <350.
- Presence of unusual pathology, e.g. Kaposi's sarcoma, hairy leukoplakia.

Treatment
Combination anti-retroviral therapy is currently the mainstay of treatment. However, increasing resistance and severe side effects can limit effectiveness. Side effects include facial lipo-atrophy. Individual pathologies are treated as they arise.

Acute necrotizing ulcerative gingivitis

Definition
Acute anaerobic infection of gingival tissues.

Epidemiology
- <0.1% population.
- More common in young ♂ and young children in developing countries.

Risk factors
- Smoking.
- Immunosuppression.
- Malnutrition.
- Poor oral hygiene.
- Local trauma.
- Recent systemic illness.

Cause
Mixed infection: fusiform bacteria, spirochaetes (*Borrelia vincentii*), and anaerobic rods.

Clinical
- Interdental papillae initially oedematous and haemorrhagic, then develop punched out ulcers and necrosis, spreads along gingival margin.
- Pain++.
- Foetor oris.
- If severe, may get necrosis of underlying bone and even skin → noma.

Treatment
- Remove bacterial challenge—hygienist/OHI.
- Hydrogen peroxide/chlorhexidine mouthwash.
- Metronidazole or tetracycline.
- Investigate for any underlying immune deficiency.

Noma (cancrum oris)
Thought to be an extension of ANUG, mainly affecting malnourished children in developing countries shortly after debilitating illness. The disease process extends into surrounding lingual and facial tissues, causing discoloration, then necrosis. Underlying bone may be affected. Treatment is with antibiotics, conservative debridement, and nutritional support. Reconstruction of often extensive resultant defects are commonly required once disease is quiescent for at least a year.

Tuberculosis

Definition
Caseating granulomatous infection caused by mycobacteria.

Epidemiology
At least 1 billion infected worldwide, with 3 million deaths/year. Incidence increased in the developing world, immigrants from these areas, and the immunosuppressed.

Cause
Mycobacterium tuberculosis and, more rarely, *M. bovis*.

Clinical
Droplet spread (*M. tuberculosis*) or via non-pasteurized milk (*M. bovis*).

Primary TB
- Almost always affects lungs with non-specific chronic inflammatory reaction.
- Usually asymptomatic.
- 5–10% infection reactivated, maybe many years later → active disease (secondary TB).
- Primary oral involvement very rare, often secondary to drinking infected milk.

Secondary TB
- Low-grade fever.
- Malaise.
- Anorexia.
- Weight loss.
- Night sweats.
- Lesion usually pulmonary if *M. tuberculosis* but may spread to different sites.
- Head and neck:
  - cervical lymphadenopathy (collar-stud abscess, scrofula);
  - intra-oral ulceration, fissures, or granular areas (secondary infection from infected saliva);
  - rarely osteomyelitis.

Investigation
- Mantoux test.
- Biopsy of unusual oral lesions for histology and microbiology.
- ZN stain for acid-fast bacilli.
- Need to culture for 6 weeks or longer (Lowenstein–Jensen slope).
- CXR.

Treatment
Respiratory physicians: long-term multi-agent therapy (usually isoniazid and rifampicin for 6 months (12 if extrapulmonary) + pyrazinamide and ethambutol for first 2 months). Drug resistance becoming a problem especially in HIV-related disease—in 2011, 2:100 cases drug resistant.

Syphilis

Definition

Sexually transmitted infection caused by *Treponema pallidum*.

Incidence

Increased in recent years especially in ♀.

Primary syphilis

- Primary chancre (large, painless ulcer) that heals in 1–2 months (Fig. 11.8).
- Usually solitary. Genitalia/anus is the most common site.
- Rarely occurs on upper lip or oral cavity.
- May be associated regional lymphadenopathy.

Secondary syphilis

- 4–8 weeks post infection.
- Systemically unwell with malaise, fever, headache, weight loss.
- Widespread generalized maculopapular cutaneous rash.
- Lymphadenopathy.
- Oral manifestations:
  - mucous patches—sensitive white patches on oral mucosa (30%);
  - may slough → exposed connective tissue and snail track ulcers (serpiginous ulceration);
  - may affect any mucosal surface.
- Resolves by 12 weeks but symptoms may recur for up to 1 year.

Tertiary syphilis

- Affects up to 1/3 of patients.
- Latent period of up to 30 years.
- Multi-system pathology usually secondary to endarteritis obliterans affecting vascular system including aneurysms, LVH, and CCF.
- CNS involvement.
- Gumma (granulomatous inflammation) widespread sites.
- Oral manifestations:
  - gumma tongue/palate;
  - interstitial glossitis—tongue becomes lobulated and irregular as muscles contract as gumma heal;
  - syphilitic glossitis—atrophy and loss tongue papillae;
  - malignant change.

Congenital syphilis

- Frontal bossing.
- Short maxilla.
- Saddle nose.
- High-arched palate.
- Mandibular prognathism.
- Hutchinson's triad:
  - VIII nerve deafness;
  - ocular interstitial keratitis;
  - Moon's/Mulberry molars and Hutchinson's notched, tapering incisors.

Investigation
- Smear lesion: dark ground microscopic-illumination of organisms.
- Serological testing: VDLR, TPHA, FTA-ABS.

Treatment
- Parenteral penicillin:
  - single dose early in disease, longer course if late presentation;
  - may be incomplete response if lymphadenopathy or in HIV patients.

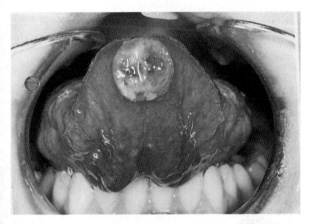

Fig. 11.8 Primary chancre on tongue.

Sarcoidosis

Definition
Systemic granulomatous disorder of unknown aetiology, can affect any organ.

Epidemiology
Affects young adults, black people, ♀>♂.

Clinical
- Lethargy, malaise.
- Bilateral hilar lymphadenopathy.
- Pulmonary infiltrates.
- Enlarged salivary glands.
- Xerostomia.
- Cervical lymphadenopathy.
- Erythema nodosum skin.
- Anterior uveitis.
- Cardiac arrhythmias.
- Hearing loss.
- Oral mucosal involvement rare but includes:
  - erythematous submucosal nodules;
  - orofacial granulomatosis.

Investigation
- CXR.
- Labial gland biopsy: show non-caseating granuloma in up to 60%.
- Bloods:
  - raised ESR;
  - hyperproteinaemia;
  - ↑ serum ACE in acute phase;
  - hypercalcaemia.

Treatment
- Most cases resolve spontaneously within 2 years but up to 1/3 may become chronic with granuloma formation.
- Systemic steroids required if lungs or eyes involved.

Heerfordt syndrome
Sarcoidosis associated with:
- Uveitis.
- Parotitis.
- VII nerve palsy.
- Lacrimal gland swelling.

Orofacial granulomatosis

Definition
Uncommon condition presenting with diffuse enlargement of the lips, cheeks or face. Appears to be due to an abnormal immune reaction (Fig. 11.9).

Epidemiology
- Presents at any age, usually teenagers/young adults.
- ?Allergic reaction to cinnamon, benzoates (E201 to E219, also found in toothpastes), cinnamaldehyde, tomatoes.
- Related to sarcoidosis or Crohn's disease in some patients.

Clinical
- Either intermittent or permanent enlargement lips or cheeks, or sometimes diffuse facial swelling.
- Intra-orally may see:
  - oedema;
  - ulcers;
  - cobblestone mucosa;
  - hyperplastic palatal tissue.

Investigation
- Patch test for allergens.
- Bloods: FBC, haematinics, ESR, albumin, calcium, ACE.
- Buccal or lip mucosal biopsy: must include underlying muscle.
- Biopsy shows non-caseating granulomas and oedema, negative stains for organisms and foreign material.

Treatment
- Referral of those with GIT symptoms or blood tests showing malabsorption.
- Avoidance diet.
- Topical corticosteroids if oral ulceration.
- Terfenadine 60mg od/bd to reduce lip swelling.

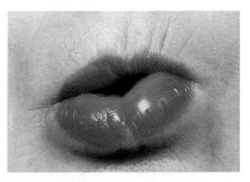

Fig. 11.9 Orofacial granulomatosis.

Crohn's disease

Definition
Chronic granulomatous disease of unknown cause that may affect any part of GIT.

Epidemiology
Usually diagnosed in young adults, often positive FH.

Clinical

Oral
- Cobblestone buccal mucosa with mucosal tags and folds.
- Oral ulceration.
- Diffuse swelling lips/cheeks.
- Raised, granulomatous gingival lesions.

GIT
- Similar appearance throughout GIT with scarring, infection, abdominal pain, obstruction, and development of fistulae.

Investigation
- In conjunction with gastroenterologists.
- Sigmoidoscopy and biopsy: shows non-caseating granulomas with macrophages, epithelioid cells, and occasional giant cells.
- Barium enema.

Treatment
- Occasionally, topical steroids may control oral lesions.
- More usually require systemic treatment including steroids, aminosalicylates, e.g. sulfasalazine, mercaptopurine, and azathioprine.
- Biological therapies such as infliximab and adalimumab increasingly used.

Candidal infections

Definition

Candida albicans is carried as an oral commensal in 75% of the population. It can, however, cause infection (candidosis). Two forms of *Candida* are seen—yeast, which is relatively benign, and hyphal, which has the ability to invade host tissue.

Risk factors

Symptomatic infection develops if there is a change in the equilibrium between the oral mucosal environment, the patient's immune status, and the strain of *Candida*. ↑ infection is seen in:

- Denture wearers, especially if poor oral hygiene.
- Immunocompromised patients, including diabetics, steroid users.
- Xerostomia.
- Broad-spectrum antibiotics.
- Malignant disease/chemotherapy/radiotherapy.
- Malnutrition.
- Smokers.

Classification

Pseudomembranous candidosis

- Acute (thrush).
- Chronic, e.g. in immunocompromised patients, inhaled steroid users:
  - creamy white plaques—can be rubbed off leaving erythematous areas;
  - bleeding points;
  - may be burning sensation and bad taste;
  - affects palate, tongue, buccal mucosa;
  - seen in neonates and patients with chronic disease.

Erythematous candidosis

- Acute (antibiotic sore tongue).
- Chronic (denture stomatitis).
- Median rhomboid glossitis (MRG): pseudoepitheliomatous hyperplasia:
  - often severe pain/burning;
  - affects mainly hard palate, buccal mucosa, dorsum tongue;
  - filiform papillae may be lost if tongue affected;
  - tongue appears smooth and red, often with macules or petechiae;
  - if denture stomatitis, screen for underlying conditions, e.g. DM.
- Angular cheilitis:
  - *Staph. aureus* also present in ~ 60%;
  - can be associated with ↓ lower face height in edentulous individuals.

Hyperplastic candidosis
- Inflammatory papillary hyperplasia.
- Candidal leukoplakia:
  - considered premalignant—occurs mainly in smokers/drinkers;
  - often deficiency in haematinics;
  - may have a high rate of malignant transformation to SCC;
  - buccal mucosa adjacent to commissures most common site;
  - varies from white plaques to speckled erythroleukoplakia;
  - candidal hyphae seen within epithelium on biopsy;
  - ↑ dysplasia in speckled lesions;
  - dysplasia may regress with fluconazole treatment;
  - some authorities consider it to be candidal infection superimposed on leukoplakia, rather than a separate entity.

Chronic mucocutaneous candidosis (CMCC)
- Rare group of immunological disorders with superficial mucocutaneous candidosis, which can affect skin, nails, and oral mucosa.
- Usually thick white plaques that cannot be removed.
- May develop endocrine abnormalities in time.

Investigation
- Oral swabs from three separate sites.
- Candidal rinse: may need to type species particularly if poor response to initial treatment.
- Biopsy: mandatory if candida leukoplakia considered.
- Check FBC and haematinics.
- Medical investigation for underlying systemic condition.

Treatment
- OHI/denture hygiene.
- Antifungal therapy:
  - polyenes, e.g. nystatin topically;
  - imidazoles, e.g. miconazole (has anti-staphylococcal action therefore use for angular cheilitis), clotrimazole topically, ketoconazole (multiple drug interactions therefore not first-line therapy);
  - triazoles, e.g. fluconazole in candidal leukoplakia (multiple drug interactions).
- Eliminate risk factors.

Trigeminal neuralgia

Definition
Disorder of the Vth cranial nerve leading to intense paroxysmal pain within one or more divisions of its sensory supply.

Epidemiology
3–6/100,000, more common in ♀, incidence and severity ↑ with age. Usual age of onset 50–70 years.

Cause
- Compression of trigeminal nerve root by artery in middle cranial fossa.
- Nerve demyelination—may suggest multiple sclerosis (MS) especially in under 50s.
- Always suspect SOL especially if <50 years of age.

Clinical
- Paroxysmal pain within one of the three divisions Vth nerve, usually maxillary or mandibular divisions.
- Intense, lancinating, burning pain, 'like an electric shock'.
- Pain lasts seconds to minutes only.
- Frequency varies, may be multiple times/hour.
- Almost always unilateral.
- Many patients have a trigger point for their pain, which may be stimulated by everyday tasks such as eating, talking, and washing.
- Patients have periods of remission and relapse but symptoms tend to worsen over time.
- Neurological examination shows no clinical abnormality.

Investigation
- Full neurological examination (look for signs/symptoms MS).
- MRI brain if:
  - atypical features;
  - patient <50 years old—possible underlying demyelinating disease or (intra-cranial space-occupying lesion;
  - considering microvascular decompression.

Medical management: first line
- Anticonvulsants such as carbamazepine, phenytoin, lamotrigine, and gabapentin or a combination. Titrate to find pain relief.
- Carbamazepine started as 100mg bd up to 1600mg/day.
- Early troublesome side effects reduce with time.
- Monitor WCC, U&Es, and LFT.
- Requires close follow-up and trial reductions of therapy once symptom free.

Surgical management
- Peripheral procedures, e.g. cryotherapy falling out of favour and being replaced by radiofrequency ablation (RFA) to affected branch under LA/GA.
- Central neurosurgical procedures:
  - open microvascular decompression (MVD)—artery causing nerve compression is separated from nerve using Teflon sheet (5% risk serious complication);
  - radiofrequency rhizotomy;
  - glycerol injection;
  - balloon compression;
  - stereotactic (Gamma knife) radiosurgery.
- All of these carry risks of permanent paraesthesia, anaesthesia dolorosa (severe continuous pain within the distribution of the nerve), and risks associated with the surgical procedure itself. Therefore, reserved for cases refractory to medical management or where medical management side effects are intolerable.

Glossopharyngeal neuralgia

Definition
Disorder of the glossopharyngeal nerve leading to intense paroxysmal pain with its area of sensory supply.

Epidemiology
Very rare. Incidence TN:GN 100:1.

Clinical
- Pain similar in character to TN.
- Often poorly localized. Affects tonsil, tongue base, ear, and intra-auricular area.
- Patients will often point to just behind angle of mandible. Symptoms often (treated as TMJ pain for some time).
- Trigger point difficult to identify—may be swallowing or yawning.

Investigation
- Topical LA to ipsilateral tonsil/pharynx immediately relieves symptoms but short-acting, therefore diagnostic only, not therapeutic.
- MRI scan: may be underlying space occupying lesion cranial cavity or at jugular foramen.

Treatment
- Medical management as for TN: pain control may be difficult.

Migraine

Definition

Primary recurrent headache disorder, more common in ♀, which usually commences on approaching adolescence.

Cause

Possibly related to abnormal 5-HT (serotonin) activity, leading initially to vasoconstriction of portions of cerebral arteries, followed by compensatory vasodilation, with cerebral oedema and pain. Postulated relationship with TMJDS. Precipitants include:

- Hormonal factors, including OCP.
- Dietary, e.g. chocolate, bananas.
- Stress.
- Sleep deprivation.
- Bright/flashing lights.

Clinical

- May have preceding aura: visual hallucinations, including flashing coloured lights, loss of colour perception, or other visual disturbances.
- Motor—temporary muscle palsies.
- Speech disorders including aphasia.
- Severe unilateral headache: initially poorly localized; becomes localized to temporal, frontal, or orbital region.
- Photophobia.
- Nausea.
- Vomiting.
- Attacks decrease in frequency with age and may totally resolve.

Treatment

- Acute attack: analgesics, sumatriptan (5-HT antagonist), ergot derivatives.
- Prophylaxis: options include pizotifen (antihistamine), propranolol, amitriptyline, topiramate.
- Botulinum toxin type A—NICE guidelines recommend only if failed three previous medications and have headaches for at least 15 days/month, of which at least 8 days are migrainous.

Cluster headaches

Definition

Recurrent headaches, also known as migrainous neuralgia and Horton's syndrome. Episodic—clusters separated by 1 month or more; chronic—separated by less than a month or not separated at all.

Epidemiology

- Less common than migraines, ♂:♀ 6:1.
- Often positive FH.
- 80% patients smoke.
- Presents in 3rd or 4th decade.
- Worse in autumn and spring.

Cause

Unknown. Possible allergic basis with mast cell release of histamine and vasodilation. Associated with:
- Sleep apnoea and ↓ oxygen saturations.
- Hypoxaemia in rapid eye movement (REM) sleep.
- Alcohol.
- Cocaine.
- GTN spray.

Clinical

- Severe, unilateral episodes of burning or lancinating pain, in and around the orbit, frontal, and temporal region.
- Abrupt onset, lasts for 15min → 3h, often awakens the patient at night.
- Begin at same time every day ('alarm clock' headaches).
- May have multiple episodes each day.
- Occur for 2–3 months, then have periods of remission that can last for years.
- May be associated autonomic problems:
  - conjunctival vessel congestion;
  - eye watering;
  - nasal stuffiness;
  - facial flushing.

Investigation

Diagnosis is clinical. However, similar symptoms may be secondary to intra-cranial pathology, so consider MRI scan of the brain.

Treatment

- Acute attack:
  - oxygen may abort an attack and its effectiveness is diagnostic;
  - sumatriptan.
- Prophylaxis:
  - verapamil;
  - nifedipine;
  - lithium;
  - indomethacin.

Temporal (giant cell) arteritis

Definition

Multifocal vasculitis affecting the cranial arteries, of unknown aetiology, with average age of onset 70 years. Most common in ♀>50 and related to poly-myalgia rheumatica (PMR). ?Genetic predisposition.

Clinical

- Unilateral headache, initially burning in character, becoming throbbing.
- Usually temporal or occipital artery.
- Lingual, facial, and maxillary arteries may also become involved →
  claudication on eating and talking.
- Affected vessels feel hard and tender and may necrose.
- Tongue may become ischaemic if lingual arteries involved.
- If untreated, 25% will develop visual problems secondary to central
  retinal artery involvement, which may be bilateral. Loss of vision may be
  the first clinical sign.

Investigation

- ↑↑ ESR: 60–100 (may be less).
- ↑ CRP also raised.
- Normocytic, normochromic anaemia.
- Artery biopsy (Fig. 11.10):
  - usually superficial temporal under LA;
  - can be ipsilateral or contralateral to symptomatic side;
  - giant cell lesions seen;
  - need to harvest >2cm as skip lesions can occur;
  - should be carried out within a week of starting steroids.

Treatment

- 60–100mg prednisolone daily.
- Start before temporal artery biopsy with aim to preserve vision.
- Treatment in conjunction with rheumatologists.
- PPI and osteoporosis cover with high-dose steroids.
- Decrease steroid dose with resolution of headache and normalization
  ESR (may take months or years).

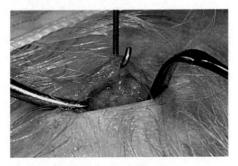

Fig. 11.10 Temporal artery biopsy.

Atypical facial pain

Definition

Diagnosis of exclusion. Constant, chronic pain in the absence of identifiable organic disease. More common in ♀. Most patients are middle aged or elderly.

Clinical

- Often difficult for patients to describe their symptoms.
- Most frequently described as deep, constant ache or burning.
- Does not stop patients sleeping but they often awake early with the pain present.
- Does not follow anatomical patterns:
  - may be bilateral;
  - can cross midline;
  - infrequently moves to another site.
- Maxilla > mandible.
- Often initiated/exacerbated by dental treatment.
- Examination entirely normal.
- Often have other complaints, such as IBS, dry mouth, and chronic pain syndromes.

Investigation

All imaging (including intracranial MRI), bloods, and biopsies normal.

Treatment

- Often unrewarding with limited response.
- Tricyclic antidepressants have some effect in some patients (no adequate (RCTs show this). Other antidepressants usually ineffective.
- ~30% will respond to gabapentin.
- The involvement of a pain team with access to cognitive behavioural therapy (CBT) or psychological input may help patients manage their pain.

Burning mouth syndrome

Definition
Burning sensation of oral mucosa, usually tongue, in absence of any identifiable clinical abnormality or cause.

Epidemiology
Common (5 per 100,000, but can be much higher in middle aged and elderly patients), ♀>♂.

Cause
Unknown, but hormonal factors, anxiety, and stress have been implicated.

Clinical
- Complain of dry mouth, with altered/bad taste.
- Burning sensation affecting tongue and anterior palate and less commonly lips.
- May be aggravated by certain foods.
- Usually bilateral.
- Does not wake patient but often present on awaking.
- Examination entirely normal.

Investigation
- FBC.
- Haematinics.
- Swab for *Candida*.
- All clinical investigations, including bloods and swabs, are normal.

Treatment
- Reassurance: patients are often cancerophobic.
- Avoidance of stimulating factors.
- Some patients may respond to tricyclic antidepressants or alpha lipoic acid.
- CBT has been shown in RCTs to help patients manage their symptoms, as medical management is often disappointing.

Eponyms in OMFS

List of eponyms in OMFS

Abbe	Robert, US Surgeon 1851–1928 Abbe flap: a pedicled full thickness flap of one lip transferred into the other
Addison	Thomas, British physician 1793–1860 Addison disease: chronic adrenal insufficiency, hypocortisolism, hypoadrenalism, and buccal mucosa pigmentation
Adson	Alfred Washington, US Neurosurgeon 1887–1951 Adson tissue forceps
Albers-Schonberg	Heinrich Ernst, German radiologist 1865–1921 Albers-Schonberg disease: osteopetrosis
Albright	Fuller, US endocrinologist 1900–1969 Albright syndrome: precocious puberty, polyostotic fibrous dysplasia, unilateral café-au-lait spots
Allen	Edgar Van Nuys, US physician 1900–1961 Allen's test for radial or ulnar artery patency
Apert	Eugene, French paediatrician, 1868–1940 Apert's syndrome: type I acrocephalosyndactyly
Battle	William H, English surgeon 1855–1936 Battle's sign: post-auricular ecchymosis in # of middle cranial fossa
Behçet	Hulusi, Turkish dermatologist 1889–1948 Behçet's syndrome: uveitis, oral, and genital ulceration
Bell	Charles, Scottish anatomist 1774–1842 Bell's palsy: idiopathic unilateral facial nerve paralysis, usually self-limiting
Binder	Karl Heinz, German dentist 1923– Binder's syndrome: nasomaxillary hypoplasia
Bowen	John T, 1857–1941 Bowen's disease: cutaneous squamous intra-epithelial carcinoma
Breslow	Alexander, US pathologist 1928–1980 Breslow thickness: melanoma depth
Burkitt	Denis P, British physician 1911–1993 Burkitt's lymphoma: EBV in African children
Caldwell	George W, US physician 1834–1918 Caldwell–Luc approach via canine fossa to maxillary sinus
Carnoy	Jean Baptiste, French biologist 1836–1899 Carnoy's solution: a fixative used in keratocystic odontogenic tumour management

Castleman	Benjamin, US physician and pathologist 1906–1982 Castleman disease: uncommon lympho-proliferative disorder (not reactive lymph node hyperplasia or malignancy)
Chvostek	František, Czecho-Austrian physician 1835–1884 Chvostek's sign: hypocalcaemia-related tapping over facial nerve elicits abnormal muscle contraction(s)
Crohn	Burrill Bernard, US gastroenterologist 1884–1983 Crohn's disease: inflammatory bowel disease, may affect any part of the gastrointestinal tract from mouth to anus
Crouzon	Octave, French physician 1874–1938 Crouzon syndrome: craniofacial dysostosis
DiGeorge	Angel Mario, US paediatrician 1921–2009 Di George syndrome: deficiency of 3rd and 4th pharyngeal pouches, cellular immunodeficiency, overlap with VCF
Epstein	Alois, Czech paediatrician 1849–1918 Epstein's pearls: cystic papules on palate
Erb	Wilhelm Heinrich, German neurologist 1840–1921 Erb's point: where the great auricular nerve crosses the SCM
Estlander	Jacob, Finnish surgeon 1831–1881 Abbe–Estlander flap: a full thickness flap reconstruction of oral commissure
Fergusson	Sir William, Scottish surgeon 1808–1877 Weber–Fergusson incision: facial access for maxillectomy
Frey	Lucie, Polish neurologist 1852–1932 Frey's syndrome: gustatory sweating following parotid surgery or trauma
Gardner	Eldon J, US physician 1909–1989 Gardner's syndrome: variant of familial adenomatous polyposis with osteomas, neuromas, lipomas, polyposis coli
Gillies	Sir Harold, English maxillofacial/plastic surgeon 1882–1960 Gillies lift: surgical approach to closed zygomatic fracture reduction Also needle holder, tissue forceps, skin hooks
Goltz	Robert William, US dermatologist 1923– Gorlin–Goltz syndrome: multiple basal cell carcinomas, odontogenic keratocysts, skeletal abnormalities

Gorlin	Robert James, US oral pathologist 1923–2006 Gorlin–Goltz syndrome: multiple basal cell carcinomas, odontogenic keratocysts, skeletal abnormalities
Guedel	Arthur Ernest, US anaesthetist 1883–1956 Guedel airway
Gunning	Thomas B, US dentist 1813–1889 Gunning splints: modified dentures for use in jaw fractures
Hand–Schüller–Christian disease	Alfred Hand Jr (US paediatrician 1868–1949), Artur Schüller (Austrian neurologist and radiologist 1874–1957), Henry Asbury Christian (US physician 1876–1951) Triad of exophthalmos, lytic bone lesions (often in the skull) and diabetes insipidus
Heck	John W, US dentist 1923– Heck's focal epithelial hyperplasia: PMOL
Heerfordt	Christian Frederick, Danish ophthalmologist 1871–1953 Heerfordt's syndrome: facial palsy, uveitis, parotid gland enlargement, fever (sarcoidosis)
Hess	Carl von, German ophthalmologist 1863–1923 Hess charting in ocular motility disorders
Highmore	Nathaniel, English anatomist 1613–1685 Maxillary antrum of Highmore
Hilton	John, English surgeon 1804–1878 Hilton's method for draining pus
Hodgkin	Thomas, English physician 1798–1866 Hodgkin lymphoma
Horner	Johan Friedrich, Swiss ophthalmologist 1831–1886 Horner's syndrome: ptosis, miosis, anhydrosis due to lesion of cervical sympathetic chain
Horton	Bayard T, US physician 1895–1980 Horton's neuralgia: cluster headache
Hounsfield	Godfrey N, English electronics engineer and Nobel Laureate 1919–2004 Hounsfield units: index of X-ray attenuation in CT scanning
Hunt	James Ramsay, US neurologist 1872–1937 Ramsay Hunt syndrome: facial palsy secondary to herpes zoster, vesicles in EAM, otalgia, deafness, vertigo
Hutchinson	Sir Jonathan, English surgeon 1828–1913 Hutchinson's melanotic freckle: lentigo maligna

Kaposi	Moritz, Hungarian dermatologist 1837–1902 Kaposi sarcoma: tumour of endothelial cells
Kelly	Adam, English ENT surgeon 1865–1941 Paterson–Brown-Kelly/Plummer–Vinson syndrome: post-cricoid web, atrophic glossitis, sideropenic dysphagia
Koebner	Heinrich, German dermatologist 1838–1904 Koebner phenomenon: skin lesions occurring in area of trauma
Koplik	Henry, US paediatrician 1858–1927 Koplik's spots: prodromic viral enanthem of measles
Lahey	Frank, US surgeon 1880–1935 Lahey pledgets: used in blunt dissection
Langenbeck	Bernhard von, German surgeon 1810–1887 Langenbeck retractor Von Langenbeck cleft palate repair
Le Fort	Rene, French surgeon 1869–1951 Le Fort levels of maxillary fracture
Luc	Henri, French ENT surgeon 1855–1925 Caldwell–Luc approach via canine fossa to maxillary sinus
Ludwig	Wilhelm Friedrich von, German surgeon 1790–1865 Ludwig's angina: bilateral sublingual and submandibular cellulitis
Malassez	Louis Charles, French physiologist 1842–1910 Epithelial cell rests of Malassez: remnants of the root sheath of Hertwig
Mohs	Frederick E, US surgeon 1910–2002 Mohs micrographic surgery
Moon	Henry, English dentist 1845–1892 Moon's mulberry molars in congenital syphilis
Paget	Sir James, English surgeon 1814–1899 Paget's disease of bone: osteitis deformans
Paterson	Donald Rose, English ENT surgeon 1863–1939 Paterson–Brown-Kelly/Plummer–Vinson syndrome: post-cricoid web, atrophic glossitis, sideropenic dysphagia
Pfeiffer	Richard FJ, German physician 1858–1945 Pfeiffer syndrome: acrocephalosyndactyly
Plummer	Henry Stanley, US endocrinologist 1874–1936 Paterson–Brown-Kelly/Plummer–Vinson syndrome: post-cricoid web, atrophic glossitis, sideropenic dysphagia

Pott	Percivall, English surgeon 1714–1788 Pott's puffy tumour: osteomyelitis of frontal bone and intracranial abscess, direct or through haematogenic spread
Ramsay Hunt	James, 1872–1937 Ramsay Hunt syndrome, see Hunt
Recklinghausen	Daniel von, German pathologist 1833–1910 Recklinghausen's neurofibromatosis Von Recklinghausen disease of bone: osteitis fibrosa cystica in secondary hyperparathyroidism
Reed	Dorothy M, US pathologist 1874–1964 Reed–Sternberg cells in Hodgkin lymphoma
Rinne	Friedrich, German otologist 1819–1868 Rinne test of hearing with tuning fork
Romberg	Mortiz, Heinrich von, German physician 1795–1873 Romberg's hemifacial atrophy
Schirmer	Otto, German ophthalmologist 1864–1918 Schirmer's test: quantifies lacrimal secretionSézary Albert, French dermatologist 1880–1956 Sézary syndrome: cutaneous T-cell lymphoma
Shiley	Donald P, US engineer 1920–2010 Shiley tracheostomy tube
Sistrunck	Walter Ellis, US surgeon 1880–1933 Sistrunck's procedure for excision of thyroglossal cysts
Sjögren	Henrik Samuel, Swedish ophthalmologist 1899–1986 Sjögren's syndrome: xerophthalmia, xerostomia, CTD
Spee	Ferdinand Graf von, German embryologist 1855–1937 Curve of Spee: AP curve of occlusal plane
Spitz	Sophie, US pathologist 1910–1956 Spitz naevus: red skin tumour mistaken for melanoma
Stafne	Edward C, US oral pathologist 1894–1981 Stafne bone cavity: ectopic submandibular salivary tissue
Stevens–Johnson	Albert Mason Stevens, Frank Chambliss Johnson 1922 Stevens–Johnson syndrome: hypersensitivity complex affecting skin and mucous membranes
Sturge	William Allen, English physician 1850–1919 Sturge–Weber syndrome: facial haemangioma in V distribution, meningeal angioma, intracranial calcification, epilepsy

Treacher Collins	Edward, English surgeon and ophthalmologist 1862–1932 Treacher Collins syndrome (mandibulofacial dysostosis): rare autosomal dominant congenital disorder characterized by craniofacial deformities
Vincent	Henri, French physician 1862–1950 Vincent's angina: ANUG
Vinson	Porter Paisley, US surgeon 1890–1959 Paterson–Brown-Kelly/Plummer–Vinson syndrome: post-cricoid web, atrophic glossitis, sideropenic dysphagia
Virchow	Rudolf, German pathologist 1821–1902 Virchow's triad in thrombosis formation
Waldeyer	Heinrich G von, German anatomist 1836–1921 Waldeyer's oropharyngeal ring of lymphoid tissue
Weber	Frederick Parks, English physician 1863–1962 Sturge–Weber syndrome: facial haemangioma in V distribution, meningeal angioma, intra- cranial calcification, epilepsy
Weber	Freidrich, German otologist 1823–1891 Weber–Fergusson incision: facial access for maxillectomy Weber test of hearing with tuning fork
Wegener	Friedrich, German pathologist 1907–1990 Wegener's granulomatosis vasculitis causing damage to lung kidneys skin and face (midline)
Whickham	Louis, French dermatologist 1861–1913 Whickham's striae in lichen planus
Whitehead	Walter, English surgeon 1840–1913 Whitehead's varnish
Whitnall	Samuel E, English anatomist 1876–1952 Whitnall's tubercle: suspensory point for lateral canthus and suspensory ligament of globe
Wolfe	John R, Scottish ophthalmologist 1824–1904 Wolfe graft: full thickness skin graft

Chapter 13

Other useful facts

Potions

Carnoy's solution
- 6 parts ethanol (absolute or 95%).
- 3 parts chloroform.
- 1 part glacial acetic acid.

Uses
- Reducing recurrence in odontogenic keratocysts.
- Applied to bony cavity following enucleation for 3min.
- Causes fixation of peripheral nerves due to neurotoxicity of ingredients.

Whitehead's varnish
- Iodoform.
- Ether.
- Balsam of tolu.
- Benzoin.
- Storax.

Tumescent solution
An example:
- Hartmann's solution (cold)—500mL.
- Hyalase—1mL.
- Adrenaline 1:1000—0.5mL.
- Bupivacaine 0.25%—25mL.
- Lignocaine 1%—25mL.
- (Triamcinolone.)

Uses
- E.g. bitemporal flap, face lift, neck dissection.

Uses of botulinum toxin in OMFS

- **Anti-wrinkle injections** (see ➔ Non-surgical aesthetic techniques, p. 332).
- **Blepharospasm:** 25 units in 10 divided doses to medial and lateral lids.
- **Frey's syndrome:** 5 units intradermally at 1cm distances.
- **Masseteric hypertrophy:** 25 units into masseter.
- **Sialorrhoea/drooling:** to submandibular/parotid glands up to 70 units total.
- **TMJ pain dysfunction/dislocation:** into lateral pterygoid muscles ± temporalis, up to 80 units each side.
- **Post-operative sialocoele:** parotidectomy—emerging evidence.
- **Migrainous headaches.**
- **Cervical dystonia** (torticollis).
- Doses relate to Botox® (Allergan).

Statistics

Sensitivity and specificity

Sensitivity
How good a test is at identifying those who have the disease.

Specificity
How good a test is at identifying those who do not have the disease.

Useful terms

- **True positives:** those with a positive test result who do have the disease.
- **True negatives:** those with a negative test result who do not have the disease.
- **False positives:** those with a positive test result who do not have the disease.
- **False negatives:** those with a negative test result who do have the disease.
- A sensitive test will therefore have few false negatives.
- A specific test will have few false positives.

For example, MRI of the neck in detection of nodal metastasis:
- Sensitivity is 75–80% (i.e. not very sensitive). It therefore has a significant number of false negatives. These are the nodes with micrometastasis that do not show up on MRI.
- Specificity is 90–100%. It has few false positives, i.e. those nodes that fit the radiological criteria for metastatic disease nearly always show disease at histology.

> Sensitivity = No. true positives/(No. true positives + No. false negatives)

> Specificity = No. true negatives/(No. true negatives + No. false positives)

- The *positive predictive value* is the proportion of patients with positive test results who are correctly diagnosed:

> PPV = No. true positives/(No. true positives + No. false positives)

The infratemporal fossa

- The infratemporal fossa is an irregularly shaped cavity, situated below and medial to the zygomatic arch.
- Previously called the pterygomaxillary space.

Boundaries

Consist of the following structures:

- **Anteriorly:** by the infratemporal surface of the maxilla and the ridge, which descends from its zygomatic process.
- **Posteriorly:** by the articular eminence of the temporal bone and the spinal angularis of the sphenoid bone.
- **Superiorly:** by the greater wing of the sphenoid below the infratemporal crest and the under-surface of the squamous temporal bone.
- **Inferiorly:** by the alveolar border of the maxilla.
- **Medially:** by the lateral pterygoid plate.
- **Laterally:** by the ramus of mandible.
- It has no floor.

Contents

Muscles

- The lower part of the temporalis muscle.
- Lateral and medial pterygoid muscle.

Vessels

- The internal maxillary vessels, consisting of the maxillary artery originating from the external carotid artery and its branches.
- Internal maxillary branches found within the infratemporal fossa including:
  - middle meningeal artery;
  - inferior alveolar artery;
  - deep temporal artery;
  - buccal artery;
  - pterygoid venous plexus.

Nerves

Mandibular nerve, inferior alveolar nerve, lingual nerve, buccal nerve, chorda tympani nerve, and otic ganglion.

Fissures

- The foramen ovale and foramen spinosum open on its roof, and the alveolar canals on its anterior wall.
- At its upper and medial part are two fissures, which together form a T-shaped fissure comprised of the inferior orbital and the pterygomaxillary fissure.

Levels of critical care

- **Level 0**: patients whose needs can be met through normal ward care in an acute hospital.
- **Level 1**: patients at risk of their condition deteriorating, or those recently relocated from higher levels of care whose needs can be met on an acute ward, with additional advice and support from the critical care team.
- **Level 2**: patients requiring more detailed observation or intervention, including support for a single failing organ system or postoperative care, and those stepping down from higher levels of care.
- **Level 3**: patients requiring advanced respiratory support alone or basic respiratory support, together with support of at least two organ systems. This level includes all complex patients requiring support for multi-organ failure.

Ionizing Radiation (Medical Exposure) Regulations

Ionizing Radiation (Medical Exposure) Regulations (IRMER) 2000: statutory regulations.

Designated members of the team include:
- Legal person to take overall responsibility.
- Radiation protection supervisor.
- IRMER practitioner who must justify risks vs benefits.
- Radiation protection advisor.

Radiation must be kept as low as reasonably practical (ALARP; Table 13.1):
- All exposure must be justified.
- A record of clinical evaluation must be kept.
- Radiographs should be provided to other practitioners.
- Quality should be audited.

Table 13.1 Effective radiation doses

Examination	Effective dose (µSv)
Intra-oral radiograph (per exposure)	<8.3
Dental panoramic radiograph	9–26
Dental cephalometric radiograph	3–6
CBCT (dento-alveolar) (focus field of view)	5–38.3
Full-mouth series	35–388
CBCT (craniofacial)	68–599
Medical fan beam CT scan (maxilla and mandible)	2000

This table was published in Stuart White & Michael Pharoah, *Oral Radiology: Principles and Interpretation*, copyright Elsevier 2008.

Piezoelectric surgery in OMFS

- Piezoelectric surgery uses ultrasonic microvibrations for the cutting of bone.
- Precise bone cuts without damaging any soft tissue, minimizing the invasiveness of surgical procedure.
- Almost totally blood-free field.
- Compared to traditional methods, it enables optimal healing because it reduces the post-surgery swelling and discomfort.
- Uses: OMFS, ENT, neurosurgery, ophthalmology, traumatology, and orthopaedics.

The main indications in oral surgery are sinus lift, bone graft harvesting, osteogenic distraction, ridge expansion, endodontic surgery, periodontal surgery, inferior alveolar nerve decompression, cyst and impacted teeth removal.

Wound care and surgical wound dressings

Problem: bleeding
- **Cause**:
  - fragile vascular condition and capillary ooze in fungating wounds;
  - dry dressings traumatize the friable tissues.
- **Prevention**: tranexamic acid 10-day oral course or applied topically.
- **Management**:
  - enough moisture to prevent adherence of dressings;
  - Kaltostat® or similar calcium alginate;
  - palliative radiotherapy—either a single fraction or short course;
  - administer blood transfusion if indicated and patient is symptomatic.

Problem: malodour
- **Cause**: fatty acids a by-product of necrotic tissue within the wound leading to malodour or due to bacterial infection.
- **Prevention**:
  - patient education;
  - essential oils infusers or metronidazole gel or oral antibiotics.
- **Management**:
  - dressings that absorb odour;
  - changing dressings when strike-through occurs;
  - autolytic debridement of necrotic tissue—*honey* (antibacterial properties) or Aquacel®.

Problem: pain
- **Cause**: general cancer burden in advanced disease or wound position.
- **Prevention**: skin barrier—Cavilon™ to prevent tapes sticking.
- **Management**:
  - continuous *analgesia* and break-through dose at change of dressing;
  - psychosocial support;
  - sometimes palliative *radiotherapy*.

Problem: heavy exudates
- **Cause**: large fungating tumours in advanced stage.
- **Prevention**: absorption via appropriate dressings.
- **Management**:
  - challenging shapes—foam dressings hold excess moisture and prevents maceration;
  - excessive—stoma bag system.

Revalidation for the new consultant

Essentials
- GMC online account.
- Know your designated body or responsible officer.
- Annual appraisal process in line with *Good Medical Practice*.
- The measurement of surgical outcomes is being introduced in the NHS across all surgical specialities.

General information about you and your professional work
- Personal details, scope of work, record of annual appraisals.
- Personal development plans and their review.
- Probity and health.

Keeping up to date—continuing professional development (CPD)
- Review of practice.
- Quality improvement activity—audit, review of outcomes, case review, and discussion.
- Significant events—clinical incidents, significant untoward incidents (SUIs), or other similar events.

Feedback on professional practice
- Colleague feedback.
- Patient and carer feedback.
- Complaints and compliments.

Some key points regarding facial transplantation

Type of facial transplantation

- Upper/lower/ full face.
- Soft tissue only or composite.

Procedure

- Timing and sequencing of surgery.
- Complex procedure involving multiple teams.
- Sentinel graft—indirect monitoring for rejection.

Donor reconstruction

- Prosthetics laboratory.

Immunosuppression problems

- Acute rejection and sepsis.
- Infections and cancers.
- Emerging evidence of tacrolimus benefits in nerve function.

Quality of life

- Recovery of facial movements ~9–12 months.
- Sensory recovery ~3–6 months.
- Aesthetics variable and secondary cosmetic procedures.
- Function depends on motor recovery and complexity of composite reconstruction.

Ethical implications

- Is it appropriate to offer a high-risk procedure and life-long immunosuppression for a non-life-threatening condition?
- To patient, facial disfigurement is life limiting + affects QOL.
- Trauma, burns, benign tumours vs malignant tumours.

Index

Armstrong's Last Goodnight

The setting of John Arden's play is the Border country
during the reign of James V. While the representatives
of England and Scotland are trying to secure peace,
there is continuous strife on the Border between
families like the Armstrongs, the Eliots and the John-
stones, and between their overlords in Scotland. The
play is concerned with the events that led up to the
hanging of one of these Border freebooters, Johnny
Armstrong of Gilnockie, in 1530, and with the part
played in them by Sir David Lindsay, Scottish diplo-
matist, Lord Lyon King of Arms and author of
The Three Estates.

*The photograph on the front of cover shows a scene
from the Glasgow Citizens' Theatre production.*
Photograph by David Sim, reproduced by courtesy of
The Observer.

by John Arden

★

SERJEANT MUSGRAVE'S DANCE

THE WORKHOUSE DONKEY

LEFT-HANDED LIBERTY

SOLDIER, SOLDIER *and other plays*

TWO AUTOBIOGRAPHICAL PLAYS

IRONHAND
(adapted from Goethe's
Goetz von Berlichingen)

by John Arden *and* Margaretta D'Arcy

★

THE BUSINESS OF GOOD GOVERNMENT

THE ROYAL PARDON

THE HERO RISES UP

THE ISLAND OF THE MIGHTY